Essentials
of Pharmacology
for
Health Occupations
5th edition

Essentials of Pharmacology for Health Occupations

5th edition

Ruth Woodrow, RN, MA

Medical Consultant for Education and Infection Control
Senior Friendship Centers, Inc.,
Health Services
Sarasota, Florida

Former Director, Staff Development
Plymouth Harbor, Inc.
Sarasota, Florida

Former Instructor, Pharmacology,
Coordinator, Continuing Education
Sarasota County Technical Institute
Sarasota, Florida

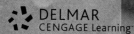 DELMAR
CENGAGE Learning

Australia   Canada   Mexico   Singapore   Spain   United Kingdom   United States

![DELMAR CENGAGE Learning]

**Essentials of Pharmacology
for Health Occupations,
Fifth edition
by Ruth Woodrow, RN, MA**

Vice President,
Health Care Business Unit:
William Brottmiller

Editorial Director:
Matthew Kane

Acquisitions Editor:
Marah Bellegarde

Editorial Assistant:
Jadin Babin-Kavanaugh

Developmental Editor:
Debra Flis

Marketing Director:
Jennifer McAvey

Health Care Channel Manager
—Education
Tamara Caruso

Marketing Coordinator:
Michele Gleason

Production Manager
Barbara A. Bullock

Art & Design Coordinator:
Alexandros Vasilakos

Production Coordinator:
Thomas Heffernan

Project Editor:
Ruth Fisher

For product information and technology assistance, contact us at
Cengage Learning Customer & Sales Support, 1-800-354-9706

For permission to use material from this text or product,
submit all requests online at **cengage.com/permissions**
Further permissions questions can be emailed to
permissionrequest@cengage.com

ExamView® and ExamView Pro® are registered trademarks of FSCreations, Inc. Windows is a registered trademark of the Microsoft Corporation used herein under license. Macintosh and Power Macintosh are registered trademarks of Apple Computer, Inc. Used herein under license.

© 2007 Cengage Learning. All Rights Reserved. Cengage Learning WebTutor™ is a trademark of Cengage Learning.

Library of Congress Control Number: 2006001536

ISBN-13: 978-1-4018-8925-8

ISBN-10: 1-4018-8925-5

Delmar Cengage Learning
5 Maxwell Drive
Clifton Park, NY 12065-2919
USA

Cengage Learning products are represented in Canada by Nelson Education, Ltd.

For your lifelong learning solutions, visit **delmar.cengage.com**

Visit our corporate website at **www.cengage.com**

Notice to the Reader

Publisher does not warrant or guarantee any of the products described herein or perform any independent analysis in connection with any of the product information contained herein. Publisher does not assume, and expressly disclaims, any obligation to obtain and include information other than that provided to it by the manufacturer. The reader is expressly warned to consider and adopt all safety precautions that might be indicated by the activities described herein and to avoid all potential hazards. By following the instructions contained herein, the reader willingly assumes all risks in connection with such instructions. The publisher makes no representations or warranties of any kind, including but not limited to, the warranties of fitness for particular purpose or merchantability, nor are any such representations implied with respect to the material set forth herein, and the publisher takes no responsibility with respect to such material. The publisher shall not be liable for any special, consequential, or exemplary damages resulting, in whole or part, from the readers' use of, or reliance upon, this material.

Printed in the United States of America
4 5 6 7 8 9 12 11 10 09

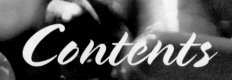

Contents

PART 1 INTRODUCTION

Chapter 1
Consumer Safety and Drug Regulations 3

Chapter 2
Drug Names and References 11

Chapter 3
Sources and Bodily Effects of Drugs 23

v

Chapter 4

Medication Preparations and Supplies   38

Chapter 5

Abbreviations and Systems of Measurement   55

Chapter 6

Safe Dosage Preparation   66

Chapter 7

Responsibilities and Principles
of Drug Administration   82

Chapter 8

Administration by the
Gastrointestinal Route   93

PART II   DRUG CLASSIFICATIONS

List of Tables

To Arlene in appreciation
for her cheerful willingness
to always give a helping hand.

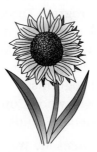

ACKNOWLEDGMENTS

I would like to acknowledge the support, encouragement, and technical assistance of my husband, Roger, for all previous editions, but especially this fifth edition.

I especially wish to thank David Smith, Registered Pharmacist for his extensive and comprehensive revision and updating of all of the drugs in this and the fourth edition. His contributions and advice have been invaluable in the development of the fourth and fifth editions.

I would also like to thank Chris Payne, RN, MA, for her technical assistance.

I wish to thank all of those at Delmar, Cengage Learning who contributed in any way to this text. Appreciation is expressed particularly to Deb Flis, Developmental Editor, for all of her guidance and support through the fourth and fifth editions, and especially for her understanding and assistance with this edition.

I and Delmar, Cengage Learning wish to thank the following reviewers for their review of the manuscript for the new edition.

Jannie R. Billue-Adams, PhD, RN, MS-HSA, BSN
Director, Medical Assisting
Clayton College and State University
School of Technology
Morrow, Georgia

Pamela deCalesta, OD, FAAO
Part-Time Faculty
Linn Benton Community College
Albany, Oregon

Donna Folmar, RN, BSN
Program Chair, Medical Assisting
Belmont Technical College
St. Clairsville, Ohio

Betty Haar, BS, RHIT
Program Director
Health Information Technology, Medical Coding, Medical Transcription Programs
Kirkwood Community College
Cedar Rapids, Iowa

Frances M. Warrick, MS, RN
Program Coordinator, Vocational Nursing
El Centro College
Dallas, Texas

I would also like to express appreciation to all of those who contributed to the previous editions.

CONTRIBUTORS

David M. Smith, RPh, MS
President, Westcoast Pharmacy Consultants, Bradenton, Florida
Pharmacist Team Leader, Pharmerica, Inc., Sarasota, Florida
Former Director of Pharmacy, Bon Secours-Venice Hospital and Health Care System, Venice, Florida

Karen DeHahn, BSN
Instructor, Practical Nursing Program
Sarasota County Technical Institute, Florida
Former Staff Nurse, Venice Hospital, Venice, Florida

Karin Ganns-Lee, MS, RD, LD
Consultant Dietitian, Hillsborough County, Florida

Julie Harman, MSN, ARNP
Former Instructor, Nursing Program, Lansing Community College
Private Practice, Obstetrics and Gynecology, Sarasota, Florida

Ann Holzheimer, RN, MSN
Clinical Nurse Specialist, Hospice of Hillsborough County
Tampa, Florida

Barbara Kirkpatrick, MEd, RRT
Assistant Professor, Respiratory Care
Manatee Community College, Bradenton, Florida

A. Christine Payne, RN, MA
Instructor, Online Coordinator, Health Science
Sarasota County Technical Institute, Sarasota, Florida
Former Instructor, Practical Nursing and Medical Assisting Programs
Sarasota County Technical Institute, Sarasota, Florida
Former Intensive Care Staff Nurse, Jess Parrish Memorial Hospital,
Titusville, Florida, Alachua General Hospital, Gainesville, Florida, and
St. Lukes Hospital, Richmond, Virginia

CONSULTANTS

Samuel L. Kalush, MD
Founder Open Heart Program, Saginaw, Michigan, Cardiologist,
Senior Friendship Center Medical Clinic, Sarasota, Florida

Leonard Kritzer, MD
Gynecologist, Senior Friendship Center Medical Clinic, and Sarasota
Memorial Hospital Community Medical Clinic, Sarasota, Florida

The Gulf Coast Glaucoma Clinic
Sarasota, Florida

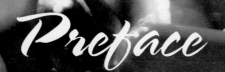

Preface

This book is designed as:

- A basic text for learners studying nursing, medical assisting, and other allied health occupations
- A continuing education update for practitioners in the health field
- Part of a refresher program for practitioners returning to health occupations
- A supplemental or reference book for practitioners wishing to extend their knowledge beyond basic training in specific health occupations

The purpose of this book is to provide an extensive framework of knowledge that can be acquired within a limited time frame. It will be especially helpful to learners in one-year training programs with limited time allotted to the study of medications. For those in longer programs, it can be used as the basis for more extensive study. It is appropriate as a required text in training those who will administer medications. It has been especially designed to meet the needs of learners in nursing and medical assistant programs. However, learners in allied health programs will find the concise format adaptable to their needs also.

This text has been field tested in several classes with learners in various health occupations. Learners who have already used this book for updating or supplemental education include registered nurses, licensed practical nurses, medical assistants, and paramedics.

Those employed in health occupations now have increased responsibilities for providing the necessary information to patients regarding the safe administration of medications, side effects, and interactions. Patient education is presented in every chapter in Part II. The quantity of information could be overwhelming and confusing to the learner unless presented in a comprehensive and concise manner.

ORGANIZATION

The text's concise format eliminates unnecessary detail that may tend to overwhelm or confuse the learner. Outdated or rarely used medications, obsolete information, and complex descriptions are eliminated. The information is both factual and functional.

Part I introduces the learner to the fascinating subject of drugs, their sources, and their uses. Calculations are simplified into two optional, step-by-step processes. *Review questions* at the end of each chapter help the learner master the information. Administration checklists allow the learner to put the knowledge into practice. Illustrations facilitate the learning process.

Part II organizes the drugs according to classifications, arranged in logical order. Each classification is described, along with characteristics of typical drugs, purpose, side effects, cautions, and interactions. Patient education for each category is highlighted.

Reference tables with each classification list the most commonly prescribed drugs according to generic and trade names, with dosage and available forms.

A **worksheet** at the end of each chapter helps the learner organize the information into outline form. When completing the worksheets, the learner is encouraged to only include those side effects from the chapter that are marked with the special side effect icon. **Case studies** within each chapter stimulate critical thinking and help learners to put into practice the information they have mastered. A review quiz follows each chapter. Comprehensive review quizzes for Part I and Part II are at the end of the book.

An extensive glossary lists and defines key terms used in the text. A comprehensive index includes both generic and trade names.

CHANGES TO THE FIFTH EDITION

More than 200 new drugs have been added. Tables and patient education boxes have been expanded. New terms have been added to the Glossary.

More than 80 illustrations have been completely revised and are now in full color. Many new photographs help to explain administration techniques, equipment, and other topics.

In Part II, a review quiz has been added to each chapter. Also in Part II, a special icon ✳ has been added that identifies the most common and/or most important side effects of drugs that the learner should be familiar with. Because the side effects for HIV/AIDS drugs are too numerous to commit to memory, there is no icon associated with these drugs. Side effects marked with an icon for the antineoplastic drugs are those common to the majority of the chemotherapy drugs. The author recognizes that opinions may differ on which side effects are the most important. This special icon is meant to serve as a valuable guide for learners. Rather than memorizing every side effect for each drug, the icon emphasizes which side effects are the most important, and those with which the learner should be familiar.

The following chapters have had significant additions with topics of current interest.

- Chapter 5: The *Abbreviations* list has been extensively revised and updated. Recommendations have been included from the *Institute for Safe Medications Practice (ISMP)* and *JCAHO* describing *dangerous* abbreviations that have been prohibited.

- Chapter 10: New protocol for *Treatment of Poisoning* has been added.

- Chapter 11: New information on *Herbal Remedies* and FDA warnings have been added, as well as new online references for herbal products.

- Chapter 12: New information regarding treatments for acne, including the *Accutane* protocol, has been included.

- Chapter 14: Many new antineoplastics are described for those specializing in the oncology field. Included are *Monoclonal Antibodies,* which target only cancer cells, and also alternatives to tamoxifen in the treatment of breast cancer.

- Chapter 15: New drugs for benign prostatic hypertrophy (BPH) have been added.

- Chapter 16: New drugs for ulcers, GERD, *Helicobacter pylori*, and inflammatory bowel disease have been added.

- Chapter 17: New information on *antimicrobial resistance* has been added. Numerous anti-infectives that were added include new agents for *VRE* and *MRSA;* new *antivirals,* especially treatment for herpes zoster (shingles); and new therapy for *HIV* and *AIDS* (for those specializing in that field).

- Chapter 19: The Table for *Opioid Analgesics* has been extensively revised, and also the section on *Sedatives* and *Hypnotics.* Other additions include *Migraine Therapy* and the *Lidoderm* patch.

- Chapter 20: New drugs added include a medicine for narcolepsy, sleep apnea, and shift-work sleep disorder. New information regarding ADHD and ADD includes extended-release drugs and a *nonstimulant noncontrolled* drug for *ADHD.* A new drug for *bipolar disorder* has also been added.

- Chapter 22: New drugs were added for Parkinson's disease and Alzheimer's.

- Chapter 23: New *Insulins* and *Oral Antidiabetic Agents* have been added.

- Chapter 24: New *Androgens* and *Impotence Agents* were added. Also included are the Women's Health Initiative (WHI) study results and recommendations regarding hormone replacement therapy (HRT) for postmenopausal women.

- Chapter 25: Many new drugs have been added, including: antihypertensives, such as, *Angiotensin Receptor Blockers* (ARBs); antilipemics, including a *Cholesterol Absorption Inhibitor;* new *Platelet Inhibitors;* and a new category called *Colony Stimulating Factors* for severe anemia.

- Chapter 26: New bronchodilators and corticosteroids, inhaled and nasal, have been added.
- Chapter 27: A new table has been added: *Potentially Inappropriate Medications for Older Adults.* This supplements the *Gray List.*

ESSENTIALS OF PHARMACOLOGY FOR HEALTH OCCUPATIONS, FIFTH EDITION STUDYWARE™

The StudyWare™ CD-ROM offers an exciting way to gain additional practice in learning pharmacology. The quizzes and activities help reinforce even the most difficult concepts. See *"How to Use the Essentials of Pharmacology for Health Occupations,* Fifth Edition StudyWARE™" for details.

STUDY GUIDE

The study guide offers additional practice with review questions corresponding to each chapter in the text including: multiple choice, fill-in-the-blank, true/false, and matching questions. Case studies encourage you to apply the knowledge you have learned about drugs in Part II. Answers to all of the questions and case studies are included in the Instructor's Manual in the Electronic Classroom Manager.
Study Guide, ISBN 1-4018-8930-1

THE ELECTRONIC CLASSROOM MANAGER

The Electric Classroom Manager is a robust computerized tool for your instructional needs! A must-have for all instructors, this comprehensive and convenient CD-ROM contains the following components.

- **Exam View® Computerized Testbank** contains over 850 questions that cover chapters 1 through 27. You can use the questions to create your own review materials or tests.
- **PowerPoint® Presentations** are designed to aid you in planning your class presentations. If a learner misses a class, a printout of the slides for a lecture makes a helpful review page.
- **Instructor's Manual** includes the following tools:
  - Review quiz with answers for every chapter
  - Alternate Comprehensive Exam Part II with answers
  - Answers to review quizzes and comprehensive review exams in the text
  - Answers to case studies and worksheets in Part II in the text
  - Answers to review questions and case studies in the Study Guide

Electronic Classroom Manager, ISBN 1-4018-8926-3

WEBTUTOR™

Designed to complement the text, WebTUTOR™ is a content-rich, Web-based teaching and learning aid that reinforces and clarifies complex concepts. The WebCT™ and Blackboard™ platforms also provide rich communication tools to instructors and students, including a course calendar, chat, e-mail, and threaded discussions.

WebTUTOR™ on WebCT™, ISBN 1-4018-8928-X

Text Bundled with WebTUTOR™ on WebCT™, ISBN 1-4180-3373-1

WebTUTOR™ on Blackboard™, ISBN 1-4018-8929-8

Text Bundled with WebTUTOR™ on Blackboard™, ISBN 1-4180-3374-X

TO THE LEARNER STUDYING PHARMACOLOGY

Other learners, such as you, have helped me put this book together. They have learned that the study of medications can be a fascinating one. They tell me that this book has helped them to develop confidence and competence in dispensing medications and information about drugs to their patients. You will find this is only the beginning, a framework upon which you will build a vast store of useful knowledge.

Learners have told me that the objectives, review questions, worksheets, and case studies were tremendously helpful to them. Organization is the key to acquiring large quantities of information. You will be amazed at all you have learned when you complete this book.

Keep growing and learning and questioning all of your life.

RUTH WOODROW

How to Use This Textbook

Essentials of Pharmacology for Health Occupations, Fifth Edition, helps you learn drug information in a concise format. Drugs are organized by classifications and include their purpose, side effects, cautions, and interactions. The following features are integrated throughout the book to assist you in learning and mastering core concepts and terms.

OBJECTIVES

The objectives alert you to core concepts you should understand after reading the chapter.

KEY TERMS

Key terms are highlighted and defined in the text the first time they are used. An extensive glossary lists and defines all key terms used throughout the book.

CLASSIFICATIONS

Drugs are organized according to classifications. Each classification is described, along with characteristics of typical drugs, purpose, side effects, cautions, and interactions.

SIDE EFFECTS OF DRUGS

A special icon identifies the most common and/or most important side effects of drugs. This special icon is meant to serve as a valuable guide for learners. Rather than memorizing every side effect for each drug, the icon emphasizes the side effects with which you should be familiar.

Chapter 3
Sources and Bodily Effects of Drugs

Objectives

Upon completion of this chapter, the learner should be able to
1. Identify the four sources of drugs
2. Differentiate between the following: drug actions and drug effects, systemic effects and local effects, loading dose and maintenance dose, and toxic dose and lethal dose
3. Define the following processes as th... drugs through the body... effectiveness...

Key Terms

Adverse drug effects
Dosage
Drug interactions
Drug processes
Effects of drugs
Sou...

Objectives

Upon completion of this chapter, the learner should be able to
1. Define the Key Terms
2. Describe side effects, contraindications, and interactions of antacids, antiulcer agents, antidiarrhea agents, antiflatulents, cathartics and laxatives, and antiemetics
3. Compare and contrast the five types of laxatives according to use, side effects, contraindications, and interactions
4. Identify examples of drugs from each of the eight categories of gastrointestinal drugs
5. Explain important patient education for each category of gastrointestinal drugs

Key Terms

Antacids
Antidiarrhea
Antiemetics
Antiflatulents
Antiulcer
GERD
Laxatives

Gastrointestinal drugs can be divided into eight categories based on the action: antacids, drugs for treatment of ulcers, antispasmodics, management of inflammatory bowel disease, antidiarrhea agents, antiflatulents, laxatives and cathartics, and antiemetics.

ANTACIDS

Antacids act by partially *neutralizing* gastric hydrochloric acid and are widely available in many over-the-counter (OTC) preparations for the relief of indigestion, heartburn, and sour stomach. Antacids are also prescribed at times (between meals and at hour of sleep) to help relieve pain and promote the healing of gastric and duodenal ulcers. Other antiulcer agents are discussed later in this chapter. Antacids are also used at times in the management of esophageal reflux.

24

250   PART II DRUG CLASSIFICATIONS

Antacid products may contain aluminum, calcium carbonate, or magnesium, either individually or in combination. Most antacids also contain sodium. Sodium bicarbonate alone is not recommended because of flatulence, metabolic alkalosis, and electrolyte imbalance with prolonged use. Calcium carbonate, for example, Tums, may cause constipation.

The choice of a specific antacid preparation depends on palatability, cost, adverse effects, acid neutralizing capacity, the sodium content, and the patient's renal and cardiovascular function. Magnesium and/or aluminum antacids are the most commonly used. Magnesium can cause diarrhea and aluminum is constipating. Therefore, combinations are frequently used to control the frequency and consistency of bowel movements, for example, Maalox, Gelusil, Mylanta.

Side effects with frequent use of antacids may include:

✱ Constipation (with aluminum or calcium carbonate antacids)
✱ Diarrhea (with magnesium antacids)
✱ Electrolyte imbalance
  Urinary calculi and renal complications
  Osteoporosis (with aluminum antacids)
  Belching and flatulence (with calcium carbonate and sodium bicarbonate)

Contraindications or extreme caution with antacids applies to:

  Congestive heart failure
  Renal pathology or history of renal calculi
  Cirrhosis of the liver or edema
  Dehydration or electrolyte imbalance

Interactions of antacids with almost any other drug administered concurrently can alter the effectiveness of the other drugs. Therefore, *antacids should not be taken within two hours of most other drugs.* With the following drug... antacids may decrease effectiveness of...

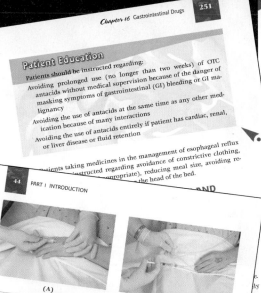

Patient Education

Patients should be instructed regarding:

Avoiding prolonged use (no longer than two weeks) of OTC antacids without medical supervision because of the danger of masking symptoms of gastrointestinal (GI) bleeding or GI malignancy

Avoiding the use of antacids at the same time as any other medication because of many interactions

Avoiding the use of antacids entirely if patient has cardiac, renal, or liver disease or fluid retention

...tients taking medicines in the management of esophageal reflux ...instructed regarding avoidance of constrictive clothing, ...ppropriate), reducing meal size, avoiding re... ...the head of the bed,

PATIENT EDUCATION

Patient education is summarized and highlighted for each classification of drugs. These special boxes will assist health care workers to instruct patients and answer their questions about the medications they are taking.

---

44 PART I INTRODUCTION

(A)

IV Solution Bag

Injection Port

(B)

IVPB

Drip Chamber

FULL-COLOR PHOTOS AND ILLUSTRATIONS

Full-color photographs and illustrations help explain and reinforce administration techniques and medication equipment.

Table 26-3 Antianxiety Medications (Anxiolytics)

GENERIC NAME	TRADE NAME	DOSAGE	COMMENTS
Benzodiazepines (short-term only)			Abrupt withdrawal may cause severe side effects
alprazolam	Xanax	PO 0.125–0.5 mg BID–TID	For panic disorder
	Xanax XR	PO 0.5–6 mg q A.M.	Larger doses IV/IM with severe anxiety or ethanol withdrawal
chlordiazepoxide	Librium	PO 5–25 mg TID or 4×/day	For older adult patients no more than 15 mg daily
chlorazepate	Tranxene	PO 15–60 mg daily div. doses	Do not mix in syringe with other medications, also used as muscle relaxant
		7.5–15 mg daily div. doses	or IV in status epilepticus
diazepam	Valium	PO 2–10 mg TID, IV	For older adults who are agitated
lorazepam	Ativan	PO or IM 2–3 mg daily div. doses	For older adults who are agitated
oxazepam	Serax	PO 10–15 mg TID or 4×/day	
Other Anxiolytics			Slow onset of action, may be used long term
buspirone	Buspar	PO 15–60 mg daily div doses	Antiemetic, antipruritic, or preoperative
hydroxyzine (antihistamine)	Atarax, Vistaril	PO 25–100 mg 4×/day or 25–100 mg deep IM	

REFERENCE TABLES

Reference tables within each classification list the most commonly prescribed drugs according to generic and trade names, with dosage and available forms.

---

36 PART I INTRODUCTION

CHAPTER REVIEW QUIZ

Fill in the blanks.

1. Drug Sources

	Example	Trade Name	Classification

2. Drugs that are distributed throughout the body have _____

3. Drugs whose action is limited to a specific location have _____ effects.

4. As drugs pass through the body, they undergo four processes: _____ effects.

Process	Definition of Process

5. Factors that may affect the passage of drugs through the body:

Primary Site of Process	Conditions Hampering Process

...ulty, or excretion in...

REVIEW QUIZZES AND COMPREHENSIVE REVIEW EXAM

Review quizzes at the end of each chapter assist learners in identifying areas for further study. Two comprehensive review exams further help learners assess understanding of material learned.

WORKSHEETS

Worksheets assist learners to become familiar with the characteristics of each classification using one or two of the most commonly used drugs in that category, including the side effects, cautions, and interactions. The worksheets help learners organize their notes in outline form, and provide a valuable study tool.

CASE STUDIES

Case studies stimulate critical thinking through the presentation of reality-based situations regarding drug usage.

WORKSHEET FOR CHAPTER 17
ANTI-INFECTIVE DRUGS

List the drugs according to category and complete all columns. Learn generic or trade names as specified by instructor.

...tions ...s	Purpose	Side Effects	Contraindications or Cautions	Interactions/ Patient Education

379

Chapter 20 Psychotropic Medications, Alcohol, and Drug Abuse

A. Case Study for Psychotropic Medications

Miss Blue, a 25-year-old secretary, presents in the physician's office with a history of depression for one month. She complains of crying frequently, loss of appetite, and insomnia. The physician prescribes Tofranil. The patient should be given the following information:

1. She should expect to feel better
   a. In a few days
   b. In a few weeks
   c. One hour after taking medicine
   d. One day after taking medicine

2. The medicine should be taken
   a. Before meals
   b. With meals
   c. In the morning
   d. At bedtime

3. She can expect all of the following side effects EXCEPT
   a. Increased appetite
   b. Improved sleep
   c. Weight loss
   d. Dry mouth

4. She should be told to report any of the following side effects EXCEPT
   a. Dizziness
   b. Palpitations
   c. Blurred vision
   d. Increased thirst

B. Case Study for Psychotropic Medication

Mr. Elzware, a 90-year-old nursing home resident with Alzheimer's, Parkinson's, and enlarged prostate, has been pacing the hall talking loudly in a confused way. He is wringing his hands. The nurse calls the physician's office and requests Haldol "to calm him down." Both the nurse in the nursing home and the medical assistant in the physician's office should be aware of the following facts about Haldol:

1. Haldol is only an appropriate medication for which condition listed below?
   a. Nervousness
   b. Confusion
   c. Uncooperativeness
   d. Combativeness

   Haldol is appropriate in which of the following conditions?
   ...Seizure disorder
   ...arkinson's disease
   d. Paranoid psychosis
   e. Depression

   ...tic hypertrophy
   ...n be caused by all of the following EXCEPT
   c. Senility
   d. Urina...

How to Use Study*WARE*™ to Accompany Essentials of Pharmacology for Health Occupations, Fifth Edition

SYSTEM REQUIREMENTS

Minimum System Requirements

Operating System: Microsoft Windows 95, 98 SE, or Windows 2000 or XP

Processor: Pentium PC 500 MHz or higher (750 MHz recommended)

RAM: 64 MB of RAM (128 MB recommended)

Screen Resolution: 800 × 600 pixels

Color Depth: 16-bit color (thousands of colors)

Macromedia Flash Player V7.x. (The Macromedia Flash Player is free, and can be downloaded from http://www.macromedia.com)

INSTALLATION INSTRUCTIONS

1. Insert disc into CD-ROM player. The *Essentials of Pharmacology for Health Occupations*, Fifth Edition StudyWare™ installation program should start up automatically. If it does not, go to step 2.

2. From My Computer, double click the icon for the CD drive.

3. Double click the *setup.exe* file to start the program.

TECHNICAL SUPPORT

Telephone: 1-800-648-7450, 8:30 A.M.–5:30 P.M. Eastern Time

Fax: 1-518-881-1247

E-mail: delmar.help@cengage.com

StudyWare™ is a trademark used herein under license.

LICENSE AGREEMENT

Refer to the license agreement in the back of the book.

The StudyWARE™ software helps you learn terms and concepts in *Essentials of Pharmacology for Health Occupations*, Fifth Edition. As you study each chapter in the text, be sure to explore the activity in the corresponding chapter in the software. Use StudyWARE™ as your own private tutor to help you learn the material in your *Essentials of Pharmacology for Health Occupations, Fifth Edition* textbook.

Getting started is easy. Install the software by inserting the CD-ROM into your computer's CD-ROM drive and following the on-screen instructions. When you open the software, enter your first and last name so the software can store your quiz results. Then choose a chapter from the menu to take a quiz or explore one of the activities.

MENUS

You can access the menus from wherever you are in the program. The menus include Quizzes, Activities, and Scores.

Quizzes. Quizzes include fill-in-the-blank and multiple choice questions. You can take the quizzes in both Practice Mode and Quiz Mode. Use Practice Mode to improve your mastery of the material. You have multiple tries to get the answers correct. Instant feedback tells you whether you're right or wrong—and helps you learn quickly by explaining why an answer was correct or incorrect. Use Quiz Mode when you are ready to test yourself and keep a record of your scores. In Quiz Mode, you have one try to get the answers right, but you can take each quiz as many times as you want.

Scores. You can view your last scores for each quiz and print your results to hand in to your instructor.

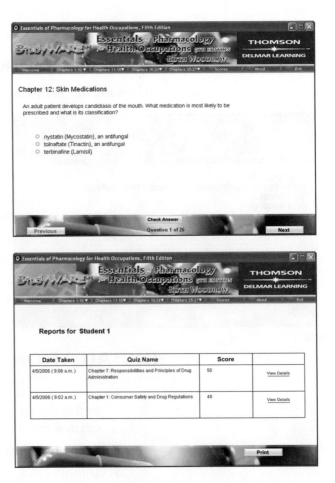

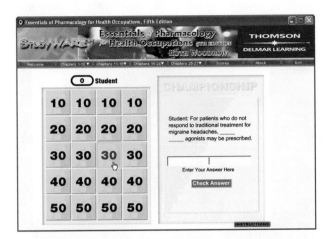

Activity. Have fun while increasing your knowledge with the Championship game!

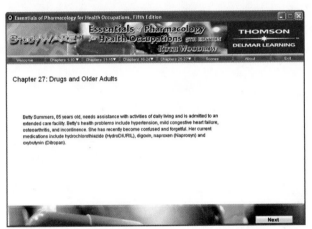

Case Studies. Case Studies stimulate critical thinking through real-world situations regarding drug usage.

PART I
Introduction

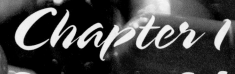

Chapter 1
Consumer Safety and Drug Regulations

Objectives

Upon completion of this chapter, the learner should be able to

1. Explain what is meant by drug standards
2. Name the first drug law passed in this country for consumer safety, and give the year it was passed
3. Summarize the provisions of the Federal Food, Drug, and Cosmetic Act of 1938, and identify the government agency that enforces the act
4. Interpret what is meant by USP/NF
5. Summarize the provisions of the Controlled Substances Act of 1970
6. Explain what is meant by a DEA number
7. Define schedules of controlled substances, and differentiate between C-I to C-V schedules
8. State several responsibilities you have in the dispensing of medications, as a direct result of the three major drug laws described in this chapter
9. Define the Key Terms

Key Terms

Controlled substances

Drug Enforcement Administration (DEA)

Drug standards

Food and Drug Administration (FDA)

Your decision to pursue a career in the health care field probably took a great deal of thought. No doubt you have questioned whether you will be able to handle the unique situations that arise in a clinic, health care facility, or physician's office. Have you ever stopped to consider the impact *you* will make on the lives of others as a health care worker? Not only can you make a tremendous difference in the efficiency of the facility, but you can have a positive impact on your friends and family, as well as the patient or client.

3

It is inevitable that you will receive phone calls and questions about medications, prescriptions, and drug therapy. A great majority of patients are far too inhibited to tell their physician that there are things they do not understand about their medications. They feel much more at ease discussing their questions with the health care worker. Your potential for informing others with knowledgeable answers about medications can be quite an asset!

The key to reaching that potential is having knowledgeable answers. A serious, responsible attitude about all aspects of drug therapy is imperative. Consider yourself a potential prime resource of medication information for your friends, family, and future patients, as you begin to examine the foundations of facts about drugs. It may be necessary for you to clarify some of the layperson misunderstandings about the legalities of dispensing medications. Consider the following misconceptions and facts.

FALLACY	FACT
Only nurses can give medications to patients.	Trained and certified health care workers who may legally give medications include physicians, physician assistants, paramedics, medical office assistants, and practical, vocational, and registered nurses.
Only physicians may write prescriptions.	Dentists, physicians, physician assistants, veterinarians, nurse practitioners, and registered pharmacists may write prescriptions for their specific field of work, within limitations. For example, veterinarians write prescriptions for animal use only.
Prescriptions are required for narcotics only.	Specific drugs ruled illegal to purchase without the use of a prescription include: • Those that need to be **controlled** *because they are addictive and tend to be abused and dangerous* (e.g., depressants, stimulants, psychedelics, and narcotics). • Those that may cause dangerous health threats from side effects if taken incorrectly (e.g., antibiotics, cardiac drugs, tranquilizers)
All drugs produced in the United States are made in federally approved laboratories.	Numerous undercover illegal laboratories exist and operate within the United States today.

DRUG LAWS

The matter of dispensing drugs in the United States is specifically addressed by laws passed in the 1900s. Scientific advances, progress, and changes in society in the last century have made it necessary for drug laws to be set for our safety. Although substances have been taken into the body for their effects for centuries, so many are being produced today that *consumer safety* is now a critical issue.

Drug standards are rules set to assure consumers that they get what they pay for. The law says that all preparations called by the same drug name must be of *uniform strength, quality,* and *purity.*

Because of drug standardization, when you take a prescription to be filled, you are assured of getting the same basic drug, in the same amount and quality, no matter to which pharmacy or to which part of the country you take the prescription to be filled. According to drug standards, the drug companies must not add other active ingredients or varying amounts of chemicals to a specific drug preparation. They must meet the drug standards (federally approved requirements) for the specified strength, quality, and purity of the drug.

Unlike our predecessors, we no longer have to wonder what ingredients, if any (other than sugar and water, or alcohol), are in the "medicinal waters" being sold.

In the market of illegal (illicit) drugs, the lack of enforcement of drug standards is the consumer's danger. With no controls on the quality of illegal drugs (because they are unapproved for safety), many deaths have occurred from overdose. Consider the heroin user, accustomed to very poor-quality heroin, who accidentally overdoses when given a much higher quality of heroin from a new source.

The laws that have evolved to provide consumer safety can be summed up by three major acts. They are described in the order in which they became necessary for consumer safety.

The importance of the timing of the Federal Food, Drug, and Cosmetic Act should be noted. It came about as the answer to a disastrous occurrence in 1937. A sulfa preparation, not adequately tested for safety, was responsible for 100 deaths that year. Thus, the need was recognized for more proof of the safety and effectiveness of new drugs.

1906   Pure Food And Drug Act

First government attempt to establish consumer protection in the manufacture of drugs and foods.

Required all drugs marketed in the United States to meet minimal standards of strength, purity, and quality.

Demanded that drug preparations containing morphine have a labeled container indicating the ingredient morphine.

Established two references of *officially* approved drugs. Before 1906, information about drugs was handed down from generation to generation. No official written resources existed. After the 1906 legislation, two references specified the official U.S. standards for making each drug. Those references, listed below, have since been combined into one book, referred to as the USP/NF:

- United States Pharmacopoeia (USP)
- National Formulary (NF)

1938 Federal Food, Drug, and Cosmetic Act and Amendments of 1951 and 1965

Established the **Food and Drug Administration (FDA)** under the Department of Health and Welfare to enforce the provisions of the act.

Established *more specific* regulations to prevent adulteration of (tampering with) drugs, foods, and cosmetics:

- All labels must be accurate and must include generic names.
- All new products must be approved by the FDA before public release.
- "Warning" labels must be present on certain preparations, for example, "may cause drowsiness," "may cause nervousness," and "may be habit-forming."
- Certain drugs must be labeled with the legend (inscription): "Caution—federal law prohibits dispensing without a prescription." Thus, the term *legend drugs* refers to such preparations. The act also designated which drugs can be sold without a prescription.
- Prescription and nonprescription drugs must be shown to be *effective* as well as *safe*.

1970 Controlled Substances Act

Established the **Drug Enforcement Administration (DEA)** as a bureau of the Department of Justice to enforce the provisions of the act.

Set much tighter controls on a specific group of drugs: *those that were being abused by society;* the name of the act indicates that such *substances needed to be controlled.* They include depressants, stimulants, psychedelics, narcotics, and anabolic steroids. The act:

- Isolated the abused and addicting drugs into five levels, or schedules, according to their degree of danger: C-I, C-II, C-III, C-IV, and C-V.
- Demanded security of **controlled substances**; anyone (e.g., pharmacists, hospitals, physicians, and drug companies) who dispenses, receives, sells, or destroys controlled substances must keep on hand special DEA forms, indicating the exact current inventory, and a two-year inventory of every controlled substance transaction.
- Set limitations on the use of prescriptions; guidelines were established for each of the five schedules of controlled substances, regulating the number of times a drug may be prescribed in a six-month period as well as for which schedules prescriptions may be phoned in to the pharmacy, and so on.
- Demanded that each prescriber of these substances register with the DEA and obtain a DEA registration number, to be present on their prescriptions of controlled substances; drug manufacturers must also be registered and identified with their own DEA numbers, as must pharmacists, physicians, veterinarians, and so on.

The five schedules of controlled substances are arranged with the potentially most dangerous at level I and the least dangerous at level V. The lower the number, the stricter are the restrictions for control by the DEA. Thus, level I is the strictest.

Drugs are frequently added, deleted, or moved from one schedule to another. If, for example, the DEA determines that drug A is becoming more of a societal problem, with an increased incidence of overdoses, drug A may be moved from the C-IV schedule to C-III. It is extremely important that the health care worker keep informed of any changes in drug scheduling. For the most part, using the most current drug reference book will keep you up to date.

You will recognize the schedule of a particular controlled substance by noting a *C* with either *I, II, III, IV,* or *V* after it. Some references show the capital C with the Roman numeral inside the curve of the C (ⓒ). Labels on controlled substances are also designated with a C and a Roman numeral to indicate its level of control. Drug inserts (information leaflets accompanying drugs) are also marked with a C and the appropriate schedule number. (See Table 1-1 and Figure 1-1.)

Table 1-1 Five Schedules of Controlled Substances

SCHEDULE NUMBER	ABUSE POTENTIAL AND LEGAL LIMITATIONS	EXAMPLES OF SUBSTANCES
1, C	High abuse potential Not approved for medical use in the United States	heroin, LSD, mescaline
2, C	High abuse potential May lead to severe dependence Written prescription only No phoning in of prescription by office health care worker No refills May be faxed, but original prescription must be handed in to pick up prescription In emergency, physician may phone in, but handwritten prescription must go to pharmacy within 72 hours	morphine, codeine, methadone, Percocet, Tylox, Dilaudid, Ritalin, cocaine, Oxycontin, meperidine (Demerol)
3, C	May lead to limited dependence Written, faxed, or verbal (phoned in) prescription, by physician only May be refilled up to five times in 6 months	Marinol, Tussionex, Tylenol with codeine
4, C	Lower abuse potential than the above schedules Prescription may be written out by health care worker, but must be signed by the physician Prescription may be phoned in by health care worker or faxed May be refilled up to five times in 6 months	Valium, Ativan, Xanax, phenobarbital, Librium, Darvocet, Restoril, Ambien
5, C	Low abuse potential compared to the above schedules Consists primarily of preparations for cough suppressants containing codeine and preparations for diarrhea (e.g., paregoric and opium tincture)	Phenergan with codeine, Robitussin-A-C, Tussi-Organidin, N.R., Donnagel-PG, Lomotil

Note: Some states may have stricter schedules than the Federal regulations. You must be aware of the regulations in your area.

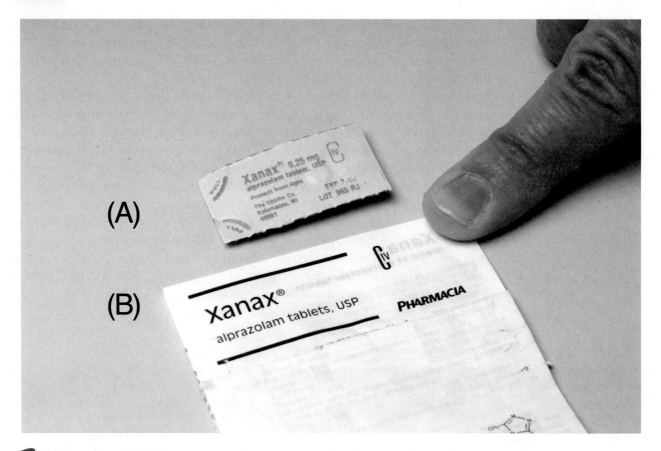

Figure 1-1 Controlled substance schedule numbers appear in a variety of drug information resources, including (A) drug packages and (B) drug inserts. Schedule numbers are also found in drug reference books.

FDA AND DEA

The increase in the number of drugs produced for marketing brought dangers to the public. The federal Food and Drug Administration (FDA) was established to assure that some basic standards would be followed. Its responsibilities include:

- Inspecting plants where foods, drugs, or cosmetics are made
- Reviewing new drug applications and petitions for food additives
- Investigating and removing unsafe drugs from the market
- Ensuring proper labeling of foods, cosmetics, and drugs

When the need for better control of addictive drugs became urgent, the FDA had its hands full just trying to enforce basic drug standards. It became imperative to set up a new department, the Drug Enforcement Administration (DEA), in 1970 to handle all the needs and safety controls for the more dangerous drugs. Thus, the two agencies—FDA and DEA—were established with their own specific areas of drug control.

As a health care worker and an informed citizen, you must be aware of the latest developments concerning these two agencies. Hardly a week goes by without mention of the activities of the FDA or the DEA in the news. You should be able to recognize their separate areas of control.

FDA
Concerned with general safety standards in the production of drugs, foods, and cosmetics Responsible for approval and removal of products on the market

DEA
Concerned with controlled substances only Enforces laws against drug activities, including illegal drug use, dealing, and manufacturing Monitors need for changing the schedules of abused drugs

HEALTH CARE WORKERS AND THE LAW

In some ways, you will be as involved as the physician in observing the restrictions of the drug laws. You will have the responsibility of keeping accurate records of the medications dispensed. You will maintain the supply of drugs at your facility. If you work in a doctor's office, clinic, or ambulatory care setting, you also will be involved with phoning in prescriptions and securing prescription forms at your facility.

The following guidelines should be followed by the health care worker involved in dispensing medications:

1. Keep a *current* drug reference book available at all times. You should be able to readily identify substances that must be controlled.

2. Keep controlled substances locked securely. Double-locking is recommended. This means:
   a. Placing the drugs in a locked safety box.
   b. Placing the locked box in a cupboard that is also locked.

3. Conceal prescription pads at your office, clinic, or facility. Do not leave pads out in the open, especially in patient examining rooms. The prescription pads, with the physician's DEA registration number, are a possible source of fraud and drug tampering when forged and used illegally. Keep the pads in a designated location (e.g., a drawer), out of the public areas of the office or nursing station.

4. Keep accurate records of each controlled substance dispensed, received, or destroyed at your facility. These records, as well as the records from the previous two years, must be available at all times.

5. Be responsible for keeping up to date with current news of the activities of the FDA and the DEA. Keep informed of any changes in the scheduling of controlled substances.

6. Establish a working rapport with a pharmacist. A local pharmacist is an excellent resource for you when you are unsure of your legal responsibilities with drugs or have any uncertainties about drug therapy.

7. If you work in an office, maintain a professional rapport with the pharmaceutical representatives who leave drug samples there. They are also excellent resources for drug information.

CHAPTER REVIEW QUIZ

Complete the following statements.

1. The first major U.S. drug law was passed in the year _____ and was called the _____.

2. USP stands for _____
   and is the title of _____.

3. NF stands for _____.

4. Which drug law established the USP and NF (which are now one)? _____

5. The agency that requires you to keep a record of each controlled substance transaction is the _____.

6. Prescriptions for schedule C-_____ drugs may be phoned in by the health care worker.

7. How long must you keep an inventory record of each controlled substance transaction at your office? _____

8. Three responsibilities of the FDA include:

   _____

   _____

   _____

9. What types of drugs are listed in the C-V schedule? _____

   _____

10. What method is recommended for securing the controlled substances at your office?_____

11. If a patient calls to request a refill of a Percocet (C-II) prescription, how would you reply?

   _____

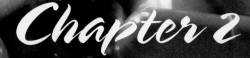

Chapter 2
Drug Names and References

Objectives

Upon completion of this chapter, the learner should be able to

1. Differentiate among the following drug names: generic name, official name, trade name, and chemical name
2. Explain what is indicated by a number included in a drug trade name (e.g., Tylenol No. 3)
3. Define and explain the restrictions of drug sales implied by the following: OTC, legend drug, and controlled substance
4. List at least two drug references available today
5. Discuss several characteristics that you consider important in choosing the best drug reference
6. Identify the types of information listed on drug cards
7. Define the following side effects: ototoxicity, nephrotoxicity, tinnitus, and photosensitivity
8. Define the Key Terms

Key Terms

Actions

Adverse reactions

Cautions

Classifications

Contraindications

Generic names

Indications

Interactions

Pharmacology

Prototype

Side effects

Trade names

Pharmacology can be defined as the study of drugs and their origin, nature, properties, and effects on living organisms. We need to know why drugs are given, how they work, and what effects to expect. The thousands of drugs products on the market would make this subject difficult to tackle if it were not for:

- Numerous drug references, geared to a variety of levels of readers, from layperson to pharmacist
- Grouping of drugs under broad subcategories
- Continuity in the use of basic identifying terms for the names and actions of drugs

11

CLASSIFICATIONS

Each drug can be categorized under a broad *subcategory*, or *subcategories*, called **classifications** (see list below). Drugs that affect the body in similar ways are listed in the same classification. Drugs that have several types of therapeutic effects fit under several classifications. For example, aspirin has a variety of effects on the body. It may be given to relieve pain (analgesic), to reduce fever (antipyretic), or to reduce inflammation of tissues (anti-inflammatory). Therefore, aspirin is categorized under three classifications of drugs (as shown in parentheses).

Another drug, cyclobenzaprine (Flexeril), however, is known to be used for only one therapeutic effect: to relieve muscle spasms. Flexeril, therefore, is listed under only one classification (muscle relaxant).

Examples of some of the other drug classifications are listed below. Are you familiar with any of them already?

adrenergics	cholinergics	hypnotics
anesthetics	decongestants	hypoglycemics
antibiotics	diuretics	laxatives
antihistamines	electrolytes	sedatives
antihypertensives	emetics	tranquilizers
antitussives	expectorants	vasoconstrictors
cardiotonics	hormones	vasodilators

The second part of this text compares the characteristics of the various major drug classifications. In each chapter, as a classification is explained, you will learn what general information to associate with drugs of that classification:

- Therapeutic uses
- Most common side effects
- Precautions to be used
- Contraindications
- Interactions that may occur when taken with other drugs or foods
- Some of the most common product names, usual dosages, and comments on administration

You will also be given a prototype of each classification. A **prototype** is a *model example,* a drug that typifies the characteristics of that classification. Hopefully, each time you learn of a new drug, you will associate the prototype and its characteristics with the new drug, based on its classification.

You can find the classification, as well as the various names of the drug, by referring to a drug reference book.

IDENTIFYING NAMES

Four terms apply to the various titles of a drug:

1. *Generic name.*   Common or general name assigned to the drug; differentiated from trade name by initial lowercase letter; never capitalized

2. *Trade name.* The name by which a pharmaceutical company identifies its product; is copyrighted and used exclusively by that company; can be distinguished from the generic name by capitalized first letter and is often shown on labels and references with the symbol ® after the name (for "registered" trademark)

3. *Chemical name.* The exact molecular formula of the drug; usually a long, very difficult name to pronounce and of little concern to the health care worker

4. *Official name.* Name of the drug as it appears in the official reference, the *USP/NF*; generally the same as the generic name

The use of generic names and trade names for drugs can be compared to the various names of grocery products. Two examples of generic names are orange juice and detergent. Corresponding trade names are Sunkist, Bird's Eye, Tropicana, and Minute Maid and Cheer, Tide, All, and Fab. While there is only one generic name, there may be many trade names.

When a company produces a new drug for the market, it assigns a generic name to the product. After testing and approval by the FDA, the drug company gives the drug a trade name (often something short and easy to remember when advertised). For 17 years, from the time the company submitts a new drug application (NDA) to the FDA for approval, the company has the exclusive right to market the drug. Once approved, the drug is listed in the USP/NF by an official name, which is usually the same as the generic name. When 17 years have passed, and the patent has expired, other companies may begin to combine the same chemicals to form that specific generic product for marketing. Each company will assign their own specific trade name to the product.

Compare the names of the following two drugs:

Generic Name	Chemical Name	Trade Name (Drug Company)
tetracycline hydrochloride	4-dimethylamino-4,12 aoctahydro-3,6,10,12,12a pentahydroxyl-6-methyl-1,11-dioxi-2 naphthacenecarboxamide hydrochloride	Achromycin V (Lederle Labs) Sumycin (Apothecon) Tetracycline HCL (Richlyn)*
propoxyphene hydrochloride	alpha-4 dimethylamino-3-methyl-1-2,2-diphyenyl-2 butanol, proprionate hydrochloride	Darvon (Eli Lilly) Propoxyphene HCL (Rexall)*

Some companies simply elect to market the product by the generic name.

Patient Education

Patients may ask you about the difference between generic and trade (brand) name products. Generally, trade name products are more expensive, although the basic active ingredients (drug contents) are the same as in the generic. The higher price helps to pay for advertisements promoting the trade name. (Can you think of certain trade names that are heavily advertised in television commercials?)

For this reason it is economically wise to compare prices of over-the-counter (OTC) products that have the same generic components and strengths. For example, several cough syrups may have exactly the same contents, but the prices may vary widely.

Read and compare all ingredients on the labels.

Concerning prescription drugs, most states have enacted legislation encouraging physicians to let pharmacists substitute less expensive *generic equivalents* for prescribed brand name drugs. Specific provisions of *drug substitution laws* vary from state to state.

The physician may indicate "no substitutions" on the prescription, usually indicated by a DAW (dispense as written). Often physicians have preferences for certain products. Even though the drug contents are the same, the "fillers," or ingredients that are used to hold the preparation together, may be slightly different. This difference in fillers may affect how quickly the drug dissolves or takes effect. Dyes in some products may alter effects in some sensitive patients by leading to an allergic response.

Many products are combinations of several generic components. You will recognize this when you see several generic names (not capitalized) and corresponding amounts listed under one trade name (capitalized). Examples are:

Trade Name	*Generic Name and Amount*
Darvocet-N-100	acetaminophen, 650 mg
	propoxyphene napsylate, 100 mg
Darvon Compound-65	aspirin, 227 mg
	propoxyphene HCL, 65 mg
	caffeine, 32 mg
Robitussin CF 5 ml	dextromethorphan 10 mg
cough syrup	guiafenesin 100 mg
	pseudoephedrine 30 mg

It should be noted that a number may be part of the trade name. The number often refers to an amount of one of the generic components and helps to differentiate it from an almost identical product. Identify the significance of the numbers in comparing the following trade names:

Trade Name	*Generic Name and Amount*
Tylenol No. 2	acetaminophen 300 mg
	codeine 15 mg
Tylenol No. 3	acetaminophen 300 mg
	codeine 30 mg
Tylenol No. 4	acetaminophen 300 mg
	codeine 60 mg

Note that each product contains the same amount of acetaminophen, with varying amounts of the controlled substance *codeine. The larger the number in the name, the greater is the amount of controlled substance present.*

Many drug errors have occurred because the trade name was misinterpreted for the number of tablets to be given. So . . .

Be certain you can clearly read and understand the order!

Another type of drug error involves preventable allergic reactions to one of the generic components of a medication. The problem stems from:

Not consulting the patient's chart for the history of allergies before a new medication is ordered or given

Not checking a reference to find out if a medication being ordered or given contains any generic components to which the patient has a known allergy

For example, if a patient has an allergy to aspirin, do not administer the first dose of any new medication to the patient without finding out if the product contains aspirin. Although the doctor is in error for ordering the medication, you are also in error for administering a medication with which you are unfamiliar. A proficient health care worker should check the history and chart for known allergies, and pick up any discrepancies. Alertness is the key to safety in any setting.

Always keep a drug reference handy, and use it when you are unfamiliar with the generic components of a drug ordered for a patient with known drug allergies. With experience, you will learn and remember the names of products most commonly used at your facility.

LEGAL TERMS REFERRING TO DRUGS

A drug may be referred to by terms other than its classification, generic name, trade name, chemical name, or official name. As mentioned in Chapter 1, the following terms imply the legal accessibility of the drug:

1. **OTC.** Over the counter; no purchasing restrictions by the FDA

2. **Legend drug.** Prescription drug; determined unsafe for over-the-counter purchase because of possible harmful side effects if taken indiscriminately; includes birth control pills, antibiotics, cardiac drugs, hormones, and so on; indicated in the *Physicians' Desk Reference* (discussed later in this chapter) by the symbol to the far right of the trade name

3. **Controlled substance.** Drug controlled by prescription requirement because of the danger of addiction or abuse; indicated in references by schedule numbers C-I to C-V (see Chapter 1)

TERMS INDICATING DRUG ACTIONS

Most references follow a similar format in describing drugs. When you research drug information, you will find the following terms as headings under each drug. You will find specific information more quickly if you understand what is listed under each heading.

Indications. A list of medical conditions or diseases for which the drug is meant to be used (e.g., diphenhydramine hydrochloride [Benadryl], is a commonly used drug; indications include allergic rhinitis, mild allergic skin reactions, motion sickness, and mild cases of parkinsonism).

Actions. A description of the cellular changes that occur as a result of the drug. This information tends to be very technical, describing cellular and tissue changes. While it is helpful to know what body system is affected by the drug, this information is geared more for the pharmacist (e.g., as an antihistamine, Benadryl appears to compete with histamine for cell receptor sites on effector cells).

Contraindications. A list of conditions for which the drug should *not* be given (e.g., two common contraindications for Benadryl are pregnancy or lactating mother).

Cautions. A list of conditions or types of patients that warrant closer observation for specific side effects when given the drug (e.g., due to atropinelike activity, Benadryl must be used cautiously with patients who have a history of bronchial asthma or hypertension, or with older adults (see Chapter 28).

Side Effects and Adverse Reactions. A list of possible unpleasant or dangerous secondary effects, other than the desired effect (e.g., side effects of Benadryl include sedation, dizziness, disturbed coordination, epigastric distress, anorexia, and thickening of bronchial secretions). This listing may be quite extensive, with as many as 50 or more side effects for one drug. Because it is difficult to know which are most likely to occur, choose a reference book that underlines or italicizes the most common side effects. Certain drugs may have side effects with which you are not familiar. Note the definitions of the following three side effects associated with specific antibiotics (Figure 2-1):

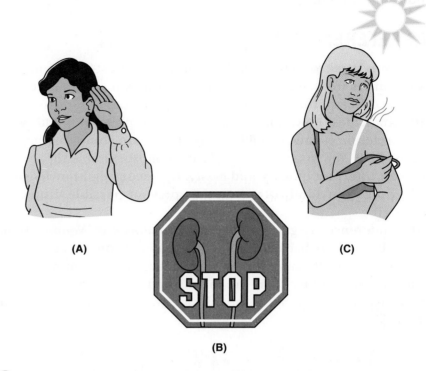

(A)

(B)

(C)

Figure 2-1 Side effects or adverse reactions can include (A) otoxicity, (B) nephrotoxicity, and (C) photosensitivity.

- Ototoxicity causes damage to the eighth cranial nerve, resulting in impaired hearing or ringing in the ears (tinnitus). Damage may be reversible or permanent.
- Nephrotoxicity causes damage to the kidneys, resulting in impaired kidney function, decreased output, and renal failure.
- Photosensitivity is an increased reaction to sunlight, with the danger of intense sunburn.

Interactions. A list of other drugs or foods that may alter the effect of the drug and usually should not be given during the same course of therapy (e.g., monoamine oxidase [MAO] inhibitors will intensify the effects of Benadryl; you will find MAO inhibitors listed under interactions for many drugs; the term refers to a group of drugs that have been used for the treatment of depression; it has been found that they can cause serious blood pressure changes, and even death, when taken with many other drugs and some foods).

Other headings often listed under information about a drug include "How Supplied" and "Usual Dosage." "How Supplied" lists the available forms and strengths of the drug. "Usual Dosage" lists the amount of drug considered safe for administration, the route, and the frequency of administration. For example:

How supplied: tablets (tabs): 20 mg and 40 mg; suppository: 20 mg

Usual dosage: 10 mg orally every 4 h (q4h)

For a listing of common abbreviations regarding drug administration and medication orders, see Tables 4-1 and 5-1.

DRUG REFERENCES*

The Physicians' Desk Reference (PDR) is one of the most widely used references for drugs in current use. It is an old standby found in every medical setting: offices, clinics, hospital units, pharmacies, and so on. As the name indicates, however, it is geared to the physician. Many new choices of references are available today. Three are compared here, including the *PDR*. You must find the reference most suitable for you, one that you can interpret quickly and easily. By becoming knowledgeable about the drugs you administer, you may prevent possible drug errors from occurring.

Other references (e.g., *The Pill Book, Handbook of Nonprescription Drugs*) may be found in bookstores, but they may not contain adequate information for the health care worker. Your school may recommend a specific drug reference other than the three listed in this text. Many new references geared to the nurse or health care worker are currently being published.

Physician's Desk Reference (PDR)[†]

PRO	CON
Distributed to practicing physicians; single hardback volume	Geared for physicians and pharmacists
Several supplements published throughout the year, with revised information or description of new products introduced after the previous edition went to press	Lengthy descriptions
	Difficult to sort out what is most important to remember
	No easily identified nursing implications
All drugs cross-referenced, by several color-coded indexes, according to one of the following:	Includes many code numbers in the description of "How Supplied," making it difficult to interpret
• Company that makes the drug (white, "Manufacturers' Index")	Contains only those drugs that manufacturers pay to have incorporated; incomplete with regard to OTC drugs, making it necessary to buy *PDR* OTC book
• Trade and generic names (pink, "Product Name Index")	
• Drug classification (blue, "Product Category Index")	
Includes photographs of many drugs for product identification	
Includes a list of all U.S. Poison Control Centers, with addresses and phone numbers	
Includes a description of substances used for medical testing (green, "Diagnostic Product Information"), for example, barium, X-ray dyes, substances used for allergy testing	

---

*References listed here were used to compile the information in this book.
[†]Published annually by Biomedical Information Corp., New York, NY

United States Pharmacopeia/Dispensing Information (USP/DI)*

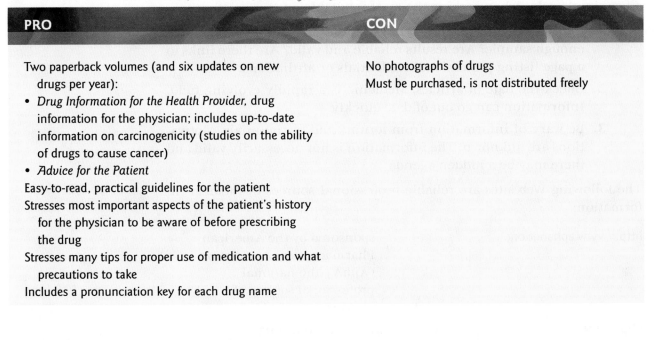

PRO	CON
Two paperback volumes (and six updates on new drugs per year):	No photographs of drugs
• *Drug Information for the Health Provider*, drug information for the physician; includes up-to-date information on carcinogenicity (studies on the ability of drugs to cause cancer)	Must be purchased, is not distributed freely
• *Advice for the Patient*	
Easy-to-read, practical guidelines for the patient	
Stresses most important aspects of the patient's history for the physician to be aware of before prescribing the drug	
Stresses many tips for proper use of medication and what precautions to take	
Includes a pronunciation key for each drug name	

AHFS Drug Information (American Health-System Formulary Service)†

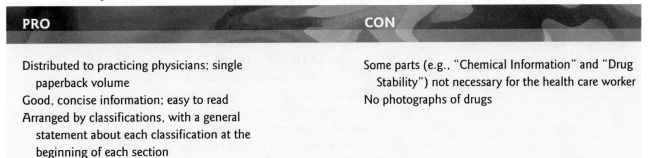

PRO	CON
Distributed to practicing physicians; single paperback volume	Some parts (e.g., "Chemical Information" and "Drug Stability") not necessary for the health care worker
Good, concise information; easy to read	No photographs of drugs
Arranged by classifications, with a general statement about each classification at the beginning of each section	

*Published annually by U.S. Pharmacopeial Convention, Inc., Rockville, Maryland.
†Published annually by American Society of Health-System Pharmacists, Bethesda, Maryland.

THE INTERNET AS REFERENCE

The Internet offers a wealth of information regarding medications and the conditions they treat. However, there can be serious dangers associated with some online sources that may not be reliable, professional, or even legitimate. Therefore, care must be taken to identify and use only Web sites that are supervised and controlled, such as those under the auspices of government agencies or sponsored by professional pharmacist groups. It is important for the health care worker to obtain accurate information and also be able to direct the patient or client to reliable sources of information regarding medicines. It is the health care worker's responsibility to caution the layperson regarding the controversial and dangerous practices of "online prescribing" without ever evaluating the patient in person, or obtaining medicines without prescriptions through the Internet.

Remember that all Web sites are not created equal. Pay attention to a few simple rules when seeking the most reputable ones.

1. Check the source. Have scientific studies been done with a large enough sample? Are results reliable and valid? Are there links to a page listing professional credentials or affiliations?

2. Check the date of articles. Medicine is a rapidly evolving field. Information can go out of date quickly.

3. Be wary of information from forums and testimonials. Motivations are unknown. The information is not necessarily valid and there may be a hidden agenda.

The following Web sites are reliable professional sources of medical information:

http://www.aphanet.org	sponsored by the American Pharmaceutical Association (AphA), the national professional society of pharmacists
http://www.fda.gov	U.S. Food and Drug Administration, includes "Human Drugs" and Center for Drug Evaluation and Research (CDER)
http://www.safemedication.com	sponsored by the American Society of Health System Pharmacists. Covers correct dosage, side effects, and optimal use of most prescriptions and over-the-counter drugs. Also offers reports on topics such as antibiotic-resistant bacteria.
http://www.uspdqi.org	U.S. Pharmacopeia/Dispensing Information (USP/DI) (See United States Pharmacopeia, previous page.)
http://www.cdc.gov/nip/	U.S. Centers for Disease Control and Prevention, National Immunization Program. Covers vaccines and immunizations.

These sites provide links to other Web sites that can be accessed through the Internet.

DRUG CARDS

As a learner of pharmacology, you may find it helpful to prepare drug cards because there are so many drugs to learn. Many educational programs require drug cards with the curriculum. You may use 3 × 5 or 5 × 7 -inch index cards stored in a recipe card box or other similar file. Included on the cards should be the information most useful to medical personnel. Although the cards should be updated periodically, using them saves valuable time compared to using the larger drug references. Preparing drug cards also reinforces learning. Certain information should be included on the drug card:

1. Generic and trade name of the drug
2. Classification or classifications of the drug
3. Forms in which the drug is available
4. Drug action
5. Indications
6. Side effects
7. Routes of administration
8. Dosage range and customary dosage
9. Any special instructions for giving the medication

In addition to making it easier and faster to locate information on drugs, drug cards constitute an ideal method of becoming more knowledgeable about drugs, classifications, and other pharmaceutical terminology.

Pharmaceutical salespeople and drug company representatives frequently have drug inserts or package brochures that are also useful. Such material can be attached to index cards or filed separately. It is especially important that drug cards be prepared on those drugs used predominantly at your medical facility.

The following is a sample drug card. Note that a number of abbreviations are used to save space. Common abbreviations regarding drug administration and medication orders appear in Tables 4-1 and 5-1.

Drug. Nitroglycerin (Nitro-Bid, Nitrostat).

Classification. Vasodilator.

Form. Sublingual tablet, timed-release tablets or capsules, ointment, dermal patches, and IV.

Action. Relaxes smooth muscles, dilates arterioles and capillaries.

Uses. Management of acute angina pectoris episodes.

Side Effects and Toxicities. Headache with throbbing, dizziness, weakness, blurred vision, dry mouth, tachycardia, and postural hypotension.

Route. Sublingual, topical, by mouth (PO), or IV.

Dosage. Sublingual, one tablet under tongue or in buccal pouch, may be repeated three times ($\times$3) if necessary; timed-release capsule, two or three times a day at 8–12-h intervals; ointment, apply to any convenient skin area and spread in thin, uniform layer 1–2 inches, may be applied every 3–4 h (q3–4h) whenever necessary (PRN).

Special Instruction. Severe headache may occur; flushing, dizziness, or weakness is usually transient; if blurred vision or dry mouth occurs, discontinue use.

CHAPTER REVIEW QUIZ

Match the definition with the term.

1. _____   List of conditions for which a drug is meant to be used

2. _____   Subcategories of drugs based on their effects on the body

3. _____   Description of the cellular changes that occur as a result of a drug

4. _____   Conditions for which a drug should not be given

   a. Contraindications

   b. Precautions

   c. Indications

   d. Prototype

   e. Actions

   f. Classifications

Refer to the following drug description to answer questions 5–8.

> Pyridium®
> (phenazopyridine HCl tablets, USP)
> Product of Warner-Lambert, Inc.
> Description: Pyridium (phenazopyridine HCl) is a urinary tract analgesic agent, chemically designated 2.6-pyridinediamine, 3-(phenylazo), monohydrochloride.

5. The generic name of the drug is _____.

6. The chemical name of the drug is _____.

7. The trade name of the drug is _____.

8. What is indicated by the ® symbol after the drug name?

   _____

9. List four drug references:

   _____

   _____

10. Explain the difference between these two medication orders:

    a. Give two Tylenol, PO.

    b. Give one Tylenol #2, PO.

    _____

    _____

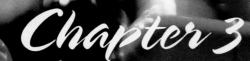

Chapter 3
Sources and Bodily Effects of Drugs

Objectives

Upon completion of this chapter, the learner should be able to

1. Identify the four sources of drugs

2. Differentiate between the following: drug actions and drug effects, systemic effects and local effects, loading dose and maintenance dose, and toxic dose and lethal dose

3. Define the following processes as they relate to the passage of drugs through the body and give conditions that may decrease the effectiveness of each: absorption, distribution, metabolism, and excretion

4. Define the following terms: selective distribution, toxicity, placebo, synergism, potentiation, and antagonism

5. List several variables that may affect the action of drugs

6. Identify the fastest route of drug administration

7. Define the following undesirable drug effects: teratogenic effect, idiosyncrasy, tolerance, dependence, hypersensitivity, and anaphylactic reaction

8. Define the Key Terms

SOURCES OF DRUGS

Any chemical substance taken into the body for the purpose of affecting body function is referred to as a drug. In earlier times, these substances were found in nature, sometimes accidentally. Plants were the primary **source of drugs** used on the human body. Berries, bark, leaves, resin from trees, and roots were found to aid the body and are still very important drug sources today (Figure 3-1).

23

Sources of Drugs	Example	Trade Name	Classification
Plants	Cinchona Bark	Quinidine	Antiarrhthymic
	Purple Foxglove Plant	Digitalis	Cardiotonic
	Poppy Plant (Opium)	Morphine, Codeine	Analgesic Analgesic, Antitussive
Minerals	Magnesium	Milk of Magnesia	Antacid, Laxative
	Zinc	Zinc Oxide Ointment	Sunscreen, Skin Protectant
	Gold	Auranofin	Anti-inflammatory; Used in the Treatment of Rheumatoid Arthritis
Animals	Pancreas of Cow, Hog	Insulin: regular, NPH, PZI	Antidiabetic Hormone
	Stomach of Cow, Hog	Pepsin	Digestive Hormone
	Thyroid Gland of Animals	Thyroid, USP	Hormone
Synthetic	Meperidine	Demerol	Analgesic
	Diphenoxylate	Lomotil	Antidiarrheal
	Co-Trimoxazole	Bactrim, Septra	Anti-infective Sulfonamide; Used in the Treatment of Urinary Tract Infections (UTI) and Some Other Infections

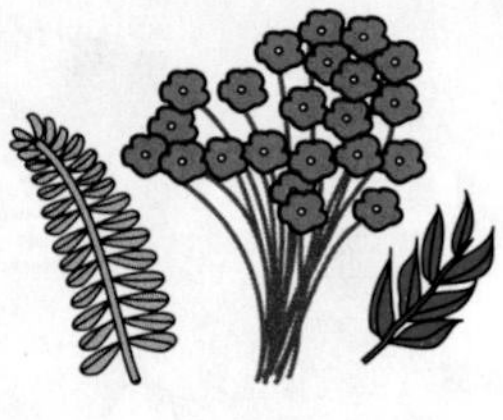

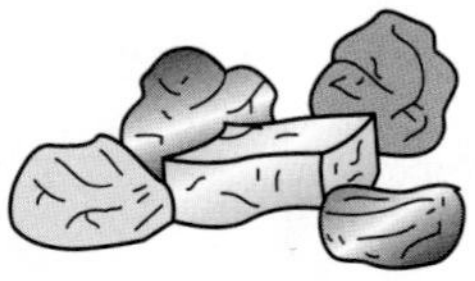

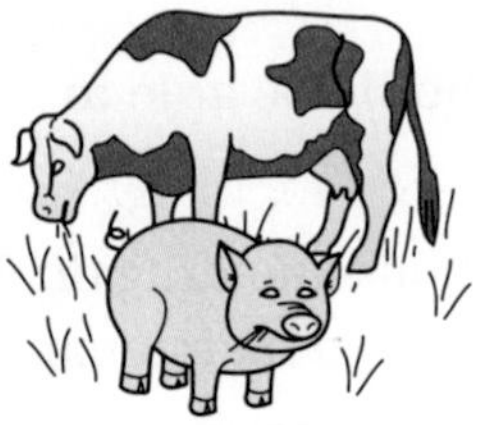

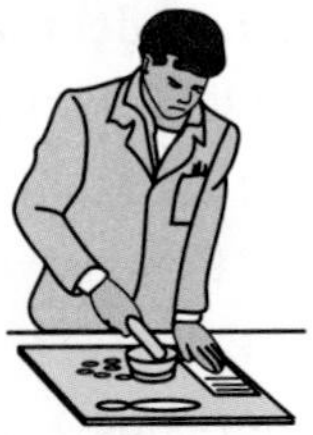

Figure 3-1 Sources of drugs: plant, mineral, animal, and synthetic sources.

Minerals from the earth and soil also found their way into human use as drugs. Iron, sulfur, potassium, silver, and even gold are some of the minerals used to prepare drugs.

More sophisticated sources of drugs emerged as human beings progressed. Research led to the use of substances from *animals* as effective drugs. Substances lacking in the human body can be replaced with similar substances from the glands, organs, and tissues of animals. The origin of drugs from an animal source even now includes human extractions. The pituitary gland from cadavers can be used to make a drug for the treatment of growth disorders.

Finally, chemists use synthetic sources to make drugs to market for human consumption. The *synthetic* (manufactured) sources evolved with human skills in laboratories and advanced understanding of chemistry. Drug compounds are produced from artificial rather than natural substances. This method is probably the most actively pursued source of drugs by major companies today. Competitive research is a big industry in experimenting with chemicals to discover cures for current medical problems. Numerous antibiotics are synthetic or semisynthetic, the results of researchers meeting the need for better treatment of infections. Someday the cure for cancer or human immunodeficiency virus (HIV) may be found from a synthetic source developed in a laboratory.

During the 1990s, the emphasis on investigational new drugs (INDs) was on the development of drugs for the treatment of life-threatening or other very serious conditions, for example, HIV infection/AIDS, various malignancies, and Alzheimer's disease. Three of the many INDs developed in the 1990s include:

- Zidovudine (AZT) (Retrovir), which slows the progression of HIV infection in some patients. It is not a cure.

- Interferon (Roferon A), which has been used to treat many different malignancies and also has been used in the management of AIDS-related Kaposi's sarcoma.

- Tacrine (Cognex), which has been used to slow the progression of dementia in some patients with Alzheimer's disease. It is not a cure.

In the twenty-first century, several of the INDs developed recently include:

- Combination drugs that treat more than one disease at a time, for example, **Caduet**®, which combines Norvasc and Lipitor for simultaneous treatment of high blood pressure and high cholesterol (two major risk factors for cardiovascular disease), was the first product to treat these conditions with a single tablet.

- **Avastin**™, an antiangiogenesis drug, is indicated as a first-line treatment for patients with metastatic colorectal cancer. A monoclonal antibody, it is the first FDA-approved product that prevents the formation of new blood vessels, a process known as angiogenesis. When tumors are unable to form new blood vessels, they are denied blood, oxygen, and other nutrients needed for their growth and metastasis. Avastin extended patient's lives longer when it was given with standard drugs for colon cancer.

- Many exciting developments are on the horizon in insulin delivery that may enhance the quality of life for insulin users. These products under development include an implantable insulin pump, a transdermal patch, and delivery by inhalation. Further studies are underway. However, the first product for insulin delivery to be approved by the FDA will probably be an inhaled nasal spray.

Research continues with these and many other INDs in the treatment of many very serious diseases.

EFFECTS OF DRUGS

No matter how different the sources, the common characteristic of all drugs is the ability to affect body function in some manner. When introduced into the body, all drugs cause cellular changes (drug actions), followed by some *physiological change* (effect of drug). Generally, drug effects may be categorized as systemic or local:

1. *Systemic effect.* Reaches widespread areas of the body (e.g., acetaminophen [Tylenol] suppository, although given rectally, has the ability to be absorbed and distributed throughout the body to cause a general reduction in fever and pain).

2. *Local effect.* Is limited to the area of the body where it is administered (e.g., dibucaine ointment [Nupercainal], applied rectally, affects only the rectal mucosa to reduce hemorrhoidal pain).

DRUG PROCESSING BY THE BODY (PHARMACOKINETICS)

Within the body, drugs undergo several changes. From start to finish, the biological changes consist of four **drug processes**:

1. *Absorption.* Getting into the bloodstream

2. *Distribution.* Moving from the bloodstream into the tissues and fluids of the body

3. *Metabolism.* Physical and chemical alterations that a substance undergoes in the body

4. *Excretion.* Eliminating waste products of drug metabolism from the body

Many variables affect how quickly or successfully substances go through the body via these four processes. If any of the four processes is hampered, the drug action and effects will be hampered. Table 3-1 lists conditions that may hamper each process.

Table 3-1 Processing of Drugs within the Body

PROCESS	PRIMARY SITE OF PROCESS	CONDITIONS THAT MAY HAMPER PROCESS
Absorption	Mucosa of the stomach, mouth, small intestine, or rectum; blood vessels in the muscles or subcutaneous tissues; or dermal layers	Incorrect administration may destroy the drug before it reaches the bloodstream or its site of action (e.g., giving certain antibiotics after meals instead of on an empty stomach).
Distribution	Circulatory system, through capillaries and across cell membranes	Poor circulation (impaired flow of blood) may prevent drug from reaching tissues.
Metabolism	Liver	Hepatitis, cirrhosis of liver, or a damaged liver may prevent adequate breakdown of drug, thus causing a buildup of unmetabolized drug.
Excretion	Kidneys, sweat glands, lungs, or intestines	Renal damage or kidney failure may prevent passage of drug waste products, thereby causing an accumulation of the drug in the body.

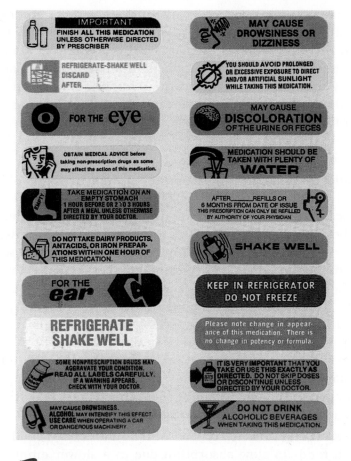

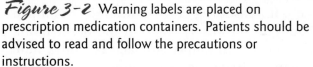

Figure 3-2 Warning labels are placed on prescription medication containers. Patients should be advised to read and follow the precautions or instructions.

Directions for the administration of one drug versus another may vary widely because the physical properties of the drugs may vary widely. The specific directions ("Usual Dosage and Administration," "Contraindications," and "Warnings") that accompany each drug are given to enhance the absorption, distribution, metabolism, and excretion of the drug. For example, directions to "Give on an empty stomach" ensure the most effective means of absorption. "Use cautiously in patients with renal dysfunction" implies possible effects on the excretion of a drug. "Decrease dose in patients with hepatic dysfunction" implies possible effects on the metabolism of a drug. *Read all labels carefully, and caution the patient to do so as well* (Figure 3-2).

ABSORPTION

The site of absorption of drugs varies according to the following physical properties of each drug:

1. *pH.* Drugs of a slightly acidic nature (e.g., aspirin and tetracycline) are absorbed well through the stomach mucosa. Drugs of an alkaline pH are not absorbed well through the stomach, but

are readily absorbed in the alkaline environment of the small intestine. The antibiotic tetracycline is recommended to be given on an empty stomach so that its pH is not altered. If given in the presence of milk, dairy products, or antacids, it will not be properly absorbed. Oral medications for infants (syrups and solutions) may not be absorbed well after infant feedings. The milk or formula neutralizes the acidity of the stomach. Thus, absorption may be enhanced when the infant is given medications on an empty stomach.

2. *Lipid (fat) solubility.* Substances high in lipid solubility are quickly and easily absorbed through the mucosa of the stomach. Alcohol and substances containing alcohol are soluble in lipids. They are rapidly absorbed through the gastrointestinal (GI) tract. Substances low in lipid solubility are not absorbed well through the stomach or intestinal mucosa and are absorbed best when given by a means other than the GI tract. An exception is the drug neomycin, which is not lipid soluble and yet is given orally. It is indicated for suppression of intestinal bacteria before intestinal or bowel surgery or in the treatment of bacterial diarrhea. By giving neomycin orally, it passes through the GI tract, unable to be absorbed. As a result, it tends to build up and accumulate in the bowel. There, the trapped antibiotic kills the bacteria in the bowel, for the desired effect.

3. *Presence or absence of food in the stomach.* Food in the stomach tends to slow absorption due to a slower emptying of the stomach. If a fast drug effect is desired, an empty stomach will facilitate quicker absorption. On the other hand, giving some medications on an empty stomach is contraindicated. Medications that are irritating to the stomach can be buffered by the presence of food. Directions may indicate "Give before meals" or "Take with food" to decrease side effects (e.g., nausea and gastric ulcers) on the GI tract.

DISTRIBUTION

The movement of a drug from the bloodstream into the tissues and fluids of the body is also affected by specific properties of the drug. Reaching sites beyond the major organs may depend on the drug's ability to cross a lipid membrane. Some drugs pass the "blood-brain barrier" or the "placental barrier," whereas others do not. You may read about drugs contraindicated for lactating mothers because the drug has the ability to pass through the cell membranes into the milk.

Some drugs have a *selective distribution* (Figure 3-3). This refers to an affinity, or attraction, of a drug to a specific organ or cells. For example, amphetamines have a selective distribution to cerebrospinal fluid (CSF). The human chorionic gonadotropin (hCG) hormone, which is used as a fertility drug, has a selective distribution to the ovaries.

By virtue of their properties, some drugs are distributed more slowly than others. Thus, while two drugs may be categorized in the same drug

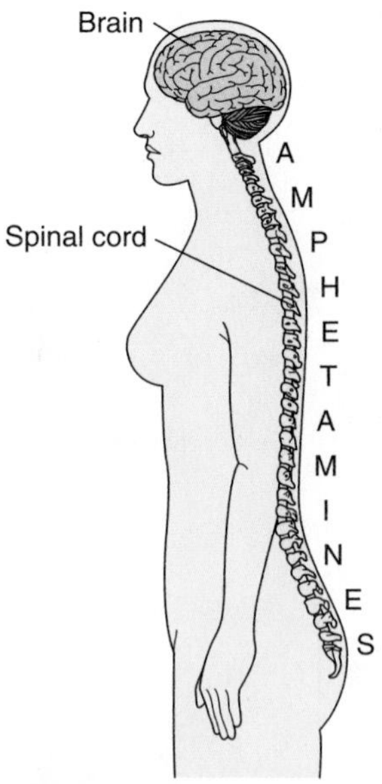

Figure 3-3
Distribution. One example of selective distribution is the attraction of amphetamines to the cerebrospinal fluid.

classification, one may be known to act on the cells and achieve the effect more quickly than the other.

METABOLISM

When transformed in the liver (biotransformation), a drug is broken down and altered to more water-soluble by-products. Thus, the drug may be more easily excreted by the kidneys.

If hepatic disease is present, a patient may exhibit toxic (poisonous) effects of a drug. This occurs because the drug is not being broken down properly by the inefficient liver. It may accumulate, unchanged by the liver, and may be unable to pass out of the body's excretory system.

It is possible for some drugs to bypass the process of metabolism. They reach the kidneys virtually unchanged and may later be detected in the urine.

EXCRETION

While it is possible for some drugs to be eliminated through the lungs (e.g., exhaled gases and anesthetics) or through perspiration, feces, bile, or breast milk, most are excreted by the kidneys.

If a drug is not excreted properly before repeated doses are given, a cumulative effect may eventually occur. A *cumulative effect* is an increased effect of a drug demonstrated when repeated doses accumulate in the body. If unnoticed, the cumulative effect may build to a dangerous, or toxic, level. This can be of particular concern with older adults. (See Chapter 27.)

Toxicity refers to a condition that results from exposure to either a poison or a dangerous amount of a drug that is normally safe when given in a smaller amount. In drug therapy, the goal is to give just enough of the drug to cause the desired (therapeutic) effect while keeping the amount below the level at which toxic effects are observed.

Digoxin is a cardiac drug that must be given cautiously because of its potential for causing a cumulative effect. Normally, digoxin slows the heart rate, but if the drug accumulates, the heart rate may slow to a dangerously low level. Circulation and renal function must be adequate, or the digoxin will accumulate, leading to digoxin toxicity.

OTHER VARIABLES

Many **variables** affect the speed and efficiency of drugs being processed by the body. The physical properties of the drugs themselves and the condition of the body systems have been discussed. Other variables affecting drug action and effect follow.

Age

Metabolism and excretion are slower in older adults, and therefore attention must be paid to possible cumulative effects. Children have a lower threshold of response and react more rapidly and sometimes in unexpected ways; therefore, frequent assessment is imperative.

Weight

Generally, the bigger the person, the greater the dose should be. However, there is great individual variation in sensitivity to drugs. Many drug dosages are always calculated on the basis of the patient's weight.

Sex

Women respond differently than men to some drugs. The ratio of fat per body mass differs, and so do hormone levels. If the female is pregnant or nursing, most drugs are contraindicated, or the dosage must be adjusted.

Psychological State

It has been proven that the more positive the patient feels about the medication he or she is taking, the more positive the physical response. This is referred to as the *placebo effect*.

A *placebo* is an inactive substance that resembles a medication, although no drug is present. For example, a sugar tablet or a saline solution for injection may be used as a placebo in a research study program.

Placebos are most often used in blind study experiments, in which groups of people are given either a drug or a placebo. The individuals, unaware of which they have been given, are studied for the effects. Often, by virtue of strong belief, the placebo-administered individuals achieve the desired effect associated with the drug they think they have received.

It is also possible to have a decreased drug effect when the attitude of a patient toward a medication is negative.

Attitudes toward medicines can also be influenced positively or negatively by cultural or religious beliefs. The caregiver needs to understand the importance of these beliefs to the patient.

> The significance for you, the health care worker, is to recognize that your attitude regarding a medication may be picked up by the patient and indirectly may affect the patient's response to the drug.

Drug Interactions

Whenever more than one drug is taken, it is possible that the *combination* may alter the normal expected response of each individual drug. One drug may interact with another to increase, decrease, or cancel out the effects of the other.

The following terms are used to describe drug interactions:

Synergism. The action of two drugs working together in which one helps the other simultaneously for an effect that neither could produce alone. Drugs that work together are said to be synergistic.

Potentiation. The action of two drugs in which one prolongs or multiplies the effect of the other. Drug A may be said to potentiate the effect of drug B.

Antagonism. The opposing action of two drugs in which one decreases or cancels out the effect of the other. Drug A may be referred to as an antagonist of drug B.

It is extremely important for the prescribing physician to know of all medications that a patient is taking in order to prevent undesirable **drug interactions**. On the other hand, it may be intentionally ordered that two drugs be taken together, because some drug interactions are desirable and beneficial. Compare the following situations, describing both desirable and undesirable drug interactions:

Desirable synergism. Promethazine (Phenergan) (a nonnarcotic sedative) and meperidine (Demerol) (a narcotic analgesic) are very effective in relieving pain. By giving small amounts of each together, pain can be relieved more safely than by giving a large amount of Demerol (which is addictive) by itself.

Undesirable synergism. Sedatives and barbiturates given in combination can depress the central nervous system (CNS) to dangerous levels, depending on the strengths of each.

Desirable potentiation. To build up a high level of some forms of penicillin (an antibiotic) in the blood, the drug probenecid (Benemid) (antigout medication) can be given simultaneously. Benemid potentiates the effect of penicillin by slowing the excretion rate of the antibiotic.

Undesirable potentiation. Toxic effect may result when cimetidine (Tagamet) (a gastric antisecretory) is given simultaneously with Tofranil (an antidepressant). Tagamet potentiates the level of antidepressant concentrations in the blood.

Desirable antagonism. A narcotic antagonist (e.g., naloxone, Narcan) saves lives from drug overdoses by canceling out the effect of narcotics.

Undesirable antagonism. Antacids taken at the same time as tetracycline alter the pH and prevent absorption of tetracycline.

Dosage

Different dosages of a drug may bring about variations in the speed of drug action or effectiveness. **Dosage** is defined as the amount of drug given for a particular therapeutic or desired effect. Terms of various dosage levels are:

1. *Minimum dose.*   Smallest amount of a drug that will produce a therapeutic effect

2. *Maximum dose.*   Largest amount of a drug that will produce a desired effect without producing symptoms of toxicity

3. *Loading dose.*   Initial high dose (often maximum dose) used to quickly elevate the level of the drug in the blood (often followed by a series of lower maintenance doses)

4. *Maintenance dose.*   Dose required to keep the drug blood level at a steady state in order to maintain the desired effect

5. ***Toxic dose.*** Amount of a drug that will produce harmful side effects or symptoms of poisoning

6. ***Lethal dose.*** Dose that causes death

7. ***Therapeutic dose.*** Dose that is customarily given (average adult dose based on body weight of 150 lb); adjusted according to variations from the norm

You may be familiar with the use of a high loading dose followed by a lesser maintenance dose. If you have taken antibiotics, you may have been instructed to take two tablets or capsules initially and then to take one tablet every six hours. It is frequently desirable to give a loading dose of antibiotics to build up a high level and get the process of killing the bacteria started.

Route

The route of administration is probably the most significant factor in the speed of drug action.

The route of drug administration can be compared to the route of travel. In planning a trip from point A to point B, you may have a map that shows several courses of travel to reach the destination. The course you select is optional, depending on your choice for the quickest, cheapest, safest, or most scenic route.

Options for routes of drug administration are much the same. There are a number of methods by which drugs may be given to reach their destination. Sometimes the route selected is based on the degree of speed, cost, or safety of administration. Sometimes there is no choice of routes because some medications can be given only by one route. Often this is because absorption occurs by that route only, or the substance is dangerous or toxic when given by another route. Insulin, for example, may be given only by injection. Much research has been done to produce an oral form of insulin, but attempts have failed because the drug is destroyed by gastric juices.

The most common routes of administration may be grouped into two main categories:

1. ***GI tract routes***
   a. Oral (PO)
   b. Nasogastric tube (NG)
   c. Rectal (R)

2. ***Parenteral routes,*** which include any other than the gastrointestinal tract
   a. Sublingual (SL) or buccal
   b. Injection routes
      i. Intravenous (IV)
      ii. Intramuscular (IM)
      iii. Subcutaneous (subQ)
      iv. Intradermal (ID)
      v. Intracardiac, Intraspinal, Intracapsular*

---

*The latter three injection routes are less common and are administered by the physician.

c. Topical (T)
   i. Dermal (D)
   ii. Mucosal
d. Inhalation

There are advantages and disadvantages in the use of each route. The doctor's choice of a particular route of administration of a drug may depend on (1) desired effects (e.g., fast or slow, local or systemic); (2) absorption qualities of the drug; and (3) how the drug is supplied. Other general points regarding the effect of the route on the drug absorption are as follows:

1. The oral route is the easiest, but the effects are slower because of the time required for disintegration of drugs in the alimentary canal before absorption.

2. The intravenous route is the fastest: Drugs enter the bloodstream immediately. Doses to be given IV are in small amounts; effects are immediate and can be quite dangerous if given in amounts recommended for other routes. Intravenous drugs can be administered by IV push or bolus (a concentrated drug solution) (Figure 3-4), or they can be diluted and solutions are then infused more slowly by IV drip.
   a. IVs are administered by a physician, registered nurse, or paramedic.
   b. IV is the best route for treatment of emergencies because of the speed of action.

3. Parenteral routes are the choice when:
   a. Patient can take nothing by mouth (NPO).
   b. The drug is not suitable for GI absorption.

4. The intramuscular route is fairly rapid because the muscles are highly vascular. If it is desirable to retard the speed of absorption, a drug to be given IM may be added to an oily base.

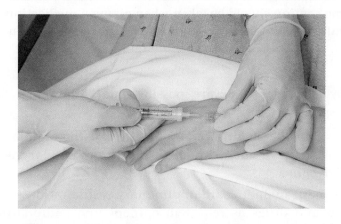

Figure 3-4 Intravenous push or bolus, IV drugs are administered slowly over a specified period of time (usually one to seven minutes).

UNEXPECTED RESPONSES TO DRUGS

Several other terms must be defined in order to complete your awareness of the bodily effects of drugs. These terms refer to **adverse drug effects**.

Teratogenic effect. Effect from maternal drug administration that causes the development of physical defects in a fetus

Idiosyncrasy. Unique, unusual response to a drug. For example, a patient may have an idiosyncrasy to a particular tranquilizer if it causes agitation and excitement rather than tranquility.

Paradoxical. Opposite effect from that expected.

Tolerance. Decreased response to a drug that develops after repeated doses are given. To achieve the desired effect, the drug dosage must be increased or the drug replaced.

Dependence. Acquired need for a drug that may produce psychological or physical symptoms of withdrawal when the drug is discontinued.

- Psychological dependence involves only a psychological craving; no physical symptoms of withdrawal other than anxiety.
- Physical dependence exists when cells actually have a need for the drug; symptoms of withdrawal include retching, nausea, pain, tremors, and sweating.

Hypersensitivity. Immune response (allergy) to a drug may be of varying degrees.

- May be mild with no immediate effects; rash or hives may appear after three to four days of drug therapy
- May develop after uneventful previous uses of a drug
- More likely to exist in patients with other known allergies

Note: Nausea, vomiting, and diarrhea are not considered signs of allergies.

> Extreme caution should be taken when giving a medication, especially antibiotics, to a patient for the first time, particularly if the patient has a history of other allergies.

Anaphylactic reaction. Severe, possibly fatal, allergic (hypersensitivity) response

- Signs include itching, urticaria (hives), hyperemia (reddened, warm skin), vascular collapse, shock, cyanosis, laryngeal edema, and dyspnea.
- Treatment includes cardiopulmonary resuscitation (CPR) if indicated and drugs as required: epinephrine (Adrenalin) to raise blood pressure; corticosteroid (Solu-Medrol) to reduce inflammation and the body's immunological response; or antihistamine

(Benadryl) to suppress histamine, thereby reducing redness, itching, and edema.

- Anaphylaxis has been noted often with the following: antibiotics, especially penicillin; X-ray dyes containing iodides (IVP [intravenous pyelogram] dye, angiogram dye, gallbladder dyes, etc.); foods (shellfish, onions, peanuts, etc.); and insect stings (bees and ants).

Knowledge of any adverse reactions to drugs should be included in the patient's history. This information can be helpful in preventing repeated episodes. Getting an accurate drug history and clearly listing known allergies is a critical function of the health care worker.

Persons who have had an anaphylactic reaction to a substance should always wear a Medic-Alert tag or bracelet to identify the substance to which they are extremely allergic. Persons who have had hypersensitivity reactions to a substance are more at risk for reactions to other substances as well. Allergies should be listed on a card and carried in the wallet of the sensitive individual.

CHAPTER REVIEW QUIZ

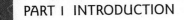

Fill in the blanks.

1.

Drug Sources	Example	Trade Name	Classification

2. Drugs that are distributed throughout the body have _____ effects.

3. Drugs whose action is limited to a specific location have _____ effects.

4. As drugs pass through the body, they undergo four processes:

Process	Definition of Process

5. Factors that may affect the passage of drugs through the body:

Process	Primary Site of Process	Conditions Hampering Process

6. If circulation is poor, metabolism faulty, or excretion inadequate, drugs may build up in the system, leading to _____ effects, causing poisonous, or _____ levels of the drug.

7. Variables affecting the efficiency of drug action include _____, _____, _____, and _____.

Match the term with the definition.

8. Synergism

9. Antagonism

10. Potentiation

11. Lethal dose

12. Toxic dose

13. Maintenance dose

14. Idiosyncrasy

15. Tolerance

16. Dependence

17. Teratogenic

_____ **a.** Amount of drug required to keep drug level steady

_____ **b.** Amount of drug that can cause death

_____ **c.** Amount of drug that can cause dangerous side effects

_____ **d.** One drug making the effect of another drug more powerful

_____ **e.** Drugs working together for a better effect

_____ **f.** Drugs working against each other or counteracting each other's effect

_____ **g.** Acquired need for a drug, with symptoms of withdrawal when discontinued

_____ **h.** Unusual response to a drug, other than expected effect

_____ **i.** Effects on a fetus from maternal use of a drug

_____ **j.** Decreased response after repeated use of a drug, increased dosage required for effect

Fill in the blanks.

18. An allergy or immune response to a drug is called

_____

19. Allergic reactions to drugs may be *mild,* with symptoms such as

_____

_____

20. Allergic reactions to drugs are more common in patients with

_____

21. *Severe* allergic reaction with shock, laryngeal edema, and dyspnea is called

_____

22. Treatment of severe allergic reactions include the following three medications in order of administration: _____, _____, and _____.

Chapter 4
Medication Preparations and Supplies

Objectives

Upon completion of this chapter, the learner should be able to

1. Differentiate between various oral drug forms: sublingual tablet versus buccal tablet, solution versus suspension, syrup versus elixir, enteric-coated tablet versus scored tablet, and timed-release capsule versus lozenge

2. Explain what is meant by parenteral

3. List four classifications of drugs that are commonly given by the rectal route

4. Define the following types of injections and explain how they differ in administration and absorption rate: IV, IM, and ID

5. Compare the IV injections referred to as IV push, IV infusion, and IV piggyback

6. List and define at least eight drug forms used for topical (both dermal and mucosal) administration

7. Explain the advantages of administering drugs via a dermal patch

8. Identify various supplies used in the preparation of medications

9. Define the Key Terms

Key Terms

Drug form

Route of delivery

The forms in which drugs are prepared are as numerous as the routes of administration. **Drug form** refers to the type of preparation in which the drug is supplied. Pharmaceutical companies prepare each drug in the form or forms most suitable for its intended **route of delivery** and means of absorption. *Drug form* and *drug preparation* are synonymous. The *PDR* lists the forms available for each drug under the heading "How Supplied." See Table 4-1 for abbreviations of some of the drug forms and routes of administration.

Table 4-1 Abbreviations for Drug Administration

DRUG FORMS		ROUTES	
cap	capsule	IM	intramuscular
elix	elixir	IV	intravenous
gtt	drop	IVPB	intravenous piggyback
supp	suppository	PO, po, per os	oral
susp	suspension	R	rectal
tab	tablet	subq	subcutaneous

A SPACE-AGE DRUG FORM

Great advances in developing a new drug form have revolutionized the way a number of drugs are administered. The more recent drug form is the dermal patch, or *transdermal delivery system*. Dermal patches were taken on the space shuttles during the 1990s for the prevention of nausea. The key to the transdermal system is that the drug molecules are present in a variety of sizes and shapes that allow for absorption through the skin at various rates. Thus, a patch can provide a constant, even flow of a drug over a long period of time—hours or days. The drug, being released at a consistent rate, remains at an effective level in the blood, as opposed to rising and falling, as happens with pills. Advantages of this method of administration include:

- Easy application, with no discomfort or undesirable taste
- Effectiveness for long periods of time, hours for some drugs and days for others
- Consistent blood level of drug because drug is released at varying rates, rather than all at one time

Dermal patches vary in size, shape, and color (Figure 4-1). They are most commonly seen today on patients for the prevention of angina. Current marketing of dermal patches also includes others for the prevention of motion sickness (may be applied before traveling), for management of chronic pain (e.g., Duragesic; see Chapter 19), as a smoking deterrent (e.g., Habitrol and Nicoderm), and for estrogen replacement (e.g., Estraderm). Research is ongoing in the development of dermal patches for birth control, high blood pressure, ulcers, allergies, and heart conditions. Probably not all drug molecules will be adaptable to this drug form, but it certainly has opened new doors in the area of drug administration.

STANDARD DRUG FORMS

You probably have received medications in many of the standard forms at some time during your life. Each form is defined and listed in the following sections according to the routes of administration (Figure 4-2). As you read in Chapter 3, drugs may be administered through the gastrointestinal

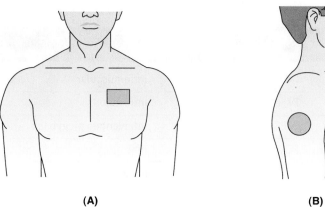
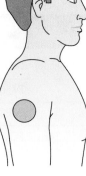
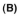

(A)

(B)

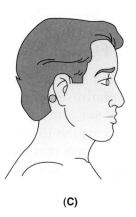

(C)

Figure 4-1 Transdermal drug delivery. Dermal patches vary in size, shape, and color (A, B). For prevention of angina pectoris, for management of chronic pain, and (C) for prevention of motion sickness.

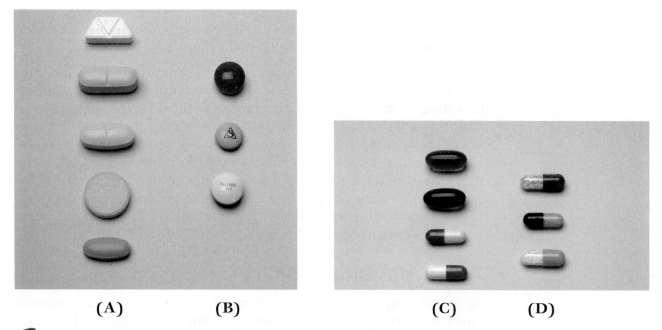

(A)   (B)   (C)   (D)

Figure 4-2 Oral drug forms. Tablets and capsules vary in size, shape, and color. (A) Tablets, scored and unscored; (B) enteric-coated tablets; (C) gelatin capsules; and (D) timed-release capsules.

(GI) tract or parenterally. GI routes include oral, nasogastric or gastrostomy tube, and rectal. Parenteral refers to any route not involving the GI tract, including injection, topical (skin or mucosal), and inhalation routes.

Oral Drug Forms

Oral drug forms include:

Tablet. Disk of compressed drug; may be a variety of shapes and colors; may be coated to enhance easy swallowing; may be *scored* (evenly divided in halves or quarters by score lines) to enhance equal distribution of drug if it has been broken.

Enteric-coated tablet. Tablet with a special coating that resists disintegration by gastric juices. The coating dissolves further down the GI tract, in the enteric, or intestinal, region. Some drugs that are irritating to the stomach, such as aspirin, are available in enteric-coated tablets. To be effective, the coating must never be destroyed by chewing or crushing when it is administered.

Capsule. Drug contained within a gelatin-type container

- Easier to swallow than noncoated tablets
- Double chamber may be pulled apart to add drug powder to soft foods or beverages for patients who have difficulty swallowing (unless specifically contraindicated for absorption).

Timed-release (sustained-release) capsule. Capsule containing drug particles that have various coatings (often of different colors) that differ in the amount of time required before the coatings dissolve. This form of drug preparation is designed to deliver a dose of drug over an extended period of time. An advantage of taking a drug in the timed-release form is the decreased frequency of administration. For example, the tranquilizer Valium may be administered in tablet form, 5 mg tid, or in the timed-release form (Valrelease, 15 mg) only once daily. (See Table 5-1 for common abbreviations.) Because of the significance of the various coatings that encapsulate the drug particles, it is important that the small colored pellets *not* be crushed or mixed with foods. Damage to the coatings of drug pellets allows the drug to be released all at one time as it is administered. Such immediate release of drug is a potential overdose. Timed-release capsules should be swallowed whole, with no physical damage to the contents of the capsule.

Lozenge (troche). Tablet containing palatable flavoring, indicated for a local (often soothing) effect on the throat or mouth.

- Patient is advised not to swallow a lozenge; it should be allowed to slowly dissolve in the mouth.
- Patient is also advised *not* to drink liquids for approximately 15 min after administration, to prevent washing of the lozenge contents from the throat or mouth.

Suspension. Liquid form of medication that must be shaken well before administration because the drug particles settle at the bottom of the bottle. The drug is not evenly dissolved in the liquid.

- A cephalosporin (Keflex) suspension is a commonly used antibiotic suspension for children. This form is more easily ingested by children than are capsules of Keflex.

Emulsion. Liquid drug preparation that contains oils and fats in water.

Elixir, fluid extract. Liquid drug forms with alcohol base.

- Should be tightly capped to prevent alcohol evaporation.
- Should not be available to alcoholics.

Syrup. Sweetened, flavored liquid drug form. Cherry syrup drug preparations are common for children.

Solution. Liquid drug form in which the drug is totally evenly dissolved. Appearance is clear, rather than cloudy or settled (as with a suspension).

Many drug forms for the oral route are commonly available over the counter and include thousands of trade name products. The oral route is the easiest and probably the cheapest for administration. It is, however, *not* the route of choice for treatment of emergencies, acute pain, NPO* patients, or patients unable to swallow. Other routes, especially the parenteral routes, produce a more rapid absorption rate and drug effect.

Rectal Drug Forms

Rectal drug forms include:

Suppository. Drug suspended in a substance, such as cocoa butter, that melts at body temperature.

Enema solution. Drug suspended in solution to be administered as an enema.

The rectal route of administration is often the choice if the patient is ordered to have nothing by mouth (NPO) or cannot swallow. The most common classifications of drugs given rectally include sedatives, antiemetics, and antipyretics. A local analgesic effect may also be achieved by this route. In the past, rectal administration of drug solutions was given for general anesthesia, but this method is not common today.

Injectable Drug Forms

Injectable drug forms include:

Solution. Drug suspended in a sterile vehicle.

- Quite often the solutions have a sterile water base and are thus referred to as *aqueous* (aq) (waterlike) solutions.
- Some solutions have an oil base, which tends to cause a more prolonged absorption time. The oily nature of these solutions makes them thick; thus they are referred to as viscous (thick) solutions.

Powder. Dry particles of drugs. The powder itself cannot be injected. It must be mixed with a sterile diluting solution (sterile water or

---

*See Table 5-1 for common abbreviations.

saline solution) to render an injectable solution. This is termed *re-constitution* of a drug. Drugs are supplied undiluted in powder form because of the short period of time they remain stable after dilution.

The various injection routes differ according to the type of tissues into which the drug is deposited and the rate of absorption.

Intravenous. Injected directly into a vein. Immediate absorption and availability to major organs renders this route a dangerous one. IV drugs are usually administered by physicians, paramedics, or registered nurses. Types of intravenous injections include:

- IV push, a small volume of drug injected through a syringe and needle into a peripheral saline lock (PRN adapter), attached to a vein (Figure 4-3A). An IV push (bolus) medication can also be injected into a port on a primary (continuous) injection line (Figure 4-3B).

- IV infusion or IV drip, a large volume of fluids, often with drugs added, that infuses continually into a vein (Figure 4-3C).

Note: When adding a medication to an IV solution bag through the injection port, take the bag down and invert it a few times to disperse the drug throughout the solution instead of concentrated at the bottom of the bag.

- IV piggyback (IVPB), a drug diluted in moderate volume (50–100 ml) of fluid for intermittent infusion at specified intervals, usually q6–8h; the diluted solution is infused (piggyback) into a port on the main IV tubing or into a rubber adapter on the IV catheter (Figure 4-3D).

Intramuscular. Injected into a muscle, by positioning the needle and syringe at a 90-degree angle from the skin (Figure 4-4). Absorption is fairly rapid due to the vascularity of muscle.

Subcutaneous. Injected into the fatty layer of tissue below the skin by positioning the needle and syringe at a 45-degree angle from the skin (Figure 4-5). This may be the route of choice for drugs that should not be absorbed as rapidly as through the IV or IM routes. Sometimes, especially with self-administration and/or a shorter needle, a 90-degree angle is used.

Intradermal. Injected just beneath the skin, by positioning the needle bevel up and the syringe at a 15-degree angle from the skin (Figure 4-6). This route is used primarily for allergy skin testing. Because of the lack of vascularity in the dermis, absorption is slow. The greatest reaction is in the local tissues rather than systemic. When a small amount (0.1–0.2 ml) of drug is injected intradermally, the amount of redness that develops around the injection site can be used to determine whether a person is sensitive to the drug. Tuberculin (TB) skin tests (PPD) are also administered intradermally, and the site is inspected 48–72 hours later for hardness (induration) and swelling. Redness (erythema) alone, *without swelling,* does not indicate a positive test result with PPD. The *raised area (induration)* is measured with a special ruler and the number of millimeters (mm) is documented. Check with

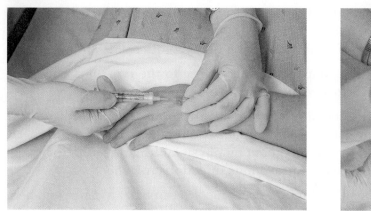

(A)

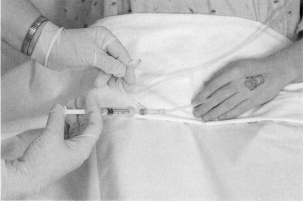

(B)

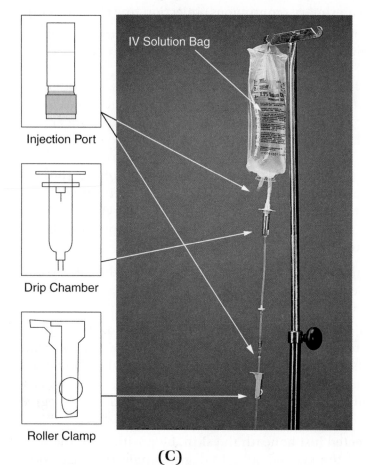

IV Solution Bag

Injection Port

Drip Chamber

Roller Clamp

(C)

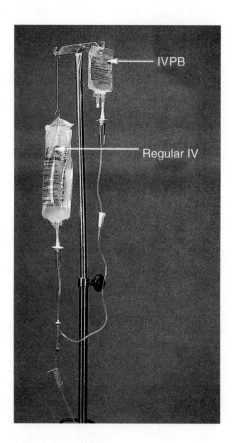

IVPB

Regular IV

(D)

Figure 4-3 Intravenous administration. Different forms of IV injection include: (A) IV push, injecting a bolus of medication into a peripheral saline lock; (B) pinch closed the IV tubing of a primary infusion line to administer an IV push medication; (C) IV infusion (continuous); and (D) IV piggyback (IVPB) intermittent.

your local Public Health Department regarding appropriate protocol with a positive PPD test result.

Epidural. Injected into a catheter that has been placed by an anesthesiologist in the epidural space of the spinal canal. Medications for pain can be administered into the catheter by bolus (a measured amount of solution in a syringe) or by continuous infusion through

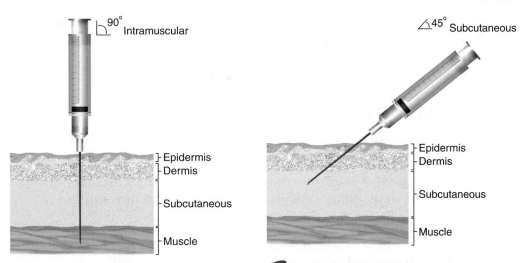

Figure 4-4 Intramuscular injection. Needle is inserted at a 90-degree angle.

Figure 4-5 Subcutaneous injection. Needle is usually inserted at a 45-degree angle. Sometimes, with a shorter needle (3/8), a 90-degree angle is used.

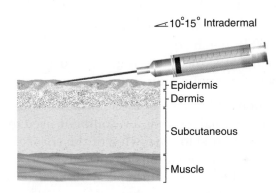

Figure 4-6 Intradermal injection. Needle is inserted just beneath the skin at a 10-15-degree angle. Bevel of needle is up.

tubing attached to a bag of solution. Epidural catheters have long been used for administration of opioid analgesics for chronic intractable pain and for chemotherapy. Epidurals have become a popular and widely accepted vehicle for the management of acute, postoperative pain.

The less common parenteral routes, which are limited to a physician's administration, are:

Intracardiac. Injected directly into the heart. This route is used to administer adrenaline as a last resort to resuscitate a patient whose heart has stopped.

Intraspinal. Injected into the subarachnoid space, which contains cerebrospinal fluid (CSF) that surrounds the spinal cord. Drugs injected by this route are frequently anesthetics, which render a lack of sensation to those regions of the body distal to the intraspinal injection.

Intracapsular (intra-articular). Injected into the capsule of a joint, usually to reduce inflammation, as in bursitis. Arthritic or bursitic joints often injected with anti-inflammatory drugs include shoulders, elbows, wrists, ankles, knees, and hips.

Topical Drug Forms

Topical drug forms include drugs for dermal application and drugs for mucosal application. Those for *dermal* application include:

Cream or ointment. A semisolid preparation containing a drug, for external application. Note: Creams and ointments are not the same. The dose used differs for each.

Rule of thumb: If skin is wet, use cream; if skin is dry, use ointment. (Follow the physician's order. Contact the physician with questions.)

Lotion. A liquid preparation applied externally for treatment of skin disorders. Unlike hand lotions, medicated lotions (e.g., calamine lotion) should be *patted,* not rubbed, on the affected skin.

Liniment. Preparation for external use that is rubbed on the skin as a counterirritant. As such, the liniment creates a different sensation (e.g., tingling or burning) to mask pain in the skin or muscles.

Dermal patch. Skin patch containing drug molecules that can be absorbed through the skin at varying rates to promote a consistent blood level between application times

Both the dermal patch and ointment are common forms for administration of nitroglycerin. Nitroglycerin is a vasodilator used for the treatment of angina (chest pain related to narrowing of the coronary arteries). The advantage of the external applications of nitroglycerin is their ability to *prevent* angina by the slow, consistent release of the drug over a period of time. Before the external applications became available, nitroglycerin was primarily available in the form of a sublingual tablet to be taken at the time of an angina attack. Now all three forms are used—the tablet, the ointment, and the patch—with the external forms focusing on the prevention of angina. They are applied at regular intervals, as follows:

Ointment: One to five inches applied q8h measured and applied on special Appli-Ruler paper (Figure 4-7).

Dermal patch: One patch (available in varied doses) usually applied every 24 hours for angina. Other types of patches are applied every 24–72 hours depending on the condition treated (Figure 4-1). (See Chapter 9 for administration instructions.)

Other drug preparations considered topical are those that are applied to *mucosal membranes.* Some are administered for local effect (at the site of application) and, in other cases, a systemic effect is desired. The *mucosal drug forms* include:

Eye, ear, and nose drops (gtt). Drugs in sterile liquids to be applied by drops (referred to as instillation of drops).

Eye ointment. Sterile semisolid preparation, often antibiotic in nature, for ophthalmic use only.

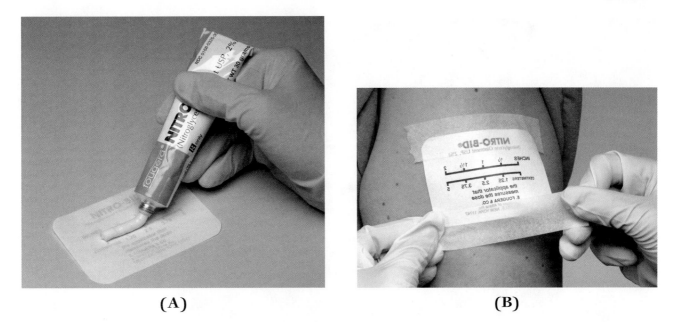

(A)   **(B)**

Figure 4-7 Topical administration. Dermal application includes creams and liquids placed on the skin. (A) Nitroglycerin ointment is measured on Appli-Ruler paper. (B) Paper containing ointment is applied to the skin and taped in place. Mark date and time on tape.

Vaginal creams. Medicated creams, often of antibiotic or antifungal nature, that are to be inserted vaginally with the use of a special applicator.

Rectal and vaginal suppositories. Drug suspended in a substance, such as cocoa butter, that melts at body temperature, for local effect. Some rectal suppositories are also used for systemic effects e.g., Tylenol suppository for fever (Figure 4-8).

Douche solution. Sterile solution, often an antiseptic such as povidone iodine solution and sterile water, used to irrigate the vaginal canal.

Buccal tablet. Tablet that is absorbed *via the buccal mucosa* in the mouth.

- Patient is told *not* to swallow tablet; it is to be placed between the cheek and gums, and allowed to dissolve slowly.
- Not commonly used today. Sublingual preferable.

Sublingual tablet. Tablet that is absorbed via the mucosa under the tongue.

- Patient is told not to swallow tablet; it is to be placed under the tongue and allowed to dissolve slowly.
- The most common sublingual tablet is nitroglycerin. Given for the treatment of angina, this drug reaches the bloodstream immediately via the sublingual capillaries. Angina may be relieved within one to five min after sublingual nitroglycerin is administered.

Inhalable Drug Forms

The drug forms used for the inhalation route include:

Spray or mist. Liquid drug forms that may be inhaled as fine droplets via the use of spray bottles, nebulizers, or metered dose inhalers.

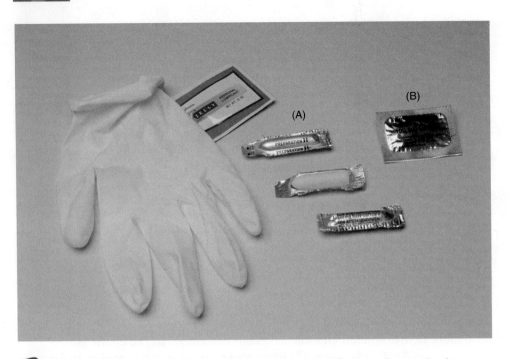

Figure 4-8 Topical administration via mucous membranes. Suppositories come in various shapes and sizes, for example, (A) rectal suppositories, wrapped in foil and unwrapped, and (B) vaginal suppository, wrapped in foil. Lubricant and a glove will be needed for administration.

- In the hospital setting, respiratory therapists instill a liquid into a chamber of a nebulizer for a patient's breathing treatment. Often the liquid contains a bronchodilator, a mucolytic agent, or sterile saline solution for moisture.

- In the home, the patient may instill sprays via nasal spray bottles, vaporizers, or inhalers. Asthma patients rely on the use of inhalers to keep their bronchioles open by inhaling the mist of a bronchodilator. A mouthpiece, through which the patient inhales, is connected to a container of liquid drug.

Gas. Anesthetics, such as nitrous oxide, that are introduced via the respiratory route for general anesthesia.

SUPPLIES

Considering the variety of drug forms you may be administering, you must become familiar with various **supplies** to be used.

Medicine cup. Two types of disposable cups are commonly used. Paper cups are used for dispensing tablets and capsules. Plastic 1-oz medicine cups with measurements (ml, tsp, tbsp, dr, or oz) marked on the side are used for dispensing oral liquid medications. (See Table 5-1 for a list of common abbreviations used in medication orders.)

Metal pillcrusher. Used in most institutions (Figure 4-9).

Mortar. Glass cup in which tablets (excluding enteric-coated tablets) may be placed to be crushed. Various other pill-crushing devices are available.

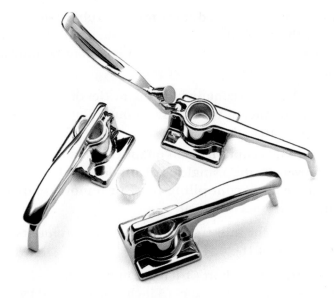

Figure 4-9 Metal pillcrusher. Place paper soufflé cup in well of the device and place tablet to be crushed in the paper cup. Then place another paper cup on top of the tablet before bringing down handle. (Reprinted with permission from *Creative Living Medical*, Brainerd, Minnesota.)

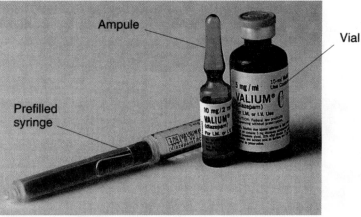

Figure 4-10 Medication for injection. Various premeasured containers include ampules, vials, and prefilled syringes. (Courtesy of Roche Laboratories.)

Note: In some areas, a physician's order is required for pill crushing. Check the regulations in your area.

Pestle. Club-shaped glass tool used as the crushing device to pulverize tablets.

Medication for injection is contained in an ampule, vial, or prefilled syringe. (Figure 4-10):

Ampule. Small glass container that holds a single dose of sterile solution for injection. The ampule must be broken at the neck to obtain the solution.

Vial. Glass container sealed at the top by a rubber stopper to enhance sterility of the contents. Contents may be a solution or a powdered drug that needs to be reconstituted. Vials may be multiple dose or unit dose.

- Multiple-dose vials contain large quantities of solution (up to 50 ml) and may be entered repeatedly through the rubber stopper to remove a portion of the contents.
- Unit-dose vials contain small quantities of solution (1–2 ml) that are removed during a single use. Unit-dose vials are widely used today as a means of controlling abuse or removal of excess amounts of solution from a drug vial.

Needles. Needles for injections have two measurements that must be noted (Figure 4-11).

- Length varies from short (3/8 inch) to medium (1–1½ inch for standard injections. Long needles (5 inch) may be used by the physician for intraspinal or intracardiac routes. Needles 2–5 inches long are used by the physician for intra-articular injections (into the joint).
- Gauge is a number that represents the diameter of the needle lumen. Needle gauges vary from 16 (largest) to 27 (smallest), with the higher gauge number representing the smaller lumen.

Syringes. The three most common disposable **syringes** for parenteral administration of drugs are the standard hypodermic syringe, the tuberculin (TB) syringe (Figure 4-12), and the insulin syringe (Figure 4-13).

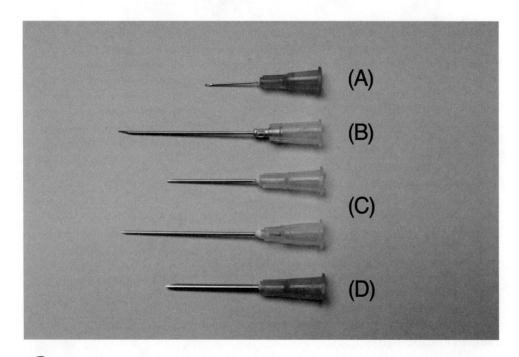

Figure 4-11 Needles commonly used for injections. Sizes vary in length and gauge. (A) 5/8 inch, 25 gauge; (B) 1½ inches, 21 gauge; (C) 1 inch and 1½ inches, 20 gauge; and (D) 1 inch, 16 gauge.

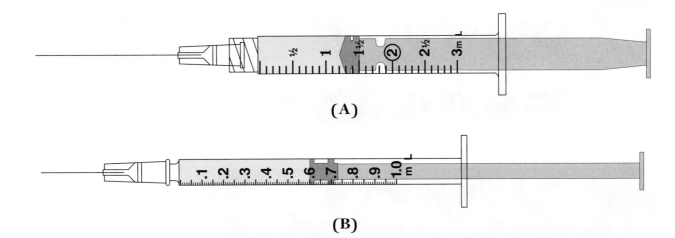

(A)

(B)

Figure 4-12 Syringes for injection. Type of syringe varies with type and quantity of medication. (A) 3 ml syringe, (B) tuberculin syringe, 1-ml capacity.

- The standard hypodermic syringe has a capacity of 2–3 ml. Most companies prepackage this type of syringe with a needle attached. You may use this type of syringe for either subcutaneous or intramuscular injections, so you must choose the package with the needle length and gauge appropriate for the route and depth of injection you will give. All hypodermic syringes are marked with 10 calibrations per milliliter (ml). Thus, each small line represents 0.1 ml. When preparing for an injection with this syringe, you must know the amount of solution needed to the nearest 0.1 ml (an additional scale on the syringe shows calibrations in minims, which is discussed in Chapter 9).

- The TB syringe is very narrow and is finely calibrated. The total capacity is only 1 ml. There are 100 fine calibration lines marking the capacity. Thus, each line represents 0.01 ml. Every tenth line is longer, to indicate 0.1-ml increments. Very precise small amounts of solution may be measured with the TB syringe. It is most commonly used for newborn and pediatric dosages and for intradermal skin tests. When preparing for an injection with this syringe, you must know the amount of solution needed to the nearest 0.01 ml.

- The insulin syringe is used strictly for administering insulin to diabetics. Insulin should be measured *only* in an insulin syringe. Like the TB syringe, the standard insulin syringe has only a 1-ml capacity, which is equivalent to 100 units of U-100 insulin. The standard U-100 syringe has a dual scale: even numbers on one side and odd numbers on the other side. Look carefully at the calibrations on each side. Count each calibration (on one side only) as *two* units (Figure 4.13).

There are also smaller insulin syringes to more accurately measure small amounts of insulin, such as for children (Figure 4.13B for Lo-Dose Insulin Syringes 50 Units and 30 Units). Look carefully at the calibrations. In these Lo-Dose syringes, each calibration counts only *one* unit.

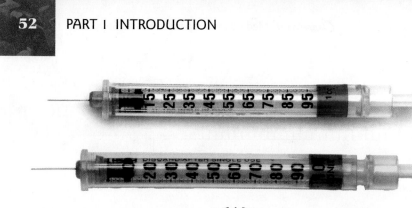

(A)

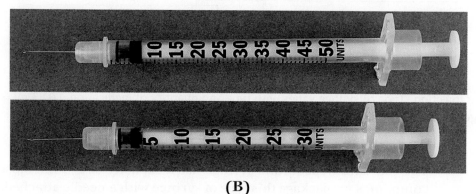

(B)

Figure 4-13 Insulin syringes. (A) Opposite sides of the same standard U-100 insulin syringe; note the numbers; (B) Lo-Dose insulin syringes, 50 units and 30 units. (Courtesy of Becton Dickson and Company.)

It is extremely important that you can interpret the value of the calibrations on each of the syringes. Study the calibrations each time you prepare for an injection to prevent a medication error from negligent misinterpretation. ***All insulin dosages should be double-checked by two caregivers before administration.***

Oral syringes. Health care workers should be aware that some oral liquid medications are dispensed from the pharmacy in disposable plastic syringes with rubber or plastic covers on the tip. These syringes are labeled "Not for injection" or "For oral use only."

Safety Devices

The Occupational Safety and Health Administration (OSHA) has mandated that every effort must be made to reduce the risk of needle-stick injuries that could lead to exposure to bloodborne pathogens, such as the human immunodeficiency virus (HIV), hepatitis B (HBV), or hepatitis C (HCV). Therefore, the following equipment is included in OSHA recommendations:

- Safety needles with a protective sheath that covers the needle automatically immediately after administration, or others that retract into the syringe upon administration
- Needleless devices that can be used to access intravenous tubing for the administration of IV push medications or IV piggybacks.

Safety devices vary depending on the company manufacturing the equipment. Therefore, it is important that you familiarize yourself with the safety equipment used in your facility.

CHAPTER REVIEW QUIZ

Fill in the blanks.

1. a. Which route of administration is used most often? Why?

_____

  b. Which route is fastest? _____

Complete with the appropriate drug form.

2. A tablet placed under the tongue: _____

3. A tablet placed in the cheek pouch: _____

4. A tablet dissolved in the mouth for local action: _____

5. A coated tablet that dissolves in the intestines instead of in the stomach:

_____

6. A capsule that has delayed action over a longer period of time:

_____

7. A liquid drug form with an alcohol base: _____

8. A liquid medication that must be shaken before administration:

_____

9. Drugs given by the rectal route include _____ _____.

10. The parenteral route refers to any route other than the gastrointestinal route. Name four parenteral routes:

_____

_____

_____

_____

Fill in the blanks.

11. Topical drug forms include those applied to the _____ and

_____.

12. To administer a rectal suppository, you need a _____ and

_____.

13. Medicine for injection is contained in two types of glass containers:

   a. With rubber stopper on top: _____

   b. All glass to be broken at the neck: _____

14. Needles are selected according to two measurements: _____ and _____.

15. The three most commonly used syringes for injections are: _____, _____, and _____.

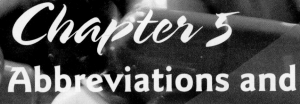

Chapter 5
Abbreviations and Systems of Measurement

Objectives

Upon completion of this chapter, the learner should be able to

1. Identify common abbreviations and symbols used for medication orders

2. List the six parts of a medication order and the two additional items required on a prescription blank

3. Describe the responsibilities of the health care worker regarding verbal and telephone orders for medications

4. Interpret medication orders correctly

5. Compare and contrast the three systems of measurement

6. Convert dosages from one system to another by use of the tables for metric, apothecary, and household equivalents

7. Describe appropriate patient education for those who will be measuring and administering their own medications

8. Define the Key Terms

ABBREVIATIONS

Interpretation of the medication order is the first responsibility when preparing medication for administration. Knowledge of abbreviations and symbols is essential for accurate interpretation of the physician's order. The abbreviations and symbols in Table 5-1 must be memorized. Orders may vary in the use of capital versus lowercase letters. You may occasionally see other abbreviations not included in this list. *When in doubt, always question the meaning. **Never guess!***

Table 5-1 Common Abbreviations For Medication Orders

Note: Abbreviations should be written without periods.

a	before	NPO, npo	nothing by mouth
ac	before meals	NS, N/S	normal saline (sodium
ad lib	as desired		chloride, 0.9%)
AM, am	morning	Ø	none
amp	ampule	OTC	over the counter
bid	twice a day	oz	ounce
c̄	with	p	after
cap	capsule	pc	after meals
Cl	chloride	PCA	patient controlled analgesia
cm	centimeter	PM, pm	afternoon
DC	discontinue	po, PO	by mouth, orally
DS	double strength	PRN, prn	whenever necessary
DW	distilled water	pt	pint, patient
D5W	dextrose, 5% in water	qh	every hour
EC	enteric coated	q2h	every 2 hours
elix	elixir	q3h	every 3 hours
ER	extended release	q4h	every 4 hours
Fe	iron	QNS	quantity not sufficient
fl	fluid	qs	quantity sufficient
gr	grain	qt	quart
Gm, g	gram	R	rectal
gtt	drop	RL, R/L	Ringer's lactate
h, hr	hour	s̄	without
IM	intramuscular	SubQ, subq	subcutaneous
IV	intravenous	SL	sublingual
IVPB	intravenous piggyback	sol	solution
K	potassium	SR	sustained release
KCL	potassium chloride	stat	immediately and once only
kg, Kilo	kilogram	supp	suppository
KVO	keep vein open	tab	tablet
L	liter	tbsp, T, tbs	tablespoon
LA	long acting	tid	three times a day
lb	pound	TO	telephone order
mEq	milliequivalent	tsp, t	teaspoon
mcg	microgram	vag	vaginal
mg	milligram	Vit	vitamin
ml, mL	milliliter (equivalent to cc)	VO	verbal order
mm	millimeter		
Na	sodium		
NaCl	sodium chloride		
NEB	nebulizer		
NG	nasogastric		
noc	night		

The Institute for **Safe Medication Practice (ISMP)** monitors medication administration and identifies practices that have contributed to medication errors. The ISMP has published a list of problematic abbreviations, **ISMP List of Error-Prone Abbreviations, Symbols, and Dose Designations** (Figure 5-1). Additionally, the **Joint Commission on Accreditation of Healthcare Organizations (JCAHO)** has approved a minimum list of "dangerous" abbreviations that have been prohibited effective January 1, 2004. Items required to be on an organization's DO NOT USE list are highlighted with a double asterisk (**) in the ISMP List. (Figure 5-1).

Another safety practice requires the avoidance of periods with all medical abbreviations. If poorly written the period could be mistaken as the number 1, and could cause an error in dosage.

Medication orders contain six parts.

1. Date
2. Patient's name
3. Medication name
4. Dosage or amount of medication
5. Route or manner of administration (if no route is specified, the oral route is usually the appropriate one). When in doubt, always check with the physician.
6. Time to be administered, or frequency

Medication orders must always be written and signed by a physician. In an emergency the physician may give a verbal order (VO). It is the responsibility of the health care worker to *repeat the order* (i.e., medication and amount) before administration and to write down medication, amount, and time of administration as soon as it is given. The physician will sign the medication order after the emergency. Always determine the policy of the agency before taking a telephone order (TO). Most agencies require a registered nurse to take telephone orders. In some facilities, licensed practical (vocational) nurses are allowed to take telephone orders. When taking a telephone order, always obtain the name of the person calling in the order and write the name of that person and the time the call was made next to the medication ordered, for example, "TO Dr. A. Smith, per Mary Jones, CMA @ 1300." Also repeat all of the details regarding the medication, dosage, frequency, and so on, as you write down the order. If you are the medical assistant, or nurse, calling in the prescription to the facility for the physician, be sure to *repeat the name of the drug, dosage, frequency, and route* to the physician as you write it on the patient's office record, adding the time the call was made and the name of the nurse receiving the call in the facility. This documentation is extremely important in preventing medication errors and legal complications. The physician must sign all verbal and telephone orders within 24 hours usually.

Note: Regulations vary from state to state regarding phone orders. Check the rules in your state regarding who can call in an order and who can receive a phone order and regarding time frame for physician's signature.

ISMP List of Error-Prone Abbreviations, Symbols, and Dose Designations

It's been over 2 years since we published a list of abbreviations, symbols, and dose designations that have contributed to medication errors. Now, with the 2004 JCAHO National Patient Safety Goals calling for organizational compliance with a list of prohibited "dangerous" abbreviations, acronyms and symbols, we thought an updated list would be useful. Since JCAHO has specified that certain abbreviations must appear on the organization's list, we've highlighted these items with a double asterisk (**). Also, effective April 1, 2004, each organization must include at least three additional items on their list. However, we hope that you will consider others beyond the minimum JCAHO requirement. Selections can be made from the attached list. These items should be considered for handwritten, preprinted, and electronic forms of communication.

Abbreviations	Intended Meaning	Misinterpretation	Correction
μg	Microgram	Mistaken as "mg"	Use "mcg"
AD, AS, AU	Right ear, left ear, each ear	Mistaken as OD, OS, OU (right eye, left eye, each eye)	Use "right ear," "left ear," or "each ear"
OD, OS, OU	Right eye, left eye, each eye	Mistaken as AD, AS, AU (right ear, left ear, each ear)	Use "right eye," "left eye," or "each eye"
BT	Bedtime	Mistaken as "BID" (twice daily)	Use "bedtime"
cc	Cubic centimeters	Mistaken as "u" (units)	Use "mL"
D/C	Discharge or discontinue	Premature discontinuation of medications if D/C (intended to mean "discharge") has been misinterpreted as "discontinued" when followed by a list of discharge medications	Use "discharge" and "discontinue"
IJ	Injection	Mistaken as "IV" or "intrajugular"	Use "injection"
IN	Intranasal	Mistaken as "IM" or "IV"	Use "intranasal" or "NAS"
HS	Half-strength	Mistaken as bedtime	Use "half-strength" or "bedtime"
hs	At bedtime, hours of sleep	Mistaken as half-strength	
IU**	International unit	Mistaken as IV (intravenous) or 10 (ten)	Use "units"
o.d. or OD	Once daily	Mistaken as "right eye" (OD-oculus dexter), leading to oral liquid medications administered in the eye	Use "daily"
OJ	Orange juice	Mistaken as OD or OS (right or left eye); drugs meant to be diluted in orange juice may be given in the eye	Use "orange juice"
Per os	By mouth, orally	The "os" can be mistaken as "left eye" (OS-oculus sinister)	Use "PO," "by mouth," or "orally"
q.d. or QD**	Every day	Mistaken as q.i.d., especially if the period after the "q" or the tail of the "q" is misunderstood as an "i"	Use "daily"
qhs	At bedtime	Mistaken as "qhr" or every hour	Use "at bedtime"
qn	Nightly	Mistaken as "qh" (every hour)	Use "nightly"
q.o.d. or QOD**	Every other day	Mistaken as "q.d." (daily) or "q.i.d. (four times daily) if the "o" is poorly written	Use "every other day"
q1d	Daily	Mistaken as q.i.d. (four times daily)	Use "daily"
q6PM, etc.	Every evening at 6 PM	Mistaken as every 6 hours	Use "6 PM nightly" or "6 PM daily"
SC, SQ, sub q	Subcutaneous	SC mistaken as SL (sublingual); SQ mistaken as "5 every;" the "q" in "sub q" has been mistaken as "every" (e.g., a heparin dose ordered "sub q 2 hours before surgery" misunderstood as every 2 hours before surgery)	Use "subcut" or "subcutaneously"
ss	Sliding scale (insulin) or ½ (apothecary)	Mistaken as "55"	Spell out "sliding scale;" use "one-half" or "½"
SSRI	Sliding scale regular insulin	Mistaken as selective-serotonin reuptake inhibitor	Spell out "sliding scale (insulin)"
SSI	Sliding scale insulin	Mistaken as Strong Solution of Iodine (Lugol's)	
t/d	One daily	Mistaken as "tid"	Use "1 daily"
TIW or tiw	3 times a week	Mistaken as "3 times a day" or "twice in a week"	Use "3 times weekly"
U or u**	Unit	Mistaken as the number 0 or 4, causing a 10-fold overdose or greater (e.g., 4U seen as "40" or 4u seen as "44"); mistaken as "cc" so dose given in volume instead of units (e.g., 4u seen as 4cc)	Use "unit"

Dose Designations and Other Information	Intended Meaning	Misinterpretation	Correction
Trailing zero after decimal point (e.g., 1.0 mg)**	1 mg	Mistaken as 10 mg if the decimal point is not seen	Do not use trailing zeros for doses expressed in whole numbers
No leading zero before a decimal dose (e.g., .5 mg)**	0.5 mg	Mistaken as 5 mg if the decimal point is not seen	Use zero before a decimal point when the dose is less than a whole unit

ISMP Medication**Safety**Alert!®

Figure 5-1 ISMP List of Error-Prone Abbreviations, Symbols, and Dose Designations. (Reprinted with the permission of the Institute for Safe Medication Practices.)

Dose Designations and Other Information	Intended Meaning	Misinterpretation	Correction
Drug name and dose run together (especially problematic for drug names that end in "L" such as Inderal40 mg; Tegretol300 mg)	Inderal 40 mg Tegretol 300 mg	Mistaken as Inderal 140 mg Mistaken as Tegretol 1300 mg	Place adequate space between the drug name, dose, and unit of measure
Numerical dose and unit of measure run together (e.g., 10mg, 100mL)	10 mg 100 mL	The "m" is sometimes mistaken as a zero or two zeros, risking a 10- to 100-fold overdose	Place adequate space between the dose and unit of measure
Abbreviations such as mg. or mL. with a period following the abbreviation	mg mL	The period is unnecessary and could be mistaken as the number 1 if written poorly	Use mg, mL, etc. without a terminal period
Large doses without properly placed commas (e.g., 100000 units; 1000000 units)	100,000 units 1,000,000 units	100000 has been mistaken as 10,000 or 1,000,000; 1000000 has been mistaken as 100,000	Use commas for dosing units at or above 1,000, or use words such as 100 "thousand" or 1 "million" to improve readability
Drug Name Abbreviations	Intended Meaning	Misinterpretation	Correction
ARA A	vidarabine	Mistaken as cytarabine (ARA C)	Use complete drug name
AZT	zidovudine (Retrovir)	Mistaken as azathioprine or aztreonam	Use complete drug name
CPZ	Compazine (prochlorperazine)	Mistaken as chlorpromazine	Use complete drug name
DPT	Demerol-Phenergan-Thorazine	Mistaken as diphtheria-pertussis-tetanus (vaccine)	Use complete drug name
DTO	Diluted tincture of opium, or deodorized tincture of opium (Paregoric)	Mistaken as tincture of opium	Use complete drug name
HCl	hydrochloric acid or hydrochloride	Mistaken as potassium chloride (The "H" is misinterpreted as "K")	Use complete drug name unless expressed as a salt of a drug
HCT	hydrocortisone	Mistaken as hydrochlorothiazide	Use complete drug name
HCTZ	hydrochlorothiazide	Mistaken as hydrocortisone (seen as HCT250 mg)	Use complete drug name
MgSO4**	magnesium sulfate	Mistaken as morphine sulfate	Use complete drug name
MS, MSO4**	morphine sulfate	Mistaken as magnesium sulfate	Use complete drug name
MTX	methotrexate	Mistaken as mitoxantrone	Use complete drug name
PCA	procainamide	Mistaken as Patient Controlled Analgesia	Use complete drug name
PTU	propylthiouracil	Mistaken as mercaptopurine	Use complete drug name
T3	Tylenol with codeine No. 3	Mistaken as liothyronine	Use complete drug name
TAC	triamcinolone	Mistaken as tetracaine, Adrenalin, cocaine	Use complete drug name
TNK	TNKase	Mistaken as "TPA"	Use complete drug name
ZnSO4	zinc sulfate	Mistaken as morphine sulfate	Use complete drug name
Stemmed Drug Names	Intended Meaning	Misinterpretation	Correction
"Nitro" drip	nitroglycerin infusion	Mistaken as sodium nitroprusside infusion	Use complete drug name
"Norflox"	norfloxacin	Mistaken as Norflex	Use complete drug name
"IV Vanc"	intravenous vancomycin	Mistaken as Invanz	Use complete drug name
Symbols	Intended Meaning	Misinterpretation	Correction
℥	Dram	Symbol for dram mistaken as "3"	Use the metric system
℔	Minim	Symbol for minim mistaken as "mL"	
x3d	For three days	Mistaken as "3 doses"	Use "for three days"
> and <	Greater than and less than	Mistaken as opposite of intended; mistakenly use incorrect symbol; "< 10" mistaken as "40"	Use "greater than" or "less than"
/ (slash mark)	Separates two doses or indicates "per"	Mistaken as the number 1 (e.g., "25 units/10 units" misread as "25 units and 110" units)	Use "per" rather than a slash mark to separate doses
@	At	Mistaken as "2"	Use "at"
&	And	Mistaken as "2"	Use "and"
+	Plus or and	Mistaken as "4"	Use "and"
°	Hour	Mistaken as a zero (e.g., q2° seen as q 20)	Use "hr," "h," or "hour"

** Identified abbreviations above are also included on the JCAHO's "minimum list" of dangerous abbreviations, acronyms and symbols that must be included on an organization's "Do Not Use" list, effective January 1, 2004. An updated list of frequently asked questions about this JCAHO requirement can be found on their website at www.jcaho.org.

ISMP Medication**Safety**Alert!®

Figure 5-1 continued

Medication orders can be written on the patient's record in the physician's office, clinic, or institution, or on a prescription blank (Figure 5-2). It is the responsibility of the health care worker to check the medication order for completeness by noting the six items—date, patient name, medication name, dosage, route, and frequency (plus additional items if using the prescription blank)—and to question any discrepancy, omission, or unusual order. The prescription blank contains two additional items: the physician's Drug Enforcement Administration registration number if the medication is a controlled substance and the number of times that the prescription can be refilled. If there are to be no refills, write the word "NO," "NONE," or "0" after Refill. Never leave a blank space in that area on the prescription blank.

COMMUNITY MEDICAL CLINIC

1700 South Tamiami Trail, Sarasota, FL 34239,   (813) 952-2577

Patient Name: ___ **Mary Chase** ___ Date: __May 12, 2007__

Address: _____

Rx   Cephalexin 250 mg
          twenty-eight (28)
          one q6h

Refill: __0__   Physician Signature: ___*J. Brown*___ M.D.

Physician Name (printed): ___J. Brown___

Physician DEA#: _____

Figure 5-2 Prescription blank. Check for completeness, legibility and accuracy, including date, patient's name, medication name, dosage, route, frequency or time, number of refills, and DEA number for controlled substances. All prescriptions must be printed.

To reduce the incidence of medication errors due to misinterpretation of the prescription, some states have passed legislation* requiring *the name of the medication to be legibly printed or typed.* In addition, these regulations require the *quantity of the drug prescribed to be in both textual and numerical formats,* for example, "ten (10)". *The prescriber must also print his or her name under the signature* (Figure 5-2).

SYSTEMS OF MEASUREMENT

To carry out a medication order accurately, the person administering medications must have an understanding of the different systems of measurement. The original system of weights and measures for writing medication orders was the *apothecary system.* An apothecary is a pharmacist or druggist. A few drugs are still ordered by the apothecary system. However, the metric system is the preferred system of measurement and is used at the present time. The third system of measurement is the *household system,* which is the least accurate. However, this system is more familiar to the layperson and is therefore used in prescribing medications for the patient at home. The health care worker must understand all three systems of measurement for accurate administration of medicines and for patient education as well. Medication orders are concerned with only two types of measurement: (1) measuring fluids, or liquid measure, and (2) measuring solids, or solid weight.

The apothecary system of liquid measurement includes the minim, fluid dram, fluid ounce, pint, quart, and gallon. The apothecary system for measuring solid weights includes the grain, dram, ounce, and pound (Table 5-2).

Table 5-2 Abbreviations for the Apothecary System

grain	gr
minim*	m, min
drop*	gtt
dram	dr
ounce	oz
pint	pt
quart	qt

*A drop is approximately equivalent to 1 minim of water, but the type of solution may cause variation. When minims are ordered, they should always be measured with a minim glass or in a tuberculin syringe for accuracy. If the order specifies drops, they may be measured with a medicine dropper.

A few drugs *sometimes* ordered by the apothecary system in grains can include aspirin, acetaminophen, iron, and phenobarbital.

The metric system was invented by the French in the late 18th century and is the international standard for weights and measures. The

---

An example of such legislation is the "Legible Prescription Law," Section 456.42, Florida Statutes, which became effective in Florida on July 1, 2003.

metric system of liquid measurement includes the liter and the milliliter, which is approximately equivalent to the cubic centimeter. The metric system for measuring solid weights includes the gram and the milligram as the measures most commonly used for medication prescriptions.

At times you will find it necessary to convert a dosage from the apothecary system to the metric or household system. It is important to memorize the few basic equivalents most commonly used. Table 5-3 lists commonly used approximate equivalents for liquid measurement. These figures are easily committed to memory. When **conversions** are necessary in the measurement of solids, you will find it useful to consult Table 5-4 for metric and apothecary equivalents. If it is necessary to convert

Table 5-3 Common Approximate Equivalents for Liquid Measurement

METRIC	APOTHECARY	HOUSEHOLD
I ml	15 m	
5 ml	I dr	**I tsp**
15 ml	4 dr	I tbsp
30 ml	I oz	2 tbsp
240 ml	8 oz	I measuring cup (240 ml)
500 ml	I pt (16 oz.)	I pt
1,000 ml	I qt (32 oz)	I qt

Table 5-4 Metric and Apothecary Approximate Equivalents for Solid Measurement

METRIC (GRAMS)	METRIC (MILLIGRAMS)	APOTHECARY
I g	**1,000 mg**	**15 gr**
0.6 g	600 mg	10 gr
0.5 g	**500 mg**	7½ gr
0.3 g	300–325 mg*	**5 gr**
0.2 g	200 mg	3 gr
0.1 g	100 mg	1½ gr
0.06 g	**60–65 mg***	**I gr**
0.05 g	50 mg	3/4 gr
0.03 g	**30 mg**	**1/2 gr**
	0.4 mg	1/150 gr

Note: Memorize all equivalents in boldface.

Pounds–Kilograms (kg) Conversion

I pound = 0.453592 kg

I kg   = 2.2 pounds (lb)

To convert pounds to kilograms, divide number of pounds by 2.2.

Warning: Be very careful in calculating the weight in kilograms. The slightest error, especially in pediatric doses, could result in serious or fatal consequences.

*****Note** that metric equivalents of apothecary are not precise. Be very careful with conversions. Consult a pharmacist when in doubt.

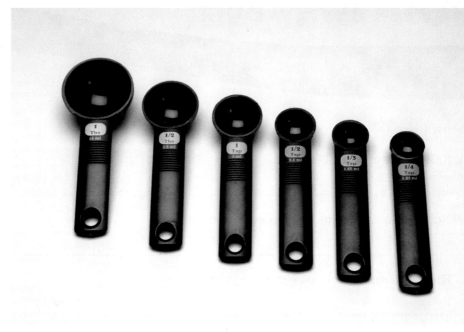

Figure 5-3 For accurate household measurement, standard measuring spoons are used.

from the apothecary system to the metric, always consult a conversion table or a pharmacist to avoid dangerous errors.

Equipment most commonly used for measuring medications includes the medicine cup and various syringes calibrated in milliliters and/or minims.

Patient Education

When explaining dosage preparation, always speak directly to the patient and observe the patient for comprehension. Many older adult patients have difficulty hearing but are reluctant to admit lack of understanding. Ask them to repeat the directions.

Many older adult patients also have vision problems. Be sure the directions for dosage preparation are written clearly. If a family member will be assisting in preparation and administration of medications, include that person in the instruction. Be sure that any measuring equipment to be used is clearly marked.

Measuring spoons and clearly marked measuring cups should be used when available for household measurement. Such calibrated utensils are more accurate than tableware (Figure 5-3). Teaspoons, tablespoons, teacups, and drinking glasses vary in size and capacity, and therefore measurements are inaccurate with such utensils.

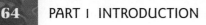

CHAPTER REVIEW QUIZ

Interpret the following orders.

1. Keflex 250-mg cap PO q6h

_____

2. Neosporin ophth sol 2 gtt in each eye tid

_____

3. Feosol 65 mg tab bid pc c̄ orange juice

_____

4. Diuril 500 mg PO qAM

_____

5. Dyazide 1 cap bid

_____

6. Demerol 50 mg IM q4h prn for pain

_____

7. Metamucil 1 tsp mixed c̄ 8 oz H₂O bid pc

_____

8. Dulcolax supp R prn for constipation

_____

9. Actifed syr 1 tsp q4h prn for cough

_____

10. Nitrostat 1 tab SL prn for angina attack, may repeat q5min 3 times

_____

11. Compazine supp 25 mg prn q6h for nausea

_____

12. DC Phenergan 48h post-op

_____

13. Tolinase 250 mg daily c̄ breakfast

_____

14. Mandol 0.5 g IVPB q8h

_____

15. Potassium chloride 20 mEq in NS 1L ql2h

_____

16. NPH insulin 20 units SubQ daily ac breakfast

_____

17. Tylenol 325 mg supp R prn T over 101

_____

18. Vasocidin ophth sol 1 gtt q3h in the right eye

_____

19. Ceclor 20 mg/kg/daily in 2 equal doses q12h

_____

20. Ambien 5 mg for sleep prn, may repeat once q noc

_____

Fill in the blanks.

21. Which is the oldest system of measurement for medication?

_____

22. Which system of drug measurement is used most frequently throughout the world?

_____

23. Which is the least accurate system for measuring medicine?

_____

24. Two different types of equipment used to measure drugs are _____
and _____.

Use Tables 5-3 and 5-4 to complete the following conversions and place the correct answer in the blank.

25. 1 gr = _____ mg

26. 7½ gr = _____ mg

27. 1 kg = _____ pounds

28. 1 pound = _____ kg

29. 1 tsp = _____ mL

30. 1 tbl = _____ mL

31. 5 gr = _____ mg

32. 15 gr = _____ g

33. 0.5 g = _____ mg

34. 1 g = _____ mg

35. ½ gr = _____ mg

Chapter 6
Safe Dosage Preparation

Objectives

Upon completion of this chapter, the learner should be able to

1. Identify the three steps for calculation of the dosage ordered when it differs from the dose on hand

2. Write the formula for each of the two methods of dosage calculation presented in this chapter

3. Convert from one system of measurement to another using the ratio and proportion method

4. Solve dosage problems using the basic calculation method

5. Solve dosage problems using the ratio and proportion method

6. List the cautions with the basic calculation method

7. List the cautions with the ratio and proportion method

8. Calculate safe dosages for infants and children

9. List the variables when assessing geriatric patients for safe dosage

10. List some steps to reduce medication errors

11. Define the Key Terms

"First, do no harm." Health care workers are dedicated to the principle of helping others, not harming them. Nowhere is this principle more important than in the calculation, preparation, and administration of safe dosages. One careless moment can lead to a catastrophe. It is the responsibility of the health care worker to be absolutely certain that the medication administered is exactly as prescribed by the physician *and* is also an **appropriate** dose for that particular patient. Doses for children and older adults can vary significantly from the average dose. Therefore, it may be necessary to compute a partial dose from the dose on hand for the average patient.

Many medications are dispensed by the pharmacist in unit-dose form, in which each individual dose of medicine is prepackaged in a separate packet, vial, or prefilled syringe. Although much of the mixing and measuring of medications is now completed by the pharmacist, the person who is administering medications must understand the preparation of dosages in order to ensure accuracy. On occasion the dosage ordered differs from the dose on hand. Consequently, it may be necessary to calculate the correct dosage. Calculations can be a simple procedure if you follow the necessary steps in sequential order.

A working knowledge of basic arithmetic is required for accurate calculation of drug dosage. To understand the calculation of correct dosage, you must evaluate your basic arithmetic skills by completing the following mathematics pretest.

BASIC ARITHMETIC TEST

1. $6\frac{1}{4} + 3\frac{2}{3}$
2. $4\frac{2}{3} - 2\frac{1}{2}$
3. $2\frac{2}{3} \times 3\frac{2}{5}$
4. $\frac{2}{5} \div \frac{3}{4}$
5. $2\frac{2}{3} \div 5$
6. Write six and a third as a decimal.
7. $6.67 + 0.065 + 0.3$
8. $10.4 - 0.037$
9. 0.223×0.67
10. $46.72 \div 6.4$
11. Write 8% as a fraction and reduce.
12. Change $\frac{2}{5}$ to a decimal.
13. Write 0.023 as a percent.
14. Express 12% as a decimal.
15. Express 0.4 as a fraction and reduce.
16. Change $\frac{3}{5}$ to a percent.
17. Change $12\frac{1}{2}$% to a decimal.
18. What is 75% of 160?
19. What is 9.2% of 250?
20. What is $37\frac{1}{2}$% of 192?
21. Which fraction is the largest: $\frac{1}{2}$, $\frac{2}{5}$, or $\frac{3}{10}$?
22. Which is the largest: $\frac{1}{3}$, 0.4, or 60%?
23. Write the Roman numeral XXV as an Arabic numeral.
24. Write 154 as a Roman numeral.
25. The label on the bottle reads 0.5 g per tablet. The doctor orders 0.25 g. How many tablets should you give?

After completing the quiz, check your answers (see following). If there is an error, review mathematics for that area until all problems can be solved accurately and easily. A minimum score of 80% is recommended as indicating readiness for dosage calculations. Those not meeting this criterion should seek remedial assistance in review of basics before beginning calculations.

Answers to Basic Arithmetic Test

1. $9^{11}/_{12}$	**8.** 10.363	**14.** 0.12	**20.** 72
2. $2^1/_6$	**9.** 0.14941	**15.** $^2/_5$	**21.** $^1/_2$
3. $9^1/_{15}$	**10.** 7.3	**16.** 60%	**22.** 60%
4. $^8/_{15}$	**11.** $^2/_{25}$	**17.** 0.125	**23.** 25
5. $^8/_{15}$	**12.** 0.4	**18.** 120	**24.** CLIV
6. 6.333	**13.** 2.3%	**19.** 23	**25.** $^1/_2$
7. 7.035			

CALCULATION GUIDELINES

Remember, there is no margin of error in administration of medications. It is possible for a small error in arithmetic to seriously harm a patient. A misplaced decimal point could cause a fatality. Safe dosage preparation requires (1) a working knowledge of basic arithmetic and (2) meticulous care with all calculations.

Calculations can be as simple as 1, 2, 3. When the dosage ordered differs from the dosage on hand, the problem can be solved simply by completing three basic steps:

1. Check whether all measures are in the same system. Convert if necessary by using Tables 5-3 and 5-4 or use the ratio and proportion method.

2. Write the problem in equation form using the *appropriate formula and labeling all parts,* and complete the necessary calculations.

3. *Check the accuracy* of your answer for reasonableness, and have someone else verify your calculations.

There are several different methods of calculating dosage. Either of the methods presented in this book may be used, or both methods may be used to verify accuracy. The two methods presented here are *basic calculation* and *ratio and proportion.* Basic calculation requires only simple arithmetic; ratio and proportion requires the ability to determine an unknown, X.

METHOD I: BASIC CALCULATION

Use the following formula:

$$\frac{\text{desired dose}}{\text{on-hand dose}} \times \text{quantity of on-hand dose}$$

In short form

$$\frac{D}{OH} \times Q$$

EXAMPLE 1

The physician orders aspirin gr 10 q4h PRN for fever over 101°. On hand are aspirin gr 5 tabs.

Step 1.   Check to see if all measures are in the same system. No conversion is necessary. Both measures are in grains.

Step 2.   Use the formula $\dfrac{D}{OH} \times Q$ and label all parts:

$$\frac{10 \text{ gr}}{5 \text{ gr}} \times 1 \text{ tab} = 10 \div 5 = 2$$

$$2 \times 1 = 2 \text{ tabs}$$

Note: The labels of the desired and on-hand doses must be the same. The label of the answer must be the same as the quantity.

Step 3.   Check for reasonableness. A dose of 2 tabs is within normal limits.

    If the calculations resulted in an answer such as 1/4 tablet or five tablets, the answer is not reasonable and the calculations should be rechecked. If calculations are correct after recheck, any unusual dosage should be checked with the person in charge: the pharmacist or the physician. *When in doubt, always question.*

EXAMPLE 2

The order reads Ampicillin 0.5 g. The unit dose packet reads 250 mg/cap.

Step 1.   Check to see if all measures are in the same system. Convert grams to milligrams:

$$1 \text{ g} = 1{,}000 \text{ mg}$$

$$0.5 \text{ g} = 0.5 \times 1{,}000 = 500 \text{ mg}$$

Step 2.   Use the formula $\dfrac{D}{OH} \times Q$ and label all parts:

$$\frac{500 \text{ mg}}{250 \text{ mg}} \times 1 \text{ cap} =$$

Reduce fraction to lowest terms:

$$\frac{500}{250} = 50 \div 25 = 2$$

$$2 \times 1 = 2 \text{ caps}$$

Step 3.   Check for reasonableness. A dose of 2 caps is within normal limits.

EXAMPLE 3

The narcotics drawer contains vials of meperidine (Demerol) labeled 75 mg in 1 ml. The preoperative order reads Demerol 60 mg IM on call.

Step 1. Check to see if all measures are in the same system. No **conversion** is necessary.

Step 2. Use the formula $\dfrac{D}{OH} \times Q$ and label all parts:

$$\frac{60 \text{ mg}}{75 \text{ mg}} \times 1 \text{ ml} =$$

Reduce fractions to lowest terms:

$$\frac{60}{75} = \frac{12}{15} = \frac{4}{5}$$

Convert fractions to decimals:

$$\frac{4}{5} = 5\overline{)4.0}^{\,0.8}$$

Multiply by quantity.

$$0.8 \times 1 \text{ ml} = 0.8 \text{ ml}$$

Note: Fractions must be converted to decimals and rounded off to one decimal place to coincide with the markings on the syringe.

Step 3. Check for reasonableness. A dose of 0.8 ml is within normal limits.

EXAMPLE 4

The physician orders Versed 3 mg IM preoperatively. On hand are vials labeled 5 mg per ml.

Step 1. Check to see if all measures are in the same system. No conversion is necessary.

Step 2. Use the formula $\dfrac{D}{OH} \times Q$ and label all parts:

$$\frac{3 \text{ mg}}{5 \text{ mg}} \times 1 \text{ ml} = 3 \div 5 = 5\overline{)3.0}^{\,0.6}$$

$$0.6 \times 1 \text{ ml} = 0.6 \text{ ml}$$

Step 3. Check for reasonableness. A dose of 0.6 ml is within normal limits.

EXAMPLE 5

The order reads atropine sulfate 0.6 mg IM on call to surgery. Available ampules are labeled atropine sulfate 0.4 mg/ml.

Step 1. Check to see if all measures are in the same system. No conversion is necessary.

Step 2. Use the formula $\dfrac{D}{OH} \times Q$ and label all parts:

$$\frac{0.6 \text{ mg}}{0.4 \text{ mg}} \times 1 \text{ ml} = 0.6 \div 0.4 = 0.4\overline{)0.6}^{\,1.5}$$

$$1.5 \times 1 \text{ ml} = 1.5 \text{ ml}$$

Step 3. Check for reasonableness. A dose of 1.5 ml is within normal limits.

Cautions for the Basic Calculation Method

1. *Label* all parts of the formula.
2. Use the *same label* for desired and on-hand doses.
3. Use the *same label* for the quantity and the answer (the amount to be given).
4. *Reduce fractions* to lowest terms before dividing.
5. *Multiply by the quantity* after dividing.
6. Take *extra care* with *decimals*.
7. *Convert* fractions to decimals.
8. *Round off* decimals to one decimal place after computation is complete.
9. *Verify the accuracy* of calculations with an instructor.
10. Question the answer if not within normal limits (e.g., less than ½ tab, more than two tabs, or more than 2 ml for injection).

METHOD 2: RATIO AND PROPORTION

A **ratio** describes a relationship between two numbers. Example:

$$1 \text{ g} : 15 \text{ gr}$$

A **proportion** consists of two ratios that are equal. Example:

$$1 \text{ g} : 15 \text{ gr} = 2 \text{ g} : 30 \text{ gr}$$

Always label each term in the equation. The terms of each ratio must be in the same sequence. In the previous examples, the first term of each ratio is labeled g and the second term of each ratio is labeled gr.

To solve a problem with the ratio and proportion method, set up the formula with the known terms on the left and the desired and unknown terms on the right. Use *X* to represent the unknown. Label all terms.

For example, we know that 1,000 mg is equal to 1 g (known). We need to administer 500 mg (desired) and do not know how many grams are equivalent (unknown = *X*). To convert a dosage from one system to another when a table of metric and apothecary equivalents (such as Table 5-4) is unavailable, set up the problem as a proportion

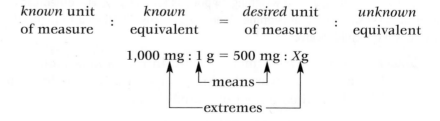

known unit   *known*   *desired* unit   *unknown*
of measure   :   equivalent   =   of measure   :   equivalent

$$1{,}000 \text{ mg} : 1 \text{ g} = 500 \text{ mg} : X\text{g}$$

means — extremes

To solve the problem, multiply the two outer terms, or extremes, and then multiply the two inner terms, or means. Using our example

$$1{,}000\,X = 500 = 1{,}000\overline{)500.0}^{\;0.5}$$

$$X = 0.5 \text{ g}$$

We now know that our desired dose, 500 mg, is equal to 0.5 g.

When the dose ordered differs from the dose on hand, the problem can be solved simply by completing three basic steps:

1. Verify that all measures are in the same system. Convert if necessary by using a table of metric and apothecary equivalents if available or by using the ratio and proportion method if the equivalent is unknown.

2. Set up the problem as a proportion, *label all terms,* and complete the calculations. Use the following formula:

$$\frac{\text{dose}}{\text{on hand}} : \frac{\text{known}}{\text{quantity}} = \frac{\text{dose}}{\text{desired}} : \frac{\text{unknown}}{\text{quantity}}$$

Note: The answer should be stated as a whole number or a decimal. Convert fractions to decimals and round off to one decimal place.

3. Check the accuracy of your answer for reasonableness and also have someone else verify your calculations.

EXAMPLE 1

The preoperative order reads Demerol 60 mg IM on call. The narcotics locker contains ampules labeled meperidine (Demerol) 100 mg/2 ml.

Step 1.   Verify that all measures are in the same system. No conversion is necessary.

Step 2.   Set up the problem as a proportion and label all terms:

$$\frac{\text{dose}}{\text{on hand}} : \frac{\text{known}}{\text{quantity}} = \frac{\text{dose}}{\text{desired}} : \frac{\text{unknown}}{\text{quantity}}$$

$$100 \text{ mg} : 2 \text{ ml} = 60 \text{ mg} : X \text{ ml}$$

$$100X = 120 = 100\overline{)120.0}^{\,1.2}$$

$$X = 1.2 \text{ ml}$$

Step 3.   Check for reasonableness. A dose of 1.2 ml is within normal limits.

EXAMPLE 2

The physician is treating a child weighing 44 pounds for epilepsy. The order reads phenobarbital elixir 3 mg/kg at bedtime. Phenobarbital elixir is labeled 15 mg/5 ml. How many ml will the child receive?

Step 1.   Verify that all measures are in the same system. Pounds must be converted to kilograms (kg). To convert lbs to kg, divide the number of pounds by 2.2.

The child weighs 20 kg.

The order reads 3 mg/kg. Therefore, 3 mg $\times$ 20 kg = 60 mg dose.

Step 2.   Set up the problem as a proportion. Label all terms.

$$\frac{\text{dose}}{\text{on hand}} : \frac{\text{known}}{\text{quantity}} = \frac{\text{dose}}{\text{desired}} : \frac{\text{unknown}}{\text{quantity}}$$

$$15 \text{ mg} : 5 \text{ ml} = 60 \text{ mg} : X \text{ ml}$$

$$15X = 300 = 15\overline{)300}^{\,20}$$

$$X = 20 \text{ ml}$$

Step 3.   Check for reasonableness. An oral dose of 20 ml is a large amount for a young child to take at one time. The physician might want to divide the daily dose. If so, the order would be written: phenobarbital 30 mg BID.

EXAMPLE 3

Meperidine Oral Solution is available as Demerol Syrup 50 mg/5 ml. The order reads Demerol liquid 150 mg PO q6h PRN.

Step 1.   Verify that all measures are in the same system. No conversion is necessary.

Step 2.   Set up the problem as a proportion. Label all terms.

$$\begin{array}{c} \text{dose} \\ \text{on hand} \end{array} : \begin{array}{c} \text{known} \\ \text{quantity} \end{array} = \begin{array}{c} \text{dose} \\ \text{desired} \end{array} : \begin{array}{c} \text{unknown} \\ \text{quantity} \end{array}$$

$$50 \text{ mg} : 5 \text{ ml} = 150 \text{ mg} : X \text{ ml}$$

$$50X = 750 = 50\overline{)750}^{\,15}$$

$$X = 15 \text{ ml}$$

Step 3.   Check for reasonableness. An oral dose of 15 ml is appropriate for an adult.

EXAMPLE 4

An 88-lb child with cancer has an order for pain medication that reads morphine liquid PO 0.2 mg/kg q 4 h PRN. Available Morphine Solution is labeled 20 mg/5 ml.

Step 1.   Verify that all measures are in the same system. Pounds must be converted to kilograms (kg). To convert lb to kg, divide number of pounds by 2.2. The child weighs 40 kg.

The order reads 0.2 mg/kg. Therefore, 0.2 mg $\times$ 40 = 8-mg dose.

Step 2.   Set up the problem as a proportion. Label all terms.

$$\begin{array}{c} \text{dose} \\ \text{on hand} \end{array} : \begin{array}{c} \text{known} \\ \text{quantity} \end{array} = \begin{array}{c} \text{dose} \\ \text{desired} \end{array} : \begin{array}{c} \text{unknown} \\ \text{quantity} \end{array}$$

$$20 \text{ mg} : 5 \text{ ml} = 8 \text{ mg} : X \text{ ml}$$

$$20X = 40 = 20\overline{)40}^{\,2}$$

$$X = 2 \text{ ml}$$

Step 3.   Check for reasonableness. An oral dose of 2 ml is appropriate for a terminally ill child.

EXAMPLE 5

The physician orders Benadryl elixir 25 mg q12h. The bottle in the medicine cupboard is labeled 12.5 mg/5 ml.

Step 1. Verify that all measures are in the same system. No conversion is necessary.

Step 2. Write the problem as a proportion and label each term

$$\begin{matrix} \text{dose} \\ \text{on hand} \end{matrix} : \begin{matrix} \text{known} \\ \text{quantity} \end{matrix} = \begin{matrix} \text{dose} \\ \text{desired} \end{matrix} : \begin{matrix} \text{unknown} \\ \text{quantity} \end{matrix}$$

$$12.5 \text{ mg}: 5 \text{ ml} = 25 \text{ mg} : X \text{ ml}$$

$$12.5X = 125 = 12.5\overline{)125.00} = 125\overline{)1250}^{10}$$

$$X = 10 \text{ ml}$$

Step 3. Check for reasonableness. The dose 10 ml is within normal limits for oral solution.

Cautions for the ratio and proportion method

1. *Label* all parts of the equation.
2. The ratio on the *left* contains the *known* quantity, and the ratio on the *right* contains the *desired* and *unknown* quantities.
3. Terms of the second ratio must be in the same sequence as those in the first ratio.
4. *Multiply* the *extremes first* and then the means.
5. Take *extra care* with *decimals*.
6. *Convert* fractions to decimals. *Round off* decimals to one decimal place.
7. *Label* the answer.
8. *Verify the accuracy* of calculations with an instructor.
9. *Question* any unusual dosage not within normal limits (e.g., less than 1/2 tab, more than two tabs, or more than 2 ml for injection).

PEDIATRIC DOSAGE

Children are not miniature adults. You cannot merely take part of an adult dose and give it to a child. There are many other variables to consider. There are numerous formulas available for computing *approximate* child's dose based on either body surface area, weight, or age. However, other factors must be taken into consideration as well. In neonates, renal function and some enzyme systems needed for drug absorption and metabolism are not fully developed. The neonate's blood-brain barrier is more permeable and his total body water contributes a greater percentage of his body weight, also affecting drug absorption.

Appropriate dosage for children, as well as adults, must take into consideration variables such as age, weight, sex, and metabolic, pathological, or psychological conditions. Recommended pediatric drug dosages are derived from data obtained in clinical trials utilizing sick children. When preparing drug dosages for children, it is important to always refer to recommended dosages as listed in drug inserts, *Physicians' Desk Reference (PDR),* or *AHFS Drug Information (Formulary).*

Recommended dosages of drugs are often expressed in the references as a number of milligrams per unit of body weight, per unit of time. For example, the recommended dose for a drug might be 6 mg/kg/24 h. This information can then be used to

1. Calculate the dose for the individual patient
2. Check on the appropriateness of the prescribed dose, watching particularly for possible overdoses

EXAMPLE 1

The recommended dose of meperidine (Demerol) is 6 mg/kg/24 h for pain, in divided doses every four to six hours, as necessary. Demerol is available in ampules or cartridges labeled 50 mg/ml. How much Demerol would be appropriate for a 33-pound child as a single dose every six hours?

Step 1.   Convert pounds to kilograms (divide number of pounds by 2.2).

$$33 \text{ pounds} = 15 \text{ kg}$$

6 mg per kg in 24 hr is recommended.

$$6 \text{ mg} \times 15 \text{ kg} = 90 \text{ mg in 24 hr}$$

Step 2.   Calculate the number of *milliliters needed in 24 h.* Write the problem as a proportion and label each term.

$$\frac{\text{dose}}{\text{on hand}} : \frac{\text{known}}{\text{quantity}} = \frac{\text{dose}}{\text{desired}} : \frac{\text{unknown}}{\text{quantity}}$$

$$50 \text{ mg} : 1 \text{ ml} = 90 \text{ mg} : X \text{ ml}$$

$$50X = 90 = 50\overline{)90.0}^{\;1.8}$$

$$X = 1.8 \text{ ml in 24 h}$$

Then, calculate the number of *milliliters needed in six hours.* Remember, the unknown quantity is always the last term in the equation.

$$24 \text{ h} : 1.8 \text{ ml} = \text{six hours} : X \text{ ml}$$

$$24X = 10.8 = 24\overline{)10.80}^{\;0.45}$$

$$X = 0.45 \text{ ml dose every six hours}$$

Step 3.   The appropriateness of this dose can be checked by applying *Clark's Rule:*

$$\frac{\text{child's wt in lb}}{\text{average adult wt}} \times \text{adult dose} = \text{child's } \textit{approximate} \text{ dose}$$

$$\frac{33}{150} \times 100 \text{ mg} = 22 \text{ mg approximate child's dose}$$

Demerol is available in ampules labeled 100 mg/2 ml

$$100 \text{ mg}: 2\text{ml} = 22 \text{ mg} : X \text{ ml}$$

$$100X = 44 = 100\overline{)44.00}$$
$$\underline{400}$$
$$\underline{400}$$

with quotient 0.44

$$X = 0.44 \text{ ml dose to be administered}$$

Remember, this is a *general* rule and other variables must be considered when assessing for appropriateness of dosage.

GERIATRIC DOSAGE

Special consideration must be given to preparation and administration of safe dosage to older adults. As with children, the dose frequently needs to be reduced. Factors leading to possible dangerous cumulative effects can include slower metabolism, poor circulation, or impairment of liver, kidneys, lungs, or central nervous system. Any chronic disease, debility, dehydration, or electrolyte imbalance can affect assimilation of drugs and interfere with therapeutic effect. Many drugs can impair mental status of older adults, leading to confusion. Any older adult taking many drugs is also at risk for potentially lethal interactions. There is no formula to guide you in safe geriatric dosage. Careful assessment on an *individual* basis, constant monitoring, and reduction of dosage, whenever possible, are the rules to follow. Each individual reacts differently to drugs, and changes occur over time. You have the responsibility to question the appropriateness of any drug, and especially as the patient's condition changes. See also Chapter 28, Drugs and Older Adults.

PREVENTION OF MEDICATION ERRORS

Medication errors can occur for a number of reasons: administering the wrong drug, the wrong amount, at the wrong time, by the wrong route, or to the wrong patient. The Rights of Medication Administration will be discussed in the next chapter. However, we will consider here errors that can occur when the drug order is misinterpreted.

- Never leave the decimal point naked. Writing .2 instead of 0.2 could cause the decimal point to be missed and could result in an overdose. Always place a zero *before* a decimal point; for example, 0.2, 0.5.

- Never place a decimal point and zero after a whole number. The decimal point could be missed and the zero could be misinterpreted, for example, 5.0 mg could be read as 50 mg. The correct way is to write 5 mg.

- Avoid using decimals whenever whole numbers can be used as alternatives; for example, 0.5 g can be expressed as 500 mg.

- If you have difficulty interpreting the spelling of a drug name or the number used for the dosage, or the dosage seems inappropriate, *always question* the order. This is not only your duty, but you have an ethical and legal responsibility to be sure that the drugs you administer are safe. If a medication error results in legal action, you could be held accountable, even though the order was written incorrectly. You are expected to recognize inappropriate dosage, to check reference books with unfamiliar drugs, and to ask the physician or pharmacist about any questionable dosage.

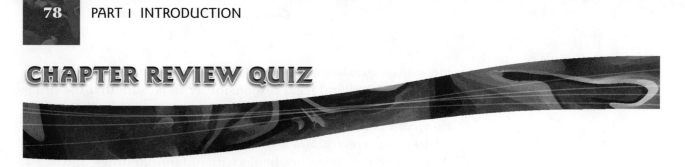

CHAPTER REVIEW QUIZ

Section A

The available dosages are listed with each drug. Choose the most appropriate available form to deliver the dosage ordered. Use only *one* form of each drug. Indicate the *amount* and *which drug form* you should give for the following orders. *Use the smallest number of tablets possible.*

Drug and Dose Ordered	Amount to Administer
1. atenolol (Tenormin) 75 mg Available 50 mg and 100 mg tablets of Tenormin	_____ of _____ mg tab
2. buspirone (Buspar) 25 mg Available 5 mg and 10 mg tablets of Buspar	_____ of _____ mg tab
3. alprazolam (Xanax) 0.75 mg Available 0.25 mg, 0.5 mg, and 1 mg tablets of Xanax	_____ of _____ mg tab
4. bumetanide (Bumex) 2 mg Available 0.5 mg and 1 mg tablets of Bumex	_____ of _____ mg tab
5. cimetidine (Tagamet) 200 mg Available 300 mg and 400 mg tablets of Tagamet	_____ of _____ mg tab
6. furosemide (Lasix) 60 mg Available 20 mg and 40 mg tablets of Lasix	_____ of _____ mg tab
7. levothyroxine (Synthroid) 0.3 mg Available 0.05 mg, 0.1 mg, and 0.15 mg tablets of Synthroid	_____ of _____ mg tab
8. propranolol (Inderal) 15 mg Available 10 mg, 20 mg, and 40 mg tablets of Inderal	_____ of _____ mg tab
9. prednisone (Deltasone) 15 mg Available 5 mg, 10 mg, and 20 mg tablets of Deltasone	_____ of _____ mg tab
10. sertraline (Zoloft) 75 mg Available 50 mg and 100 mg tablets of Zoloft	_____ of _____ mg tab

Section B

Show your work. Label and circle your answers.

1. The physician orders Lovenox 1 mg/kg subq q12h. The patient weighs 176 lb. Lovenox is available 100 mg in 1 ml.

    a. What is the patient's weight in kilograms? _____

    b. What is the dose of Lovenox to be administered? _____ mg in _____ ml

2. The medication order reads Demerol 60 mg IM. The narcotic drawer contains syringes labeled meperidine (Demerol) 75 mg/ml.

    a. How many ml would you administer? _____

    b. How many ml would you discard and mark as "wasted" on the narcotic record?

    _____

3. Lasix is available in 40 mg tablets. The order reads Lasix 60 mg PO qAM. How many tablets should you give?

4. Phenergan 12.5 mg is ordered. Available vials of phenergan are labeled 25 mg/ml. How many ml would you administer?

5. Acetaminophen elixir 650 mg is ordered. The container is labeled 325 mg/5 ml.

    a. How many ml would you administer? _____

    b. How many teaspoons per dose? _____

6. Morphine sulfate PO 30 mg liquid is ordered. Morphine oral solution is labeled 20 mg/ml. How many ml would you administer?

7. The medication order reads heparin 5,000 units. Vials available in the medication cupboard are labeled heparin 10,000 units/ml. How many milliliters should you draw into the syringe?

8. Digoxin elixir is available in 50 mcg/ml. The physician orders 125 mcg Lanoxin daily. How many milliliters should you give?

9. The physician orders prednisone 7.5 mg daily. Prednisone is available in 5-mg and 10-mg scored tablets, which can be broken in half. Which strength tablet and how many tablets should you give?

10. Amoxicillin suspension 750 mg q8h is ordered. Liquid medication available is labeled 250 mg/5 ml. How many milliliters should you give?

11. Calcium carbonate 1,000 mg daily is prescribed, to be given in divided doses bid. Available tablets contain calcium 250 mg/tab. How many tablets should be taken each time?

12. Robitussin A-C contains 10 mg of codeine in each teaspoon (5 ml). If 2 tsp Robitussin A-C is prescribed q4h, how much codeine would be contained in each dose?

13. The physician orders Ivermectin tablets for a 200-lb adult with scabies. The recommended dose is 0.2 mg/kg. Ivermectin tablets are labeled 6 mg. How many tablets should be given for the dose?

14. The physician orders Ceclor Suspension 200 mg q8h for a 44-lb child. Ceclor Suspension is available 250 mg/5 ml.

    a. How many ml should be administered each time? _____

    b. Recommended dosage of Ceclor is 30 mg/kg/daily. How many mg would be appropriate for this child daily? _____

15. List five variables to consider in determining a child's dose:

_____, _____, _____, _____,

and _____

16. List five factors that could lead to serious cumulative effects with medicines in the elderly:

_____, _____, _____, _____,

and _____

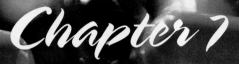

Chapter 7
Responsibilities and Principles of Drug Administration

Objectives

Upon completion of this chapter, the learner should be able to

1. Describe four responsibilities of the health care provider in safe administration of medications
2. List the six Rights of Medication Administration
3. Explain moral, ethical, and legal responsibilities regarding medication errors
4. Cite three instances of medication administration that require documentation
5. Explain the rights of the health care worker to question or refuse to administer medications
6. Define the Key Terms

Key Terms

Documentation

Reporting

Responsibilities

Rights of Medication Administration

RESPONSIBLE DRUG ADMINISTRATION

The safe and accurate administration of medications requires knowledge, judgment, and skill. The **responsibilities** of the health care provider in this vital area include:

1. Adequate, up-to-date *information* about all medications to be administered, including purpose, potential side effects, cautions, and contraindications, and possible interactions.
2. *Wisdom* and judgment to accurately *assess* the patient's needs for medications, to *evaluate* the response to medications, and to *plan* appropriate interventions as indicated.
3. *Skill in delivery* of the medication accurately, in the best interests of the patient, and with adequate documentation.

4. *Patient education* to provide the necessary information to the patient and family about why, how, and when medications are to be administered and potential side effects and precautions with administration by the layperson.

Responsibility for safe administration of medications requires that the health care worker be familiar with every medication before administration. Knowledge of the typical and most frequently used drugs of the systems (as described in Part II of this text) is imperative. However, this is only a framework upon which to build and add other knowledge of new drugs or new effects as changes in medicine become known. Unfamiliar drugs should never be administered. Resources such as the *PDR,* the *AHFS Drug Information,* the *USP/DI,* package inserts, and pharmacists must be consulted *before* administration in order to become familiar with the desired effect, potential side effects, precautions and contraindications, and possible interactions with other drugs or with foods.

Responsibility for safe administration of medications requires *complete planning* for patient care, including prior *assessment, interventions,* and *evaluations* of the results of drug therapy. Assessment involves taking a complete history, including all medical conditions (e.g., pregnancy or illness), allergies, and all other medications in use, including over-the-counter drugs, vitamins, and herbal remedies. Assessment also involves careful observation of the patient's vital signs, posture, skin temperature and color, and facial expression before and after drug administration. Appropriate interventions require judgment in timing, discontinuing medicine if required, and taking steps to counteract adverse reactions, as well as knowing what and when to report to the physician. Evaluation and documentation of results also play a vital role for all health care providers, including the physician, in planning effective drug therapy.

The safe administration of medications necessitates training to develop skills in delivery of medications. The goal is to maximize the effectiveness of the drug with the least discomfort to the patient. Sensitivity to the unique needs of each patient is encouraged (e.g., awareness of difficulty swallowing or impaired movement that could affect administration of medications).

Patient education is an essential part of the safe administration of medicines. If the patient is to benefit from drug therapy, she must understand the importance of taking the medicine in the proper dosage, on time, and in the proper way. Information for patients should be in language they understand, with instruction both verbal and written, as well as demonstrations of techniques when indicated.

Administration of medication carries moral, ethical, and legal responsibilities. Some rules and regulations vary with the institution, agency, or office. When in doubt, consult those in authority—supervisors or administrators—and/or policy and procedure books. However, documentation on the patient's record is always required for all medicines given, as well as for patient education provided. In addition, controlled substances given must also be recorded in a narcotics record.

MEDICATION ERRORS

Medication errors can and do occur in all health care settings. More errors are reported from acute care settings, where the risk is greatest. However, outpatient facilities, ambulatory care sites, home health care, and long-term care facility practitioners have challenges unique to their practice as well. Patients in these settings often are older adults and likely to have several chronic conditions requiring multiple medications (see Chapter 28, Drugs and Older Adults). Increasing the number of medications an individual receives not only increases the risk of interactions and adverse side effects, but also increases the risk of error.

Meticulous care in preparation and administration of medications reduces the chances of error. However, if a mistake is made, it is of the utmost importance to **report it** immediately to the one in charge so that corrective action can be taken for the patient's welfare. The patient's record should reflect the corrective action taken for justification in case of legal proceedings. An incident report must also be completed as a legal requirement. Failure to report errors appropriately can jeopardize the patient's welfare, as well as increase the possibility of civil suits against the health care provider and/or the risk of loss of professional license or certificate. Honesty is not only the best policy, it is the *only* policy for moral, ethical, and legal reasons.

Health care practitioners have a responsibility to provide quality care and provide for patient safety at all times. Remember, *"First, do no harm."* This challenge includes prevention of medication errors and also **reporting** errors so that corrective steps can be taken. As part of this goal, the U.S. Pharmacopoeia (USP) has established a Medication Errors Reporting (MER) program. Confusion over the similarity of drug names, either written or spoken, accounts for approximately one-quarter of all reports to this agency. Therefore, the MER has published a USP Quality Review report, *Use Caution—Avoid Confusion,* listing many similar drug names that have led to medication errors. This list is reproduced in the Appendix for your convenience and reference.

PRINCIPLES OF ADMINISTRATION

When preparing to administer medications, several basic principles should always be kept in mind

1. *Cleanliness.* Essential to safe administration of medicines. Always wash hands before handling medicines, and be sure preparation area is clean and neat.

2. *Organization.* Necessary for safe administration of medicines. Always be sure medications and supplies are in the appropriate area and in adequate supply. When stock drugs are used, they should be reordered immediately.

3. *Preparation area.* Should be well lighted and away from distracting influences.

Guidelines to review before giving medicines are called the six **Rights of Medication Administration** (Figure 7-1):

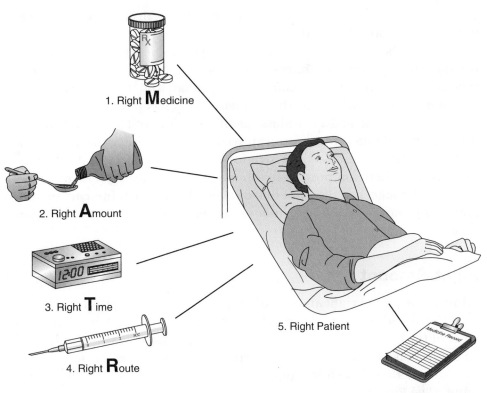

1. Right **M**edicine

2. Right **A**mount

3. Right **T**ime

4. Right **R**oute

5. Right Patient

6. Right Documentation

Figure 7-1 The six Rights of Medication Administration. Using the acronynm MATR, read down, saying, "It matters to the patient." Don't forget #6, the right documentation.

1. Right medication
2. Right amount
3. Right time
4. Right route
5. Right patient
6. Right documentation

Right Medication

You can confirm that you have the right medication by carefully comparing the name of the drug prescribed (on the physician's order sheet, prescription blank, medication record, or medicine card) with the label on the package, bottle, or unit-dose packet (medications with each dose separately sealed in an individual paper, foil, plastic, or glass container). *Never* give medication when the name of the medication is obscured in any way. Some drugs have names that sound or look similar (e.g., digoxin and digitoxin, or Inderal and Isuprel), and therefore it is essential to scrutinize every letter in the name when comparing the medicine ordered with the medicine on hand. Accuracy can be facilitated by placing the unit-dose packet next to the name of the drug ordered on the patient's record, while comparing the drug ordered with the drug on hand. (See Figure 8-2 in Chapter 8, Administration.)

If there is any question about the drug order because of handwriting, misspelling, inappropriateness, allergies, or interactions, you have the *right* and *responsibility to question* the physician and/or the pharmacist.

Never give medications that someone else has prepared. *Never* leave medications at the bedside unless specifically ordered by the doctor (e.g., nitroglycerin tablets and contraceptives are frequently ordered to be left with the patient for self-administration). If the patient is unable to take a medication when you present it, the medication must be returned (in an unopened packet) to the patient's drawer in the medicine cart or medicine room. Never open the unit-dose packet until the patient is prepared to take the medicine.

Right Amount

Administering the right amount of drug is extremely important. The drug dosage ordered must be compared *very carefully* with the dose listed on the label of the package, bottle, or unit-dose packet. Here again, accuracy can be facilitated by placing the unit-dose packet next to the written order on the patient's record while comparing the dose ordered with the dose on hand. (See Figure 8-2.)

The three different systems of measurement (household, apothecary, and metric) were discussed in Chapter 5. It is important to consult a table of equivalents (Table 5-4), if necessary, to convert from one system to another. Directions for calculation of different drug doses were presented in Chapter 6. Drug calculations are infrequent with unit-dose packaging. However, if it is necessary to compute calculations, such calculations must be checked by another trained health care worker, pharmacist, or doctor to verify accuracy. Be especially careful when the dose is expressed in decimals or fractions. Always recheck the dose if less than one tablet or more than one tablet is required, or with less than 1 ml or more than 1 ml for injection. An unusual dosage should alert you to the possibility of error. Those who administer medications have the right, as well as the responsibility, to question any dosage that is unusual or seems inappropriate for the individual patient. Remember that drug action is influenced by the condition of the patient, metabolism, age, weight, sex, and psychological state (see Chapter 3). The health care worker has the responsibility of reporting the results of careful assessment and observations in order to assist the physician in prescribing the right dosage for each patient.

Directions for measurement and preparation of the right dose are described in Chapters 8 and 9. An important part of the patient education includes complete instructions about the importance of preparing and taking the right amount of medicine prescribed by the physician.

Right Time

The time for administration of medications is an important part of the drug *dosage,* which includes the amount, frequency, and number of doses of medication to be administered. For maximum effectiveness, drugs must be given on a prescribed schedule. The physician's order specifies the number of times per day the medicine is to be administered (e.g., bid, or twice a day). Some medications need to be maintained at a specific level in the blood and are therefore prescribed at regular intervals around the clock (e.g., q4h, or every 4 hours). Some medications, such as some antibiotics, are more effective on an empty stomach and are therefore prescribed ac (before meals). Medications that are irritating to the stomach are ordered pc (after meals). Drugs that cause sedation are more frequently prescribed at hour of sleep. If the physician does not prescribe a specific time for administration of a drug, the health care worker arranges an appropriate schedule, taking into consideration the purpose, action, and side effects of the medication. Patient education includes instruction about the right time to take specific medicines and why.

Right Route

The route of administration is important because of its effect on degree of absorption, speed of drug action, and side effects. Many drugs can be administered in a variety of ways (see Chapter 4). The physician's order specifies the route of administration. If no route is specified, the oral route is used unless conditions warrant otherwise (e.g., nausea, vomiting, or difficulty swallowing). Those administering medications have the right and responsibility to question the appropriateness of a route based on assessment and observation of the patient. Change of route may be indicated because of the patient's condition. However, the route of administration may not be changed without the physician's order.

Right Patient

The patient who is to receive the medication must be identified by use of certain techniques to reduce the chance of error. In health care facilities, the patient's wrist identification band should be checked *first,* and then the patient should be called by name or asked to state her name, *before* administering the medication. In the ambulatory care setting, the patient can be asked to give name and date of birth; this can be verified with the chart before administering medications. If the patient questions the medication or the dosage, recheck the order and the medicine before giving it.

Right Documentation

Another essential duty is **documentation**. Every medication given must be recorded on the patient's record, along with *dose, time, route,* and *location* of injections. If the medication is given on a PRN (as necessary) basis (e.g., for pain), notation should also be made on the patient's record of the effectiveness of the medication. The person administering the medication must also sign or initial the record after administration (the policy of each facility determines the exact procedure to be followed). The accuracy of medication documentation is a very important legal responsibility. At times, patients' records are examined in court, and the accuracy of medication documentation can be a critical factor in some legal judgments.

Documentation also includes the recording of narcotics administered on the special controlled substances record kept with the narcotics. If narcotics are destroyed because of partial dosage, cancellation, or error, two health care workers must sign as witnesses of the disposal of the drug (the policy about documentation of narcotics may vary with the agency).

In summary, safe and effective administration of medications involves current drug information; technical and evaluation skills; and moral, ethical, and legal responsibilities. Guidelines include the six Rights of Medication Administration. In addition, the health care worker has the right and responsibility to question any medication order that is confusing or illegible or that seems inappropriate, and the right to refuse to administer any medication that is not in the best interests of the patient. The welfare of the patient is the primary concern in administration of medications.

Med Watch

The Food and Drug Administration (FDA) issued a form in 1993 to assist health care professionals in reporting serious, adverse events or product quality problems associated with medications, medical devices, or nutritional products regulated by the FDA, for example, dietary supplements or infant formulas. Even the large, well-designed clinical trials that precede FDA approval cannot uncover every problem that can come to light once a product is widely used. Or a drug could interact with other drugs in ways not revealed during clinical trials. Reports by health care professionals can help ensure the safety of drugs and other products regulated by the FDA.

In response to these voluntary reports from the health care community, the FDA has issued warnings, made labeling changes, required manufacturers to do postmarketing studies, and ordered the withdrawal of certain products from the market. Such actions can prevent injuries, suffering, disabilities, congenital deformities, and even deaths.

You are not expected to establish a connection or even wait until the evidence seems overwhelming. The agency's regulations will protect your identity and the identities of your patient and your facility. With your cooperation, MED WATCH can help the FDA better monitor product safety and, when necessary, take swift action to protect your patients and you. MED WATCH encourages you to regard voluntary reporting as part of your professional responsibility. See Figure 7-2 for a MED WATCH form, which can be reproduced, and for instructions for completing and submitting this form to the FDA.

ADVICE ABOUT VOLUNTARY REPORTING

Report experiences with:
- medications (drugs or biologics)
- medical devices (including in-vitro diagnostics)
- special nutritional products (dietary supplements, medical foods, infant formulas)
- other products regulated by FDA

Report SERIOUS adverse events. An event is serious when the patient outcome is:
- death
- life-threatening (real risk of dying)
- hospitalization (initial or prolonged)
- disability (significant, persistent or permanent)
- congenital anomaly
- required intervention to prevent permanent impairment or damage

Report even if:
- you're not certain the product caused the event
- you don't have all the details

Report product problems – quality, performance or safety concerns such as:
- suspected contamination
- questionable stability
- defective components
- poor packaging or labeling

How to report:
- just fill in the sections that apply to your report
- use section C for all products except medical devices
- attach additional blank pages if needed
- use a separate form for each patient
- report either to FDA or the manufacturer (or both)

Important numbers:
- 1-800-FDA-0178   to FAX report
- 1-800-FDA-7737   to report by modem
- 1-800-FDA-1088   for more information or to report quality problems
- 1-800-822-7967   for a VAERS form for vaccines

If your report involves a serious adverse event with a device and it occurred in a facility outside a doctor's office, that facility may be legally required to report to FDA and/or the manufacturer. Please notify the person in that facility who would handle such reporting.

Confidentiality: The patient's identity is held in strict confidence by FDA and protected to the fullest extent of the law. The reporter's identity may be shared with the manufacturer unless requested otherwise. However, FDA will not disclose the reporter's identity in response to a request from the public, pursuant to the Freedom of Information Act.

The public reporting burden for this collection of information has been estimated to average 30 minutes per response, including the time for reviewing instructions, searching existing data sources, gathering and maintaining the data needed, and completing and reviewing the collection of information. Send your comments regarding this burden estimate or any other aspect of this collection of information, including suggestions for reducing this burden to:

Reports Clearance Officer, PHS
Hubert H. Humphrey Building,
Room 721-B
200 Independence Avenue, S.W.
Washington, DC 20201
ATTN: PRA

and to:
Office of Management and Budget
Paperwork Reduction Project
(0910-0291)
Washington, DC 20503

Please do NOT return this form to either of these addresses.

U.S. DEPARTMENT OF HEALTH AND HUMAN SERVICES
Public Health Service • Food and Drug Administration

FDA Form 3500-back   **Please Use Address Provided Below – Just Fold In Thirds, Tape and Mail**

**Department of
Health and Human Services**

Public Health Service
Food and Drug Administration
Rockville, MD 20857

Official Business
Penalty for Private Use $300

NO POSTAGE
NECESSARY
IF MAILED
IN THE
UNITED STATES
OR APO/FPO

BUSINESS REPLY MAIL
FIRST CLASS MAIL   PERMIT NO. 946   ROCKVILLE, MD

POSTAGE WILL BE PAID BY FOOD AND DRUG ADMINISTRATION

MEDWATCH
**The FDA Medical Products Reporting Program
Food and Drug Administration
5600 Fishers Lane
Rockville, MD 20852-9787**

Figure 7-2 MED WATCH form. The FDA Medical Products Reporting Program for voluntary reporting by health professionals of adverse events and product problems.

MEDWATCH
THE FDA MEDICAL PRODUCTS REPORTING PROGRAM

For **VOLUNTARY** reporting
by health professionals of adverse
events and product problems

Page _____ of _____

Form Approved: OMB No. 0910-0291 Expires: 12/31/94
See OMB statement on reverse

FDA Use Only (EPHO)

Triage unit
sequence #

PLEASE TYPE OR USE BLACK INK

A. Patient information

1. Patient Identifier	2. Age at time of event: or _____ Date of birth:	3. Sex ☐ female ☐ male	4. Weight _____ lbs or _____ kgs
In confidence			

B. Adverse event or product problem

1. ☐ **Adverse event** and/or ☐ **Product problem** (e.g., defects/malfunctions)

2. **Outcomes attributed to adverse event** (check all that apply)

☐ death _____ (mo/day/yr)
☐ life-threatening
☐ hospitalization -- initial or prolonged

☐ disability
☐ congenital anomaly
☐ required intervention to prevent permanent impairment/damage
☐ other: _____

3. Date of event (mo/day/yr)	4. Date of this report (mo/day/yr)

5. **Describe event or problem**

6. **Relevant tests/laboratory data,** including dates

7. **Other relevant history, including preexisting medical conditions** (e.g., allergies, race, pregnancy, smoking and alcohol use, hepatic/renal dysfunction, etc.)

C. Suspect medication(s)

1. **Name** (give labeled strength & mfr/labeler, if known)

#1 _____

#2 _____

2. **Dose, frequency & route used**	3. **Therapy dates** (if unknown, give duration) from/to (or best estimate)
#1	#1
#2	#2

4. **Diagnosis for use** (indication)	5. **Event abated after use stopped or dose reduced**
#1	#1 ☐ yes ☐ no ☐ doesn't apply
#2	#2 ☐ yes ☐ no ☐ doesn't apply

6. **Lot #** (if known)	7. **Exp. date** (if known)	8. **Event reappeared after reintroduction**
#1	#1	#1 ☐ yes ☐ no ☐ doesn't apply
#2	#2	#2 ☐ yes ☐ no ☐ doesn't apply

9. **NDC #** (for product problems only)
_____ - _____ - _____

10. **Concomitant medical products** and therapy dates (exclude treatment of event)

D. Suspect medical device

1. **Brand name**

2. **Type of device**

3. **Manufacturer name & address**	4. **Operator of device** ☐ health professional ☐ lay user/patient ☐ other: _____
6. model # _____ catalog # _____ serial # _____ lot # _____ other # _____	5. **Expiration date** (mo/day/yr)
	7. **If implanted, give date** (mo/day/yr)
	8. **If explanted, give date** (mo/day/yr)

9. **Device available for evaluation?** (Do not send to FDA)
☐ yes ☐ no ☐ returned to manufacturer on _____ (mo/day/yr)

10. **Concomitant medical products** and therapy dates (exclude treatment of event)

E. Reporter (see confidentiality section on back)

1. **Name, address & phone #**

2. **Health professional?** ☐ yes ☐ no	3. **Occupation**	4. **Also reported to** ☐ manufacturer ☐ user facility ☐ distributor

5. **If you do NOT want your identity disclosed to the manufacturer, place an "X" in this box.** ☐

Mail to: MEDWATCH
5600 Fishers Lane
Rockville, MD 20852-9787

or FAX to:
1-800-FDA-0178

FDA Form 3500

Submission of a report does not constitute an admission that medical personnel or the product caused or contributed to the event.

Figure 7-2 continued

CHAPTER REVIEW QUIZ

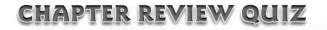

Complete the statements by filling in the blanks.

1. Before administering any medication, you should have the following information about the drug:

   _____

   _____

   _____

   _____

2. Before administering any medication, you should have the following three pieces of information about the patient:

   _____   _____

   other _____

3. Assessment of the patient's need for pain medication and reactions to drugs includes observation of the following four signs:

   _____

   _____

   _____

   _____

4. Patient education about medication should include the following four pieces of information:

   _____

   _____

   _____

   _____

5. When administering a controlled substance, documentation is necessary in two places:

   _____

   _____

6. Documentation of an injection given for pain should include the following five pieces of information:

_____

_____

_____

_____

_____

7. Name the six Rights of Drug Administration:

_____

_____

_____

_____

_____

_____

8. Medication errors must be reported immediately, and documentation includes recording the information in the following two areas:

_____

_____

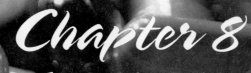

Chapter 8
Administration by the Gastrointestinal Route

Key Terms

Dysphagia

Gastric tube administration

Nasogastric tube administration

Oral medication administration

Rectal medication

Objectives

Upon completion of this chapter, the learner should be able to

1. Describe the advantages and disadvantages of administering medications orally, by nasogastric or gastrostomy tube, and rectally

2. Explain appropriate action when patient is NPO, has dysphagia, refuses medication, vomits medication, or has allergies

3. List special precautions in preparation of timed-release capsules, enteric-coated tablets, and oral suspensions

4. Demonstrate measurement of liquid medications with medicine cup and syringe

5. Demonstrate proficiency in administering medications orally, by nasogastric or gastric tube, and rectally

6. Satisfactorily complete all of the activities listed on the checklists

7. Define the Key Terms

Medications are administered by the gastrointestinal route more often than any other way. Gastrointestinal administration includes four categories: oral, nasogastric tube, gastric tube, and rectal.

*Advantages of the **oral route** include:*

- Convenience and patient comfort

- Safety, because medication can be retrieved in case of error or intentional overdose

- Economy, because there are few equipment costs

Disadvantages of the oral route include:

- Slower onset of absorption and action
- Rate and degree of absorption that vary with gastrointestinal contents and motility
- Some drugs (e.g., insulin and heparin) destroyed by digestive fluids and must be administered by injection
- Cannot be used with nausea or vomiting
- Dangerous to use if patient has difficulty swallowing (**dysphagia**), because of possible aspiration
- Cannot be used for unconscious patients
- Cannot be used if patient is NPO (e.g., before surgery or while fasting for a laboratory test or X-ray examination)

Administration of medications by nasogastric tube is sometimes ordered when the patient is unable to swallow for prolonged periods of time because of illness, trauma, surgery, or unconsciousness. Medications are usually administered intravenously when these conditions exist for short periods of time.

*Advantages of the **nasogastric tube*** include:

- Ability to bypass the mouth and pharynx when necessary
- Elimination of numerous injections

The *disadvantage of the nasogastric tube* with a conscious patient is the discomfort of the tube in the nose and throat for prolonged periods of time.

When a patient is unable to take nourishment by mouth for a very extended period of time, the surgeon will sometimes insert a *gastric tube* through the skin of the abdomen, directly into the stomach. This G-tube, or peg tube, as it is sometimes called, is secured in place and can remain there for feeding purposes indefinitely. Medication can be administered via the G-tube, directly into the stomach.

Medications are sometimes administered by the rectal route when nausea or vomiting is present, or the patient is unconscious or unable to swallow. *Advantages of the **rectal route*** include:

- Bypassing the action of digestive enzymes
- Avoidance of irritation to the upper GI tract
- Usefulness with dysphagia

Disadvantages of the rectal route include:

- Many medications are unavailable in suppository form
- Some patients have difficulty retaining suppositories (e.g., older adults and children)
- Prolonged use of some rectal suppositories can cause rectal irritation (e.g., aminophylline)
- Absorption may be irregular or incomplete if feces are present

ADMINISTRATION OF MEDICATIONS ORALLY
Guidelines for Oral Medications Administration

1. Wash your hands (Figure 8-1).

2. Locate appropriate medication sheet and check for completeness of the order (i.e., date, patient's name, medication name, dosage, route, and time).

3. Check for special circumstances (e.g., allergies or NPO).

4. Be sure that you know the purpose of the drug, possible side effects, contraindications, cautions, interactions, and normal dosage range. If unfamiliar with the drug, consult a reference book for this information.

5. Select appropriate receptacle in which to place medication (i.e., paper medicine cup for tablets or capsules and plastic medicine cup for liquids).

6. Locate medication in medication cupboard or medication cart drawer and compare the label against the medication sheet for the five Rights of Medication Administration: right medicine, right amount, right time, right route, and right patient (Figure 8-2).

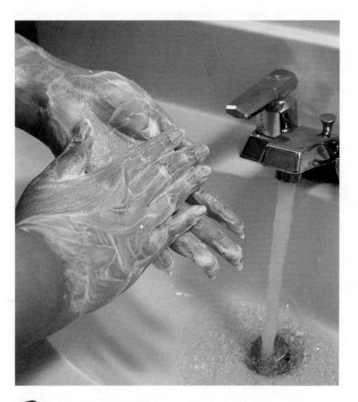

Figure 8-1 Medical asepsis handwash.

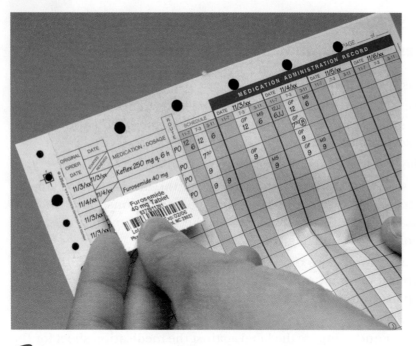

Figure 8-2 Compare name and dosage on medication package with the Medication. Administration Record.

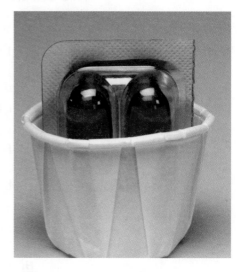

Figure 8-3 Keep the unit-dose packet intact until you are with the patient.

7. If the dose ordered differs from the dose on hand, complete calculations on paper and check for accuracy with instructor or coworker in clinical setting.

8. Prepare the dosage as ordered. Do not open unit-dose packages until you are with the patient (Figure 8-3). If medication is liquid, see "Preparation of Liquid Medications" later in this section.

9. Take medication in cup to patient and place it on table nearby.

10. Check patient's identification bracelet (Figure 8-4). Ask the patient to *tell you* his name and date of birth (DOB). Compare this information with the medication record to verify that you have the right patient.

11. Call patient by name and explain what you are doing. Answer any questions. Recheck medication order if patient expresses any doubts. Use this opportunity for patient education about the medication.

12. Monitor patient's vital signs if required for specific medication (e.g., blood pressure, apical pulse, or respiration). Blood pressure should always be taken and recorded *before* administering antihypertensives.

13. Open unit-dose package and place container in the patient's hand. Avoid touching the medication (Figure 8-5).

14. Provide full glass of water and assist the patient as necessary (e.g., raise the head of the bed and provide drinking straw if required).

15. Stay with the patient until the medication has been swallowed. Make the patient comfortable before you leave the room.

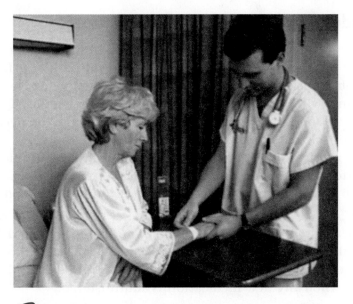

Figure 8-4 Check identification to be sure it is the right patient. Also ask the patient for name and date of birth and verify with the Medication Record. Always check for allergies.

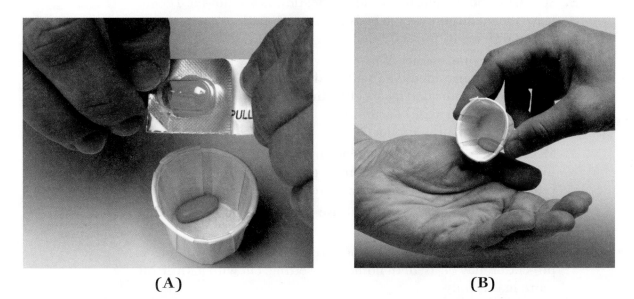

(A)   **(B)**

Figure 8-5 Do not touch medicine. (A) Open the unit-dose packet and drop the tablet in a cup. (B) Place the cup containing the medicine in the patient's hand.

16. Discard used medicine cup and wrappers in wastebasket.

17. Record the medication, dosage, time, and your signature or initials in the correct place on patient's record according to rules of the facility. ("Documentation, sixth right.")

18. Document on patient's record and report if a medication is withheld or refused and the reason. Record *and report* any unusual circumstances associated with administration or any adverse side effects.

Special Considerations for Oral Administration

1. If patient is NPO, check with the person in charge regarding appropriate procedure, based on reason for NPO. If patient is fasting for laboratory X-ray tests, medication can usually be given at a later time with possible modification of time schedule. If patient is NPO for surgery, nausea, or dysphagia, it may be necessary to consult the doctor regarding a change of route. Do not omit the medications completely without specific instructions to that effect. Abrupt withdrawal of some medications, for example, phenytoin (Dilantin) or diazepam (Valium), may lead to seizures.

2. *Always check the patient's record carefully for allergies* and be aware of the components of combination products. Patients with a history of allergy should be watched carefully for possible drug reactions when any new medication is administered.

3. Give the most important medicine first, e.g., cardiac medicine before vitamin.

4. Elevate the patient's head, if not contraindicated by the patient's condition, to aid in swallowing.

5. Stay with the patient until the medication is swallowed. *Do not* leave the medication at the bedside or in the patient's possession unless ordered by physician.

6. Administer oral medications with water, unless ordered otherwise. *Do not* give medicine with fruit juice, milk, or any other liquid unless indicated by specific directions. The absorption of many medicines (e.g., antibiotics) is inhibited by interaction with acid or alkaline products.

7. Medications whose action depends on contact with the mucous membranes of the mouth or throat (e.g., topical anesthetics or fungicides) *should not* be administered with any fluid or food.

8. *Do not* open or crush timed-release capsules or enteric-coated tablets.

9. If tablets must be divided, *do not* break by hand. If available, a pill-cutter may be used. In home care setting, cut with a knife on score marks only.

10. When removing tablets or capsules from a stock bottle, pour into lid and from there into medicine cup. *Do not* touch tablets or capsules.

11. *Do not* administer any medication that is discolored, has precipitated, is contaminated, or is outdated.

12. If a patient is NPO, refuses the medication, or vomits within 20–30 min of taking the medication, always report this to the person in charge. A written order from the physician is required to change either the medication or the route of administration. Document on the patient's record the time of emesis and appearance of the emesis, for example, medication remained intact.

13. If the patient refuses a medication, determine the reason. Report the refusal and reason to the person in charge and record all information on patient's record.

14. Tablets (unless enteric coated) may be crushed with mortar and pestle or pill-crusher. Capsules (except timed-release capsules) may be opened and the contents mixed with applesauce or ice cream to facilitate administration for patients with difficulty swallowing (e.g., children and the elderly). Check diet to be sure these foods are allowed. Be sure that any equipment used to crush medication is wiped clean.

Note: In some areas a physician's order is required for pill-crushing. If available, ask for the medication to be ordered in liquid or powdered form.

Preparation of Liquid Medications

Follow the "Guidelines for Administration of Oral Medications," at the beginning of this section. Preparation of *liquid medications* requires these additional steps:

1. Shake bottle if indicated. Remove cap and place cap upside down on table.

2. Hold medicine bottle with label side upward to prevent smearing of label while pouring (Figure 8-6).

3. In other hand, hold medicine cup at eye level and place thumbnail on level to which medication will be poured (Figure 8-6).

4. While holding the medicine cup straight at eye level, pour the prescribed amount of medication.

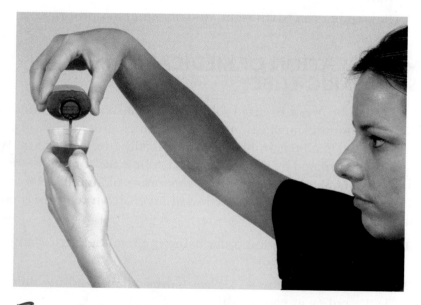

Figure 8-6 Hold the medicine bottle with label side up and medicine cup at eye level, with thumbnail marking measurement.
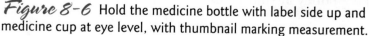

5. Replace cap on bottle.

6. Compare the information on the medication sheet against the label on the stock bottle and the quantity of drug in the cup.

7. Replace medication bottle in cupboard or medicine cart.

8. Recheck the five Rights of Medication Administration.*

9. Proceed with the "Guidelines for Administration of Oral Medications."

When administering liquid medication to someone who is unable to drink from a cup (e.g., infants and persons with wired jaws), a syringe may be used. Follow the "Guidelines for Administration of Oral Medications." Administration of *liquid medications orally via syringe* requires these additional steps:

1. Pour prescribed medication into medicine cup.

2. Withdraw prescribed amount with syringe.

3. Check medication and order using the five Rights of Medication Administration.

4. Identify the patient, verify name and DOB, and elevate the patient's head.

5. Be sure the patient is alert and able to swallow.

6. Place the syringe tip in the pocket between the cheek and the gums. (When administering large amounts of liquid via syringe, it helps to fit a 2-inch length of latex tubing on the syringe tip to facilitate instillation of the medication into the cheek pocket.)

7. Instill the medication slowly to lessen chances of aspiration.

8. Be sure all medication is swallowed before leaving the patient.

9. Proceed with "Guidelines for the Administration of Oral Medications."

10. Remember the "sixth right" and document appropriately.

ADMINISTRATION OF MEDICATIONS BY NASOGASTRIC TUBE

A nasogastric tube is not inserted solely for the purpose of administering medication. However, medications are sometimes ordered by this route when a nasogastric tube is in place for tube feeding or for suction. When medications are ordered by nasogastric tube, follow the "Guidelines for Administration of Oral Medications" and "Preparation of Liquid Medications."

Nasogastric tube administration of medication requires these additional steps:

1. Check the medication order using the five Rights of Medication Administration.

2. Wash hands (Figure 8-1). Wear gloves when handling tubes, if it is the policy at your facility.

---

*Remember the "sixth right" and document appropriately.

3. Prepare the medication as ordered and take to the patient's room. Be sure the medication is at room temperature.

4. Check identification bracelet, ask the patient his name and verify, and explain the procedure. Elevate head of bed, if not contraindicated.

5. Hold the end of the tube up and remove the clamp, plug, or adapter.

6. Make sure that the tube is properly placed in the stomach by using at least two tests (Figure 8-7).

   a. Aspirate with bulb or piston syringe for stomach contents and check the pH of the aspirated fluids. The pH of gastric juice is acid (0.9–1.5). If the aspirate does not meet these parameters or if there is any question, do *not* instill any liquids. Instead, report to the person in charge. If the criteria are met, flush the tube with normal saline solution or with water.

   b. Place a stethoscope over the patient's stomach, attach the syringe to the tube, and inject about 15 ml of air. If you hear a swooshing sound, air has entered the stomach, verifying correct placement.

7. Clamp the tube with your fingers by bending it over upon itself or by pinching it. While tube is closed, remove plunger or bulb from syringe, leaving syringe attached firmly to tubing (Figure 8-8).

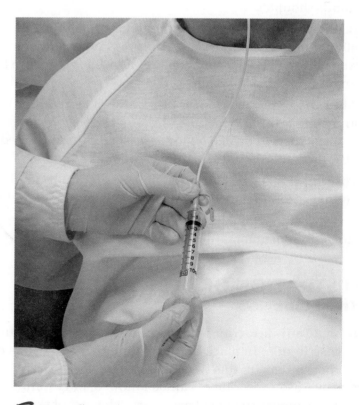

Figure 8-7 Test for correct placement of nasogastric tube. Aspirate with syringe and check the pH of aspirated fluids.

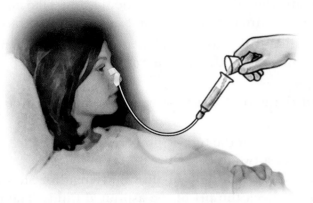

Figure 8-8 Pinch tube shut before filling syringe. Let fluid flow in by gravity. Hold syringe at level of patient's shoulder. Flush tube with water.

8. Pour medication into syringe. Release or unclamp the tubing and let medication flow through by gravity. Never force fluids down a nasogastric tube (Figure 8-8). Watch the patient during the procedure and stop immediately at any sign of discomfort, coughing, or shortness of breath by pinching the tube. Holding the syringe too high causes fluid to run in too quickly, possibly causing nausea and vomiting. Syringe should be at level of patient's shoulder.

9. Before the syringe empties completely, flush the tube by adding 60–100 ml of water, to the syringe or amount ordered, If the patient's input and output are being monitored, be sure to add this amount to the patient's record.

10. After the water has run in, pinch the tube, remove the syringe, and clamp or plug the tube. If the patient is on suction, be sure to leave suction turned *off* for at least 30 min until medication is absorbed, then restart suction as ordered.

11. Position patient on right side and/or elevate head of bed to encourage the stomach to empty. Make the patient comfortable.

12. Proceed with "Guidelines for the Administration of Oral Medications" for documentation.

ADMINISTRATION OF MEDICATIONS BY GASTRIC TUBE

Gastric tube administration of medications is a simple matter. If a patient has a **gastric tube** in place in the abdomen, medications can be administered per order in this way. Directions for "Administration of Medications by Nasogastric Tube" can be followed, only omitting number 6. No test for placement of tube is necessary. The rest of the directions regarding flushing the tube afterward and positioning the patient, and so on, should be followed carefully. Remember to document appropriately.

ADMINISTRATION OF MEDICATIONS RECTALLY

Medications are sometimes ordered to be administered by rectal route. The **rectal medication** may be in suppository form or in liquid form to be administered as a retention enema. This treatment is more effective with the patient's cooperation. Tact and consideration are required for successful administration of rectal medications. Remember to respect the patient's dignity and privacy by closing the door and curtains completely. Do not expose the patient unnecessarily.

The retention enema is administered in the same way as a cleansing enema. However, the retention enema must be retained approximately 30 min or more for absorption of the medication. Therefore, the patient is instructed to lie quietly on either side to aid in retention. If the patient is uncooperative, unconscious, or has poor sphincter control, the buttocks can be taped together with 2-inch paper adhesive for 30 min. Do not use this method unless absolutely necessary. Remember to treat the patient with dignity. Always explain everything you are doing and why. Even if patients are unconscious or unable to speak, they may be able to hear and cooperate in some way if they understand.

Administration of Rectal Suppository

1. Wash hands (Figure 8-1).
2. Check the medication order using the five rights of Medication Administration.
3. Identify medication (purpose, side effects, contraindications, cautions, and normal dose range). Research information if necessary.
4. Assemble supplies: disposable glove and water-soluble lubricant.
5. Select the medication as ordered, checking medication name and dosage again. Some suppositories are stored in a refrigerator, and some may be stored at room temperature, according to manufacturer's instructions.
6. Check patient's identification bracelet, ask patient for name and DOB and explain the procedure. Answer any questions.
7. Close door and curtain completely.
8. Lower the head of the bed if necessary and position the patient on left side with upper knee bent. Keep patient covered, exposing only the rectal area (Figure 8-9).
9. Put on disposable glove.
10. Remove suppository from wrapper and lubricate the tapered end with water-soluble lubricant.
11. With ungloved hand, separate the patient's buttocks gently so you can see anus.
12. Ask patient to take a deep breath. Insert the lubricated suppository gently into the rectum and push gently with gloved index finger until the suppository has passed the internal sphincter (Figure 8-10). With infants, use gloved *little* finger.

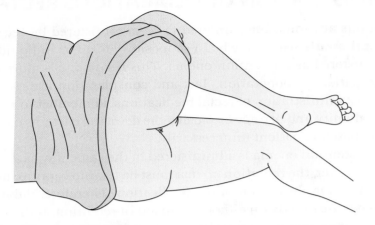

Figure 8-9 Drape and position patient on side with upper knee bent.

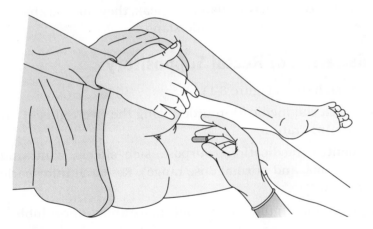

Figure 8-10 Lubricate the tip of suppository and insert it with covered index finger. Push the suppository past the sphincter.

13. Urge the patient to retain the suppository for at least 20 min. If patient is unable to cooperate, hold the buttocks together as required.

14. Remove and dispose of glove, turning it inside out as you remove it.

15. Be sure the patient is comfortable, with covers and bed adjusted appropriately.

16. Wash hands.

17. Record the medication in the appropriate place (the sixth right).

CHAPTER REVIEW QUIZ

1. Name six disadvantages of oral administration compared with administration by injection.

_____

_____

_____

_____

_____

_____

Match the column on left with the appropriate action on the right. Actions may be used more than once.

2. _____	To facilitate swallowing	**a.** Watch closely for drug reactions
3. _____	If NPO for laboratory tests	**b.** Crush tablet, mix with applesauce
4. _____	Patient vomits 15 min after medication	**c.** Administer first
		d. Cannot be opened
5. _____	Most medications	**e.** Elevate patient's head
6. _____	Patient is allergic to penicillin	**f.** Notify person in charge
7. _____	Most important medicine	**g.** Modify schedule, give medicine later
8. _____	Tablet cannot be swallowed	
9. _____	Timed-release capsules	**h.** Administer with water
10. _____	Dilantin ordered PO, patient NPO for surgery	**i.** Leave medication at bedside

Complete the following statements by filling in the blanks.

When pouring liquid medicine:

11. The bottle should be held _____.

12. The medicine cup should be held _____.

13. The bottle cap should be placed _____.

14. If medication is in suspension, the bottle should first be _____.

When administering medication by nasogastric tube:

15. Check tube placement first with two tests:

_____

_____

Check the appropriate answer.

16. _____ **a.** Medication should be pushed through the nasogastric tube by pressure on barrel of syringe.

_____ **b.** Medication should flow through the nasogastric tube by gravity.

17. _____ **a.** Medication should be cold.

_____ **b.** Medication should be at room temperature.

18. _____ **a.** Patient's head should be elevated.

_____ **b.** Patient should be placed in Trendelenburg position.

19. Name four steps in administration of a rectal suppository that are different from PO administration.

_____

_____

_____

_____

20. Medication documentation should include:

_____

_____

_____

_____

Checklist for Administration of Oral Medications

Activity	Rating S	U
1. Washed hands	___	___
2. Checked medication sheet for date, dosage, time, route, and allergies	___	___
3. Identified medication: purpose, side effects, contraindications, cautions, interaction, and normal dosage range	___	___
4. Selected appropriate medicine cup	___	___
5. Selected correct medication and checked label against medication sheet for five Rights of Medication Administration	___	___
6. Calculated correct dosage on paper if necessary and verified calculations with instructor	___	___
7. Placed medication as ordered in cup without opening packet or touching medication; prepared liquid medication by shaking if necessary, pouring away from label and measuring at eye level	___	___
8. Identified patient by checking bracelet and asking patient for name and DOB	___	___
9. Explained procedure to patient and answered any questions about medication	___	___
10. Checked patient's vital signs if necessary for specific medicine	___	___
11. Opened unit-dose packages and offered medication in container to patient	___	___
12. Provided drinking water and assisted patient as necessary	___	___
13. Made patient comfortable and left unit in order	___	___
14. Recorded medication, dosage, time, and signature or initials on patient's record (the sixth right)	___	___

Note: S, satisfactory; U, unsatisfactory.

Checklist for Administration of Rectal Suppository

Activity	Rating S	U
1. Washed hands	___	___
2. Checked the medication order for date, dosage, time, route, and allergies	___	___
3. Identified medication: purpose, side effects, contraindications, cautions, and normal dosage range	___	___
4. Assembled supplies: glove and lubricant	___	___
5. Selected correct medication and checked label with medication order for five Rights of Medication Administration	___	___
6. Identified patient by checking bracelet and asking patient for name and DOB	___	___
7. Explained procedure to patient and answered any questions about medication	___	___
8. Closed door and curtain	___	___
9. Positioned patient on left side with upper knee bent and only rectal area exposed	___	___
10. Put on disposable glove	___	___
11. Removed wrapping from suppository and lubricated tapered end	___	___
12. With ungloved hand, separated buttocks gently	___	___
13. Instructed patient to take a deep breath and inserted suppository gently, pushing it past the sphincter	___	___
14. Instructed patient about retaining the suppository	___	___
15. Removed glove correctly and disposed of it appropriately	___	___
16. Made patient comfortable and left unit in order	___	___
17. Washed hands.	___	___
18. Recorded medication, dosage, time, and signature or initials on patient's record	___	___

Note: S, satisfactory; U, unsatisfactory

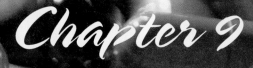

Chapter 9
Administration by the Parenteral Route

Objectives

Upon completion of this chapter, the learner should be able to

1. Define the Key Terms
2. Name four parenteral routes with systemic effects
3. Explain administration via the sublingual and buccal routes, including instructions to the patient
4. Demonstrate application of nitroglycerin ointment and the transdermal patch
5. Identify three conditions treated with transcutaneous delivery systems
6. Compare and contrast advantages and disadvantages of inhalation therapy
7. Describe patient education for those receiving inhalation therapy with hand-held nebulizers
8. List cautions when administering IPPB therapy
9. Identify the three parts of the syringe and the three parts of the needle
10. Select appropriate-length and correct-gauge needles for various types of injections
11. List three types of syringes and a purpose for each
12. Demonstrate drawing up medications from a vial and an ampule
13. Describe and demonstrate an intradermal injection
14. Describe and demonstrate a subcutaneous injection
15. Describe five sites for intramuscular injection and demonstrate intramuscular injection

Key Terms

Inhalation therapy

Intradermal

Intramuscular

Local

Parenteral

Subcutaneous

Systemic

Topical

Transcutaneous

16. Give purpose and demonstration of Z-track injection
17. List four types of administration for local effects

Parenteral routes include any route other than the gastrointestinal tract. The most common form of parenteral administration is injection. However, other routes must be considered as well: the skin, mucous membranes, eyes, ears, and respiratory tract.

Parenteral administration can be understood more easily if the *purpose* of administration or the effects desired are considered as two categories: systemic and local. **Systemic** effects are those affecting the body as a whole, the entire system. The goal of administering drugs for systemic effects is to distribute the medication through the circulatory system to the area requiring treatment. Parenteral routes with systemic effects include (1) sublingual or buccal, (2) transcutaneous (transdermal), (3) inhalations, and (4) injections.

Local effects are those limited to one particular part (location) of the body, with very little, if any, effect on the rest of the body. Medications in this category include:

1. Medications applied to the skin for skin conditions, sometimes called **topical** medications
2. Drugs applied to the mucous membranes to treat that specific tissue
3. Medication instilled in the eyes
4. Medication instilled in the ears

SUBLINGUAL AND BUCCAL ADMINISTRATION

With sublingual administration, the medication is placed under the tongue. The drug is absorbed directly into the circulation through the numerous blood vessels located in the mucosa of this area. With buccal administration, the medication is placed in the pouch between the cheek and the gum at the back of the mouth. The sublingual route is used more commonly than the buccal. Medications absorbed in this way are unaffected by the stomach, intestines, or liver. Absorption via this route is quite rapid, and therefore this method is used frequently when quick response is required (e.g., with nitroglycerin to treat acute angina pectoris). The constricted coronary blood vessels are usually dilated within a few minutes, bringing quick relief from pain.

Patient Education

For the sublingual or buccal route, include the following instructions:

1. Hold the tablet in place with mouth closed until medication is absorbed.
2. Do not swallow the medication.
3. Do not drink or take food until medication is completely absorbed.

TRANSCUTANEOUS DRUG DELIVERY SYSTEM

Transcutaneous, or transdermal, systems deliver the medication to the body by absorption through the skin. Nitroglycerin ointment, for example, is applied to the skin in prescribed amounts every few hours for prevention of angina pectoris. The absorption is slower, and therefore this method is not effective in the treatment of acute angina attacks. Other transcutaneous delivery systems utilize a patch impregnated with a particular medication, applied to the skin, and left in place for continuous absorption. Examples of transcutaneous drug delivery systems include nitroglycerin (Transderm-Nitro), in which the patch is sometimes left in place for 24 h in prophylactic treatment of chronic angina; scopolamine (Transderm-Scop), in which the patch is placed behind the ear and left in place up to 72 h, as necessary, to prevent motion sickness; and fentanyl (Duragesic), applied every 72 h in the management of chronic pain in patients requiring opiate analgesia. (See Analgesics, Chapter 19.) There are also other medications delivered transdermally, for example, Estrogen (Estraderm). Absorption by this method is slower, but the action is more prolonged than with other methods of administration.

Note: To reduce the occurrence of headaches, sometimes the physician will order the nitroglycerin ointment or the Transderm-Nitro patch to be applied at bedtime and removed the next day at noon.

Patient Education

For those applying transcutaneous systems of administration, include the following instructions. With nitroglycerin ointment (Figure 9-1):

1. Squeeze the prescribed amount of ointment onto Appli-Ruler paper. When the ointment reaches the correct marking, give the tube a slight twist to cut off the ointment and recap the tube.

2. *Do not* touch the ointment! Absorption of ointment through the skin of the fingers can cause a severe headache.

3. Carefully fold the Appli-Ruler paper lengthwise with the ointment inside.

4. Flatten the folded paper carefully to spread the ointment inside. *Do not* allow the ointment to reach the edges of the paper. Keep paper folded.

5. Rotate sites for application. Appropriate areas include chest, back, upper arms, and upper legs. *Do not* shave the area. Be sure the area is clean, dry, and free of irritation, rash, and abrasion.

6. After the area for application is exposed, open the paper carefully and apply paper to the skin, ointment side down. *Do not*

touch ointment. Fasten paper in place with paper tape. Write the date and time on the tape.

7. Remove previous paper carefully, without touching the inside, and discard in trash container. Cleanse area and inspect skin for any sign of irritation. Report and record any skin changes.

8. Wash hands immediately.

9. Report and record any skin changes or complaints of headache.

With transdermal sealed drug delivery systems (Figure 9-2):

1. Select site for administration, rotating areas. Be sure the skin is clean, dry, and free of irritation.

2. Open the packet carefully, pulling the two sides apart *without touching the inside.*

3. Apply the side containing the medication to the skin. Press the adhesive edges down firmly all around. If for any reason the adhesive edges do not stick, fasten in place with paper tape. This is usually unnecessary. Write date and time on patch.

4. Remove previous patch carefully, without touching the inside, and discard in trash container. Cleanse area and inspect skin for irritation.

5. Wash hands immediately.

INHALATION THERAPY

Medications are frequently administered by inhalation method, especially to those with chronic pulmonary conditions, such as asthma. Patients may self-administer the medication with a metered dose inhaler (MDI) or small-volume aerosol nebulizer (Figure 9-3), or the physician may prescribe intermittent positive pressure breathing (IPPB) therapy, to be administered by trained personnel.

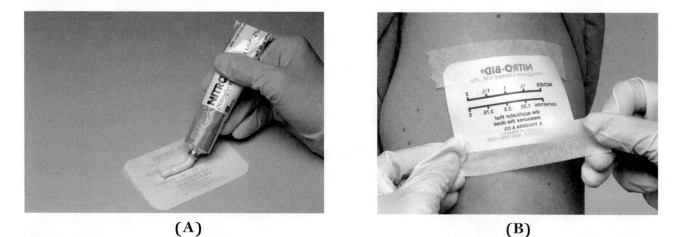

(A) **(B)**

Figure 9-1 Transdermal administration of nitroglycerin ointment. (A) Ointment is measured on Appli-Ruler paper. (B) Paper containing ointment is applied to the skin and fastened with paper tape. Write date and time on tape.

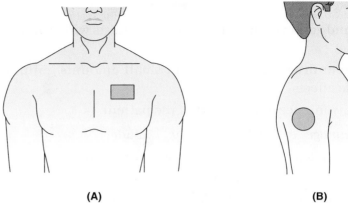
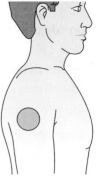

(A)   (B)

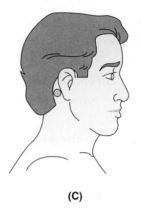

(C)

Figure 9-2 Transdermal drug delivery. Dermal patches vary in size and shape. (A,B) For prevention of angina pectoris. (C) For prevention of motion sickness. Other patches are also available for analgesia, estrogen replacement, and smoking cessation.

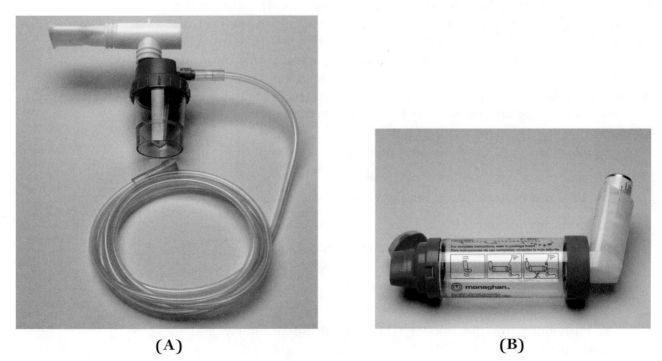

(A)   (B)

Figure 9-3 (A) Small-volume aerosol nebulizer. (B) Metered-dose inhaler (MDI) with spacer.

Advantages of **inhalation therapy** include:

1. Rapid action of the drug, with local effects within the respiratory tract

2. Potent drugs may be given in small amounts, minimizing the side effects

3. Convenience and comfort of the patient

Disadvantages of inhalation therapy include:

1. Requires cooperation of the patient in proper breathing techniques for effectiveness.

2. Adverse systemic side effects may result rapidly because of extensive absorption capacity of the lungs.

3. Improperly administered, or too frequently administered, inhalations can lead to irritation of the trachea or bronchi, or bronchospasm.

4. Asthmatic and COPD (chronic obstructive pulmonary disease) patients sometimes become dependent on a small-volume nebulizer or MDI.

5. If not cleaned properly, the small-volume nebulizer can be a source of infection.

Metered Dose Inhaler (MDI)

Metered dose inhalers (see Figure 9-3B) have become more popular in recent years. MDIs are portable and easy to use, and recently more drugs have become available in the inhaler form. Proper administration by the patient is essential for drug effectiveness. Older adult patients may have difficulty coordinating the depression of the canister and inhaling at the same time. A *spacer* may be added to act as a reservoir for the aerosol, allowing the patient to first depress the canister and then inhale. Many spacers have an audible horn or whistle to signal the patient if inspiration is too rapid. MDIs may be used in pediatric patients with a mouthpiece or a mask. A full MDI canister provides approximately 200 puffs of medication.

See Chapter 26: Bronchodilators for variations of the MDI.

Patient Education

How to Use a Metered Dose Inhaler (MDI)

1. Sit upright or stand.

2. Assemble inhaler and shake for 10 seconds.

3. Place the mouthpiece between the lips, forming a seal, or use a spacer prescribed by your physician.

4. Exhale slowly and completely.

5. Push down on the inhaler while breathing in slowly and deeply.

6. Hold your breath for at least 5–10 seconds.

7. Exhale slowly through pursed lips.

If your prescription is for more than 1 puff, rest for 1 or 2 min before the second dose.

Note: If a bronchodilator and an inhaled steroid medication are to be given at the same time, administer the bronchodilator first and then the steroid.

Important: If using an inhaled steroid (such as Azmacort, Aerobid, Beclovent, or Vanceril), rinse your mouth out with tap water after using the inhaler.

Small-Volume Nebulizers (MINI-NEBS, MED-NEBS)

Many drugs for the respiratory system may be delivered in aerosol form via a small-volume nebulizer. (see Figure 9-3A) The nebulizer is powered by a gas source, usually a small air compressor in the home care setting. For optimal drug deposition in the lung, proper breathing techniques must be used by the patient. The patient should be instructed to inhale slowly and deeply, perform a short breath, hold, and exhale slowly. In addition to the side effects of the drugs themselves (see Chapter 26), patients should be cautioned that dizziness may occur if they hyperventilate (breathing too rapidly). Proper cleaning of equipment on a daily basis is essential to avoid infection.

Patient Education

Proper Home Cleaning of Small-Volume Nebulizer

1. Disassemble the pieces of the nebulizer. Wash in mild soapy water and rinse thoroughly.
2. Place in a solution of one part vinegar to two parts water. Soak for 20–30 minutes.
3. Wash your hands with soap and water.
4. Remove the nebulizer parts from vinegar solution and rinse with warm tap water.
5. Allow to dry completely.
6. Reassemble pieces for next use.

Patient Education

With use of an inhaler or nebulizer, include the following instructions:

1. Name of the medication, dosage, and how often it is to be administered.
2. Desired effects and possible adverse side effects (e.g., palpitations, tremor, nervousness, dizziness, headache, nausea, dry mouth, irritated throat, hoarseness, or coughing).

3. Notify the physician if any adverse side effects occur or if the medication seems ineffective. The doctor may want to change the dosage or the medication.

4. Caution *not* to take any other medication, including over-the-counter drugs, without doctor's permission. Many drugs and alcohol can interact with these drugs, causing serious side effects.

5. Rising slowly from a reclining position will help prevent dizziness.

6. Rinsing the mouth after inhalation will counteract dry mouth or unpleasant taste.

7. Step-by-step demonstration with the patient, answering all questions.

8. Rinsing equipment after use and storage of medication as indicated on the package.

9. Importance of not smoking.

10. Importance of handwashing before treatments.

Intermittent Positive Pressure Breathing (IPPB)

Intermittent positive pressure breathing treatments may be ordered by the physician. IPPB combines administration of an aerosol with a mechanical breather to assist patients who are unable to take a deep breath on their own. Health care personnel, such as respiratory therapists or nurses, are specifically trained in the use of this equipment.

Cautions with IPPB therapy include:

1. Monitor vital signs closely, watching for a sudden drop in blood pressure, tachycardia, and decreased or shallow respirations.

2. Observe for nausea or distended abdomen.

3. Watch for tremors or dizziness.

4. Assure the patient that coughing after the treatment is to be expected. The goal of the treatment is to aid in coughing up the loosened secretions.

5. Record effectiveness of therapy and any side effects observed or reported by the patient.

INJECTIONS

To administer **injections,** you must be familiar with equipment.

Syringes

The syringe has three parts (Figure 9-4):

1. *Barrel.* The outer, hollow cylinder that holds the medication. It contains the calibrations for measuring the quantity of medication.

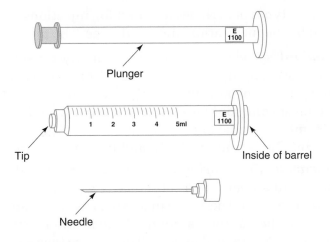

Figure 9-4 Parts of a syringe and needle that must remain sterile during preparation and administration of medication.

2. *Plunger.* The inner, solid rod that fits snugly into the cylinder. Pulling back on the plunger allows solution to be drawn into the syringe. Pushing forward on the plunger ejects solution or air from the syringe.

3. *Tip.* The portion that holds the needle. Most tips are plain. Some larger syringes contain a metal attachment at the tip, called a Luer-Lok, which locks the needle in place.

Most syringes are plastic and disposable after one use. Some syringes for special procedures are glass and must be resterilized after use.

Needles

The needle has three parts:

1. *Hub.* The flared end that fits on the tip of the syringe.

2. *Shaft.* The long, hollow tube embedded in the hub. Needles have shafts with different lengths. Shorter needles (½, ³⁄₈, and ⁵⁄₈ inches) are used for **intradermal** (into the skin) or **subcutaneous** (into the tissue just below the skin) injections. Longer needles (1½ and 2 inches) are used for **intramuscular** (into the muscle) injections. The length of the needle depends on the type of injection and the size of the patient (i.e., shorter needles for children and thin adults and longer needles for larger adults). The gauge is the size of the lumen, or hole, through the needle, or the diameter of the shaft. The gauge is numbered in reverse order (i.e., the thinner needle with the smaller diameter has the larger number, e.g., 25 gauge for subcutaneous injections, and 19–21 gauge, a thicker needle with a larger opening, for IM or IV injections. The size of the gauge is determined by the site of the injection and the viscosity of the solution (e.g., blood and oil require a thicker-gauge needle, e.g., 15–18).

3. *Tip.* The tip is the pointed end with a beveled edge.

Three main types of syringes are used for injections. The type used is determined by the medication and the dosage. The three types are:

1. *Standard syringe.* Used most frequently for subcutaneous or intramuscular injections, calibrated or marked in cubic centimeters (cc) or milliliters (ml) and minims (m) (Figure 9-5). The most commonly used size is 3 ml or 2½ ml. Larger sizes of 5–50 ml are available for other purposes (e.g., irrigations, withdrawing fluids from the body, and intravenous injections).

2. *Tuberculin (TB) syringe.* Used for intradermal injections of very small amounts of a substance (e.g., testing for tuberculosis or for allergies). The TB syringe is also used for subcutaneous injections when a small amount of medication, less than 1 ml, is ordered (e.g., in pediatrics). The TB syringe is calibrated in tenths of a milliliter and in minims and holds only a total of 1 cc, or 1 ml (Figure 9-6).

3. *Insulin syringe.* Used only for injection of insulin and is calibrated in units. The size in common use today is U-100, in which 100 units of insulin is equal to 1 ml. The standard U-100 syringe has a dual scale: even numbers on one side and odd numbers on the other side. Look carefully at the calibrations on each side. Count each calibration (on one side only) as *two* units (Figure 9-7A).

There are also smaller insulin syringes to more accurately measure small amounts of insulin, such as for children (Figure 9-7B for Lo-Dose Insulin Syringes 50 Units and 30 Units). Look carefully at the calibrations. In these Lo-Dose syringes, each calibration counts *only one* unit. It is extremely important that you study the calibrations carefully each time you prepare for an insulin injection, to prevent a medication error from negligent misinterpretation. **All insulin dosages should be double-checked by two caregivers before administration.**

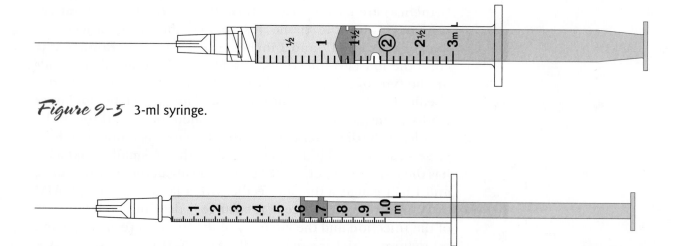

Figure 9-5 3-ml syringe.

Figure 9-6 Tuberculin syringe with 1-ml capacity.

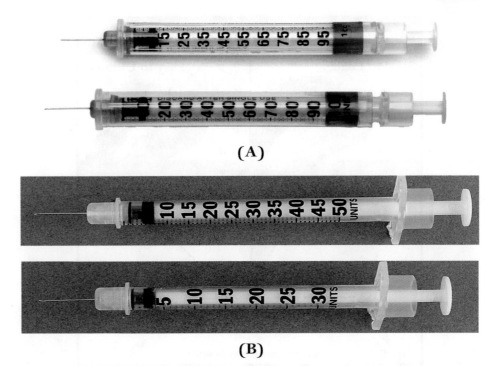

(A)

(B)

Figure 9-7 Insulin syringes. (A) Opposite sides of the same standard U-100 insulin syringe; note the numbers. (B) Lo-dose insulin syringes, 50 units and 30 units. (Courtesy of Becton Dickinson and Company.)

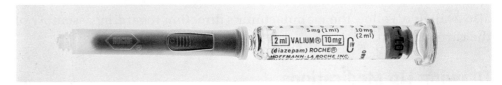

Figure 9-8 Prefilled, single-dose syringe. (Courtesy of Roche Laboratories, Inc.)

When instructing new diabetics in self-administration or administration by a family member, be sure that they can see and understand the calibrations and what they represent.

Prefilled syringes are available for certain medications (Figure 9-8). A premeasured amount of the drug is contained in the syringe. Check the dose ordered, compare with the dose in the syringe, and adjust if necessary. After injection, discard the syringe with needle attached and uncapped in the disposal bin.

Prefilled cartridges are also available, in which a premeasured amount of a medication is contained in a disposable cartridge. These prefilled units are made ready for injection by placing the cartridge in a holder. This unit can then be used to access a needleless IV system, or a needle can be attached to administer intramuscular or subcutaneous injections. After administration, the used cartridge is released from the holder and dropped into the disposal bin. If a needle is attached, it is released *uncapped* along with the cartridge into the bin. An example of such a unit is the *Carpuject,* produced by Hospira (Figure 9-9). Other units are

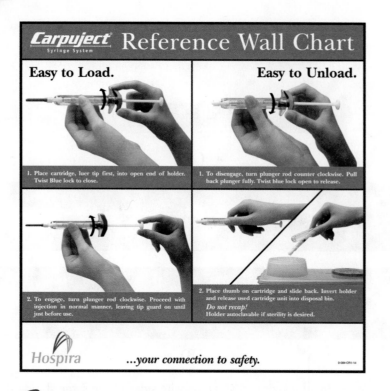

Figure 9-9 Carpuject prefilled cartridge. (Carpuject Syringe System reprinted with permission from Hospira, Inc., Lake Forest, IL.)

also available. Follow the manufacturer's direction regarding assembly of the cartridge unit.

Drawing Up Medications

1. Wash hands.
2. Assemble equipment (i.e., syringe, needle, packaged alcohol wipes, and medication ampule or vial).
3. Check the order using the five Rights of Medication Administration.
4. If medication is contained in a vial, first remove the protective cap. If the vial has been opened previously, wipe the rubber diaphragm on top with an alcohol wipe. Check vial for date and discoloration of contents (Figure 9-10).
5. Seat the needle securely on the syringe by pressing firmly downward on the top of the needle cover. Pull the needle cover straight off. *Note:* Luer-Loks require a half-turn to lock the needle in place.
6. Draw air into the syringe equal to the amount of solution you will be withdrawing from the vial. Insert needle into center of rubber diaphragm and inject air into vial (Figure 9-11). Invert vial and withdraw prescribed dosage (Figure 9-12). Be sure syringe is filled to proper level with solution and no bubbles are present. Withdraw needle from vial. For intramuscular injections, a small bubble (0.2 ml) of air may now be added to the correct dose of medicine already in the syringe.

7. The needle must now be recapped *carefully* to maintain sterility and prevent needle sticks. After withdrawing solution from an ampule or vial, the needle cap is laid horizontally on a flat surface. The syringe is held in the dominant hand, and the sterile needle is inserted carefully into the cap. The syringe with needle

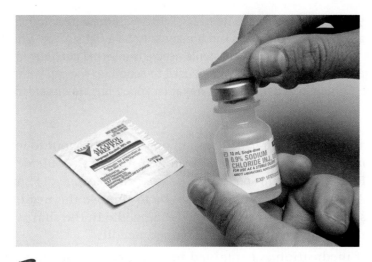

Figure 9-10 Preparing to withdraw medication from a vial. Cleanse the top with alcohol wipe.

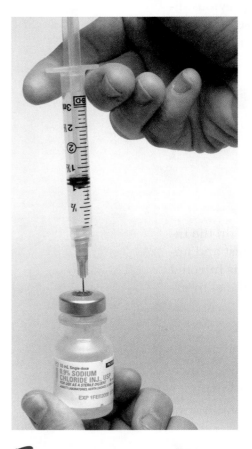

Figure 9-11 Injection of air into vial. Vial is upright so air is not injected into fluid.

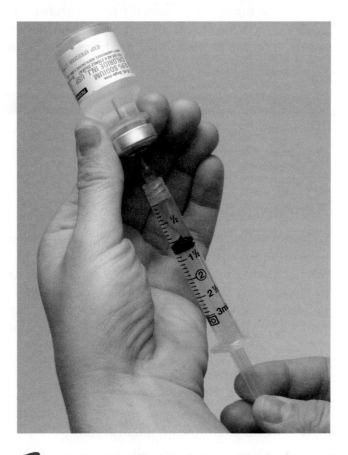

Figure 9-12 Withdrawal of prescribed amount of medication. Invert the vial. Be sure needle point is in fluid, not in the air.

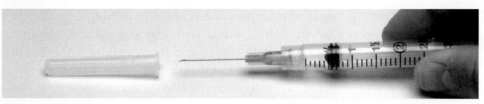

Figure 9-13 Recapping **sterile** needle. After withdrawing solution from an ampule or a vial, the needle cap is laid horizontally on a flat surface. The syringe is held in the dominant hand, and the sterile needle is inserted *carefully* into the cap. The syringe with needle attached is then used to scoop up the cap without touching it. Contaminated needles are **never** recapped but are discarded **uncapped** in sharps container.

attached is then used to scoop up the cap without touching it. *Do not contaminate the needle* by touching it to the outside of the cap. Remember, *only sterile needles are to be recapped* (Figure 9-13). An alternative method would be to remove the needle from the syringe carefully and discard the needle in the sharps container, replacing it with a sterile, capped needle.

8. If medication is contained in an ampule, hold tip with alcohol wipe to protect your fingers and break open along the scored marking at the neck. Tip vial and withdraw prescribed amount of medication. Recap needle carefully according to previous directions (Figure 9-13). Some facilities require the use of a filter needle to withdraw fluid from an ampule. Check the regulations in your area.

If two drugs are to be combined in a syringe, you must first check for compatibility of the drugs.

Administration by Injection

Intradermal injections are usually administered into the skin on the inner surface of the lower arm. For allergy testing, the upper chest and upper back areas may also be used. A small amount (0.1–0.2 ml) is injected so close to the surface that a wheal, or bubble, is formed by the skin expanding (Figure 9-14).

Technique for intradermal injection is as follows:

1. Wash hands.

2. Assemble equipment (i.e., TB syringe, 26 or 27 gauge, ⅜-inch needle, alcohol wipes, 2 × 2 gauze square and medication).

3. Check the order using the five Rights of Medication Administration and draw up medication.

4. Identify patient and explain procedure. Arm should be supported on flat surface.

5. Put on gloves.

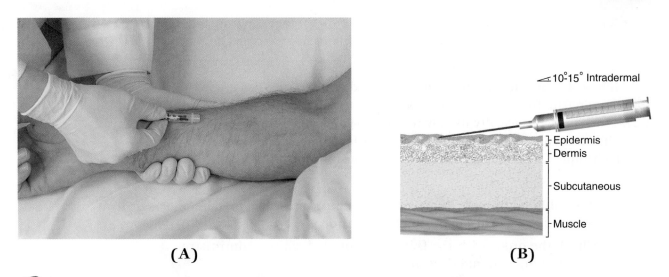

(A)   **(B)**

Figure 9-14   Intradermal injection. Hold the arm in nondominant hand and stretch the skin taut. *The needle bevel is up.* The needle is almost flat against the arm. Inject slowly just under the skin so that a bubble forms.

6. Cleanse skin with alcohol wipe on inner surface of the forearm (or other area if ordered by the physician). Allow the skin to dry thoroughly. (If you inject before the skin is dry, you might introduce alcohol into the skin and interfere with test results.) Avoid areas with hair or blemishes.

7. Hold the patient's arm in your nondominant hand and *stretch the skin taut.*

8. Hold the syringe so that *the bevel is up* and the needle is almost flat against the patient's arm. Insert the needle slowly only far enough to cover the lumen or opening in the needle. The point of the needle should be visible through the skin.

9. Inject the medication *very slowly.* You should see a small, white bubble in the skin forming immediately. If no bubble forms, withdraw the needle slightly; it may be too deep. If solution leaks out as you inject, the needle is not deep enough.

10. After correct amount of medication is injected, withdraw needle and apply gentle pressure with 2 × 2 gauze. *Do not* massage the area or you may interfere with test results.

11. Discard syringe with needle *uncapped* into sharps container immediately without touching needle. Remove gloves. Wash hands.

12. Note drug name, dosage, time, date, and site of injection on patient's record (sixth Right—Documentation).

13. Instruct the patient not to scrub, scratch, or rub the area. Provide written instructions regarding time to return for reading. Tell the patient to contact the physician immediately or report to an emergency facility if breathing difficulty, hives, or a rash appears.

Caution: Do not start allergy testing unless emergency equipment is available nearby and personnel are trained in emergency care in case of anaphylactic response. Patients receiving allergy testing should remain in office or clinical facility for 30 minutes after injection to be observed for possible anaphylactic reaction.

Subcutaneous injections are administered into the fatty tissues on the upper outer arm, front of the thigh, abdomen, or upper back (Figure 9-15). A 2½–3-ml syringe is usually used with a 24–26-gauge, ³/₈–⁵/₈-inch needle. No more than 2 ml of medication may be administered subcutaneously.

Technique for subcutaneous injection is as follows:

1. Wash hands.
2. Assemble equipment (correct-size syringe and needle, alcohol wipes, 2 × 2 gauze square, and medication).
3. Check the order with the five Rights of Medication Administration and draw up medication.
4. Identify patient, ask the patient's name, check armband, and explain procedure.
5. If patient is receiving frequent injections, be sure to rotate injection sites.
6. Put on gloves.
7. Cleanse skin with alcohol wipe.
8. Pinch the skin into a fat fold of at least 1 inch (Figure 9-15).

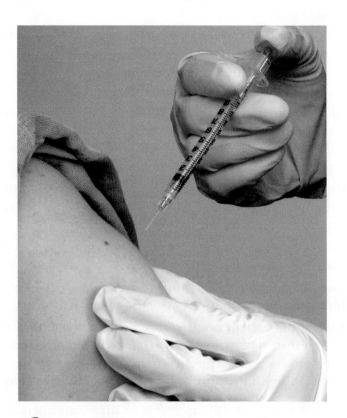

Figure 9-15 Subcutaneous injection. The tissue is pinched, and the needle is held at a 45-degree angle.

9. Insert the needle at a 45-degree angle. A 90-degree angle may be used with a ⅜ needle, if there is sufficient subcutaneous tissue, and also for insulin and heparin injections.

10. Pull back on the plunger (aspirate). If any blood appears in the syringe, withdraw the needle. Place pressure with dry 2 × 2 gauze over injection site until bleeding stops. Discard the syringe with needle *uncapped* into sharps container immediately. You will then have to draw up fresh solution with another sterile syringe and needle. (*Do not* aspirate with heparin injection.) It is also not necessary to aspirate with an insulin syringe as the needle is shorter. Therefore, there is not a danger of contacting larger blood vessels.

11. Inject the medication *slowly,* pushing the plunger all the way. Too rapid injection may cause pain.

12. Place dry 2 × 2 gauze over the entry site, applying pressure with it, as you withdraw the needle rapidly. Do not push down on the needle while withdrawing it.

13. Massage the site gently with the dry 2 × 2 gauze to speed absorption. (*Do not* massage with heparin injection.) Be sure there is no bleeding.

14. Discard syringe with needle *uncapped* into sharps container immediately.

15. Remove gloves and discard.

16. Wash hands.

17. Note the medication, dosage, time, date, site of injection, and your signature on the patient's record (sixth Right—Documentation).

18. Observe the patient for effects and record observations.

Intramuscular injections are administered deep into large muscles (Figure 9-16). There are five recommended sites.

1. *Dorsogluteal.*   Upper outer quadrant of the buttock (preferred site for adults)

2. *Ventrogluteal.*   Above and to the outside of the buttock area, on the hip

3. *Deltoid.*   Upper outer arm above the axilla

4. *Vastus lateralis.*   Front of the thigh toward the outside of the leg

5. *Rectus femoris.*   Front of the thigh toward the midline of the leg

The intramuscular route has two advantages over the subcutaneous route:

1. A larger amount of solution can be administered (up to 3 ml, or a maximum of 1 ml in children).

2. Absorption is more rapid because the muscle tissue is more vascular (i.e., contains many blood vessels).

The needle must be long enough to go through the subcutaneous tissue into the muscle. The length of the needle varies with the size of the patient. With a child or very thin, emaciated adult, a 1-inch needle is usually adequate. For most adults, a 1½-inch needle is appropriate. However, for an obese person, a 2-inch needle might be required. The needle is inserted at a 90-degree angle with the skin spread taut (Figure 9-16).

Because there are more large blood vessels and nerves in this deeper tissue, the site for injection must be chosen more precisely. Using the illustrations as a guide, follow these steps in selecting the site:

1. **Dorsogluteal site.** Most commonly used for adults, but not for children under 3 years old (Figure 9-17). Position the patient flat on the stomach (prone) with the toes pointed inward or on the side with the upper leg flexed. Identify the site by drawing an

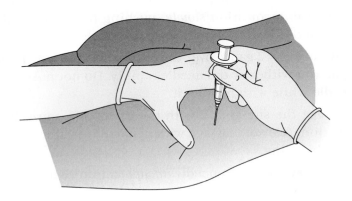

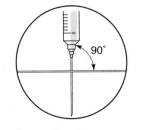

Figure 9-16 Intramuscular injection. The skin is held taut. The needle is at a 90-degree angle.

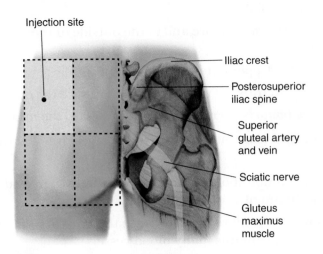

Injection site

Iliac crest

Posterosuperior iliac spine

Superior gluteal artery and vein

Sciatic nerve

Gluteus maximus muscle

Figure 9-17 Dorsogluteal site for IM injection. Most common site for adults.

imaginary line from the posterior superior iliac spine to the greater trochanter of the femur. These two bony prominences can be palpated with the thumb and forefinger. The injection is given above and to the outside of this line. Note that this site is high enough to avoid the sciatic nerve and the major blood vessels.

2. *Ventrogluteal site.*   Can be used for all patients. Position the patient on the back or side (Figure 9-18). Identify the site by placing the palm of your hand on the patient's greater trochanter. Place the index finger on the anterior superior iliac spine and the middle finger on the iliac crest. The injection is made into the center of the V formed between the index and middle fingers.

3. *Deltoid site.*   Seldom used because the muscle is smaller and is close to the radial nerve (Figure 9-19). The maximum solution

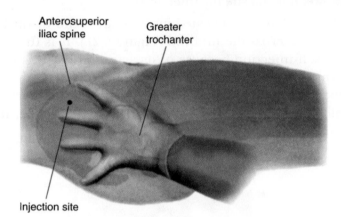

Anterosuperior
iliac spine

Greater
trochanter

Injection site

Figure 9-18 Ventrogluteal site for IM injection. Can be administered with patient on back or side.

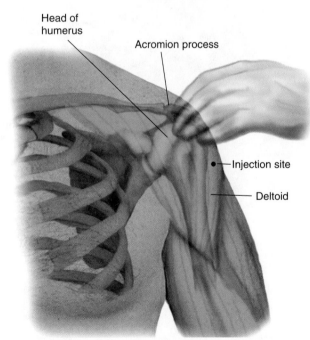

Head of
humerus

Acromion process

Injection site

Deltoid

Figure 9-19 Deltoid site for IM injection. Maximum of 1-ml of medication and 1-inch needle is used. Injected above the level of the armpit.

that can be used is 1 ml; and a shorter needle, 1 inch, is used. Caution must be exercised to avoid the clavicle, humerus, acromium, brachial vein and artery, and radial nerve. Identify the site by drawing an imaginary line across the arm at the level of the armpit. The injection is made above this line and below the acromium on the outer aspect of the arm.

4. *Vastus lateralis.* Located on the anterior lateral thigh, the preferred site for infants, since these muscles are the most developed for children under the age of three years (Figure 9-20). In the older, nonambulatory, and emaciated adult, this muscle may be wasted and insufficient for injection. Identify the mid-portion on the side of the thigh by measuring one hand breadth above the knee and one hand breadth below the great trochanter. The area between is the site for injection.

5. *Rectus femoris.* Located just medial to the vastus lateralis, but does not cross the midline (Figure 9-21). It is the preferred site for self-injection because of its accessibility. It is located in the same way as the vastus lateralis. **Caution:** Do not get too close to the midline, which is adjacent to the sciatic nerve and major blood vessels. If the muscle is not well developed, injections in this site may be painful.

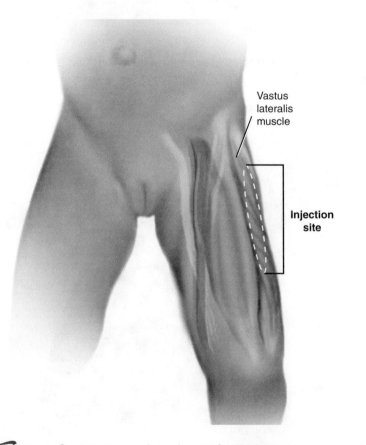

Vastus
lateralis
muscle

**Injection
site**

Figure 9-20 Vastus lateralis site for IM injection, preferred for infants. Injected on the anterior lateral thigh.

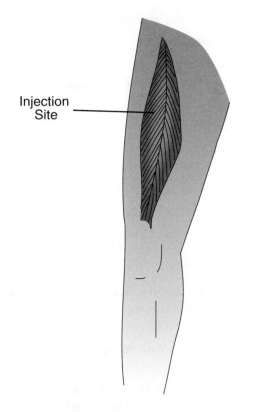

Injection
Site

Figure 9-21 Rectus femoris site for IM injection. Preferred for self-injection. Injected medial to the vastus lateralis, but not too close to midline.

Technique for intramuscular injection is as follows:

1. Wash hands.

2. Assemble equipment (i.e., correct-size syringe, needle, alcohol wipes, 2 × 2 gauze square, and medication).

3. Check the order with the five Rights of Medication Administration and draw up the medication, or insert appropriate prefilled cartridge into Tubex or Carpuject holder.

4. After measuring correct amount of medication in syringe, draw 0.2 ml air into syringe to clear needle. Recap carefully using method illustrated in Figure 9-13.

5. Identify the patient, ask the patient's name and check armband, and explain procedure.

6. If patient is receiving frequent injections, be sure to rotate sites.

7. Put on gloves.

8. Position the patient and expose area to be used for injection.

9. Cleanse skin with alcohol wipe.

10. With your nondominant hand, stretch the skin *taut* at the injection site.

11. Insert the needle at a 90-degree angle with a quick, dartlike motion of your dominant hand.

12. Pull back on the plunger (aspirate), and follow previous guidelines if blood appears.

13. Inject the medication at a slow, even rate.

14. Withdraw the needle rapidly, holding dry 2 × 2 gauze over the site.

15. Apply pressure and massage area gently with alcohol wipe.

16. Discard syringe with needle *uncapped* into sharps container immediately.

17. Discard gloves and wash hands.

18. Note the medication, dosage, time, date, site of injection, and your signature on the patient's record (sixth Right—Documentation).

19. Observe the patient for effects and record observations.

The *Z-track method* (Figure 9-22) is used for injections that are irritating to the tissue, such as iron dextran, hydroxyzine, or cephazolin. The dorsogluteal is the site for this type of intramuscular injection.

Technique for the Z-track method is as follows:

1. Draw up the medication and then add 0.3–0.5 ml of air to the syringe. Then replace the needle with a sterile one two to three inches long.

2. Stretch the skin as far as you can to the outer side and hold it there.

3. After cleansing the site, insert the needle with a dartlike motion, aspirate, and then inject the medication *slowly*. Wait ten seconds before withdrawing the needle.

4. Withdraw the needle and allow the skin to return to normal position. This seals off the needle track.

5. Press firmly on injection site with 2 × 2 gauze square. Do *not* massage the site, as this could spread the medication to the subcutaneous tissue, causing irritation.

6. Advise the patient that walking will aid absorption and to avoid tight garments, such as girdles, that cause pressure on the site.

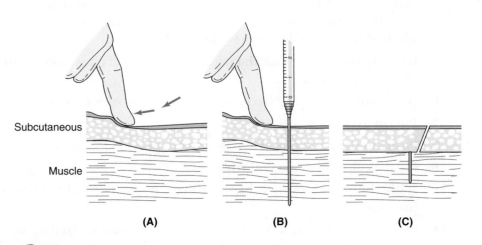

Subcutaneous

Muscle

(A)   (B)   (C)

Figure 9-22 Z-track method of IM injection of iron preparations. (A) Skin and subcutaneous tissue pulled to one side and held there. (B) Needle is placed in muscle. (C) Z-track sealed when tissue released.

SKIN MEDICATIONS

Topical medications for the skin are prescribed for a great variety of conditions and are available in a variety of forms: ointments, lotions, creams, solutions, soaks, and baths. Administration of topical medications requires knowledge of the condition being treated and the purpose of the treatment, and strict adherence to directions as prescribed by the doctor or provided by the pharmacist, or to instructions on the medication container or in a package insert. *When in doubt regarding administration techniques, always ask* a qualified person for advice. Some specific principles for skin medications are outlined in Chapter 12. In addition, good judgment is also required.

Several suggestions for applying topical medications include:

1. For burns, use sterile gloves to apply, and cover with sterile dressings because of the danger of infection. Use gentle, light touch because of pain.

2. For skin conditions in which there is irritation or itching, use cottonball or snug-fitting gloves to apply. *Never* use gauze, which can cause additional irritation and discomfort.

3. Follow physician's order regarding covering or leaving open to the air.

4. Wash old medication off before applying new, unless specifically directed to do otherwise.

APPLICATION TO THE MUCOUS MEMBRANES

Medications applied to the mucous membranes also come in a variety of forms: suppositories, ointments, solutions, sprays, gargles, and so on. Always follow the specific directions that accompany the individual medication, unless directed to do otherwise by the physician. When in doubt, always ask questions.

EYE MEDICATIONS

Technique for instillation of eye medications is as follows:

1. Wash hands (Figure 8-1).

2. Assemble eye medication (ophthalmic solution or ointment).

3. Check the order with the five Rights of Medication Administration. Pay particular attention to *percentage* on medication label and to *which eye* is to be treated (right eye, left eye, or both eyes).

4. Identify patient, ask the patient's name and explain procedure.

5. Put on gloves.

6. Position patient flat on back or upright with head back. Ask the patient to look up.

7. Carefully instill the ophthalmic solution, correct number of drops, or ointment into the lower conjunctival sac, using caution to avoid contamination of the tip of the dropper or ointment tube (Figure 9-23). Do not let solution run from one eye to the other.

8. Tell the patient to close the eye gently so as not to squeeze out the solution.

9. Press gently on the inner canthus following administration of eyedrops (Figure 9-24). Systemic absorption is thus minimized with medications such as corticosteroids, miotics, and mydriatics.

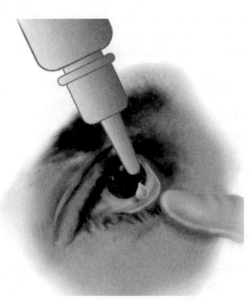

Figure 9-23 Instilling eye medication. Gently press the lower lid down and have the patient look upward. Ophthalmic solution is dropped inside lower eyelid.

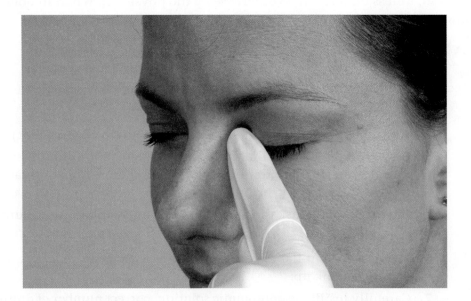

Figure 9-24 Gentle pressure on the inner canthus following administration of ophthalmic medications. Systemic absorption is thus minimized with medications such as corticosteriods, miotics, and mydriatics.

10. Remove gloves.

11. Wash hands. Replace medication in appropriate place.

12. Record the medication, dosage, time, date, and which eye was treated, on the patient's record (Sixth Right—Documentation).

13. When more than one eye medication is ordered, wait at least five minutes before instilling the second medication.

14. If eyedrops and ointment are ordered for the same time, instill eyedrops first, wait five minutes, then apply ointment.

When in doubt about administration of any medication, always ask a qualified person for advice. Never guess! Remember that the patient who is receiving the medication could be you or your loved one. By thinking of yourself in the patient's place you will have the proper attitude to administer medications with competence, good judgment, and compassion.

Checklist For Intradermal Injection

Activity	Rating	
	S	U
1. Washed hands	_____	_____
2. Checked medication order for date, dosage, time, route, and allergies	_____	_____
3. Identified medication: purpose, side effects, cautions, and normal dosage range	_____	_____
4. Assembled supplies: TB syringe, 27-gauge, ⅜-inch needle, alcohol wipes, and medication	_____	_____
5. Checked medication vial against medication sheet using the five Rights of Medication Administration	_____	_____
6. Withdrew correct dose from vial *after* cleansing top with alcohol and injecting equivalent amount of air into vial	_____	_____
7. Recapped needle using sterile technique (see Figure 9-13 for technique)	_____	_____
8. Identified patient by checking bracelet and asking the patient's name and DOB	_____	_____
9. Explained procedure to patient and answered any questions regarding procedure	_____	_____
10. Positioned patient with inner forearm exposed and supported on a flat surface	_____	_____
11. Put on gloves	_____	_____
12. Selected area without hair or blemish, cleansed skin with alcohol wipe, and allowed skin to dry	_____	_____
13. Held patient's arm with nondominant hand, stretching the skin taut	_____	_____
14. Expelled any air bubbles from syringe	_____	_____
15. Inserted needle point slowly, bevel side up, only enough to cover needle opening; point of needle visible through skin	_____	_____
16. Injected medication very slowly, with immediate formation of small bubble	_____	_____
17. Withdrew needle and applied gentle pressure to injection site with dry gauze (no massage)	_____	_____
18. Discarded syringe with needle *uncapped* into sharps container	_____	_____
19. Removed gloves	_____	_____
20. Washed hands	_____	_____
21. Recorded drug name, dosage, time, date, and site of injection on patient's record and signed or initialed entry (sixth Right—Documentation)	_____	_____
22. Observed patient for 30 min. for possible anaphylactic reaction; identified location of emergency equipment and medication if required	_____	_____
23. Provided written instructions regarding time to return for reading; instructed patient to avoid scrubbing, scratching, or rubbing the area and to report to emergency facility with dyspnea, hives, or rash	_____	_____

Note: S, satisfactory; U, unsatisfactory

Checklist For Subcutaneous Injection

Activity	Rating	
	S	U
1. Washed hands	_____	_____
2. Checked medication order for date, dosage, time, route, and allergies	_____	_____
3. Identified medication: purpose, side effects, contraindications, interactions, and normal dosage range	_____	_____
4. Assembled supplies: $2\frac{1}{2}$–3-ml, TB or insulin syringe; 24–26-gauge, $\frac{3}{8}$–$\frac{5}{8}$ inch needle; alcohol wipes; and medication vial or ampule	_____	_____
5. Checked medication against medication sheet using the five Rights of Medication Administration; also checked drug for date and discoloration	_____	_____
6. Calculated correct dosage on paper if necessary and checked calculations with instructor	_____	_____
7. If drug is contained in *vial,* withdrew correct amount after cleansing top with alcohol wipe and injecting equivalent amount of air into vial. If drug is contained in *ampule,* held tip with alcohol wipe while breaking it at neck. Withdrew correct amount of drug without bubbles in syringe	_____	_____
8. Recapped needle using proper sterile technique	_____	_____
9. Identified patient by checking identification bracelet and asking the patients' name and DOB	_____	_____
10. Explained procedure to patient and answered any questions	_____	_____
11. Selected appropriate site, using rotation if frequent injections	_____	_____
12. Put on gloves	_____	_____
13. Cleansed skin with alcohol wipe	_____	_____
14. Pinched skin into fold with nondominant hand	_____	_____
15. Expelled any air bubbles from syringe	_____	_____
16. Inserted needle at a 45-degree angle and released skin fold	_____	_____
17. While holding needle hub with nondominant hand, aspirated for blood (used new site if necessary)	_____	_____
18. Injected medication slowly	_____	_____
19. Placed alcohol wipe over entry site, and applied pressure as needle was withdrawn; massaged site gently (with heparin, pressure only, no massage)	_____	_____
20. Disposed of syringe and needle *uncapped* in sharps container	_____	_____
21. Removed and discarded gloves	_____	_____
22. Washed hands	_____	_____
23. Recorded drug name, dosage, time, date, site of injection, and signature on patient's record; also recorded effects after appropriate time (Sixth Right—Documentation)	_____	_____

Note: S, satisfactory; U, unsatisfactory

Checklist for Intramuscular Injection

Activity	Rating S	Rating U
1. Washed hands	_____	_____
2. Checked medication order for date, dosage, time, route, and allergies	_____	_____
3. Identified medication: purpose, side effects, cautions, and normal dosage range	_____	_____
4. Assembled supplies: 2½, 3-ml syringe; 1½–2 inch needle, usually 21 gauge; alcohol wipes; and medication	_____	_____
5. Checked medication against medication sheet using the five Rights of Medication Administration; if PRN medication, checked time of last dose	_____	_____
6. If narcotic, signed and checked time of last dose, on controlled substance sheet; calculated correct dosage on paper if necessary	_____	_____
7. If drug is contained in *vial,* withdrew correct amount after cleansing top with alcohol wipe and injecting equivalent amount of air into vial. If drug is contained in *ampule,* held tip with alcohol wipe while breaking it at neck. Withdrew correct amount of drug without bubbles in syringe.	_____	_____
8. *After* drug measured accurately in syringe, drew 0.2 ml air into syringe	_____	_____
9. Recapped needle using sterile technique (see Figure 9-13 for techniques)	_____	_____
10. Identified patient by checking bracelet and asking their name and DOB	_____	_____
11. Explained procedure to patient and answered any questions	_____	_____
12. Closed door to room and/or curtain around bed	_____	_____
13. Selected appropriate site, using rotation if frequent injections	_____	_____
14. Put on gloves	_____	_____
15. Positioned patient appropriately, exposing only the area for injection	_____	_____
16. Cleansed skin with alcohol wipe	_____	_____
17. With forefinger and thumb of nondominant hand, spread the skin *taut* at injection site	_____	_____
18. Inserted needle at a 90-degree angle with a quick, dartlike motion of dominant hand	_____	_____
19. Aspirated for blood (used new site if necessary)	_____	_____
20. Injected medication at a slow, even rate	_____	_____
21. Applied pressure with alcohol wipe over entry site as needle was withdrawn rapidly; massaged site gently with alcohol wipe unless medication irritating (with Ancef, Vistaril, or iron dextran, pressure only, no massage)	_____	_____
22. Made sure there was no bleeding before covering patient and making patient comfortable	_____	_____
23. Disposed of syringe and needle *uncapped* in sharps container	_____	_____
24. Discarded gloves appropriately; washed hands	_____	_____
25. Recorded drug, name, dosage, time, date, site of injection, and signature on patient's record (sixth Right—Documentation)	_____	_____

Note: S, satisfactory; U, unsatisfactory

Checklist for Instillation of Eye Medication

Activity	Rating S	U
1. Washed hands	_____	_____
2. Checked the order with the five Rights of Medication Administration; noted percent, which eye, and allergies	_____	_____
3. Identified medication: purpose, side effects, and cautions	_____	_____
4. Identified patient by checking bracelet and asking the patient's name and DOB	_____	_____
5. Explained procedure to patient and answered any questions regarding procedure	_____	_____
6. Positioned patient on back or upright with head back	_____	_____
7. Asked the patient to look up	_____	_____
8. Used aseptic technique to instill correct number of drops or ointment dosage into lower conjunctival sac	_____	_____
9. Gently closed the eyelid and applied pressure to the inner canthus (eye drops only)	_____	_____
10. Washed hands and replaced medication in appropriate place	_____	_____
11. Recorded medication, dosage, time, date, and which eye was treated, on patient's record (Sixth Right—Documentation)	_____	_____

Note: S, satisfactory; U, unsatisfactory

CHAPTER REVIEW QUIZ

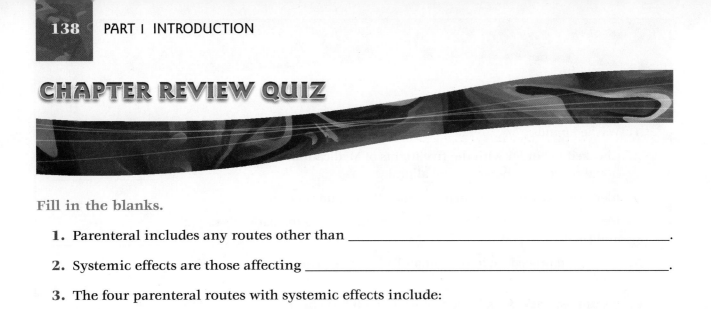

Fill in the blanks.

1. Parenteral includes any routes other than _____.

2. Systemic effects are those affecting _____.

3. The four parenteral routes with systemic effects include:

    _____   _____

    _____   _____

Label the routes according to their action. Use R for rapid and S for slow. Match each route with the appropriate definition:

	Action			Definition
4. _____	Sublingual		_____	**a.** Given with a needle
5. _____	Transcutaneous		_____	**b.** Nebulizer or IPPB
6. _____	Inhalation		_____	**c.** Under the tongue
7. _____	Injection		_____	**d.** Skin patch

8. What precautions should be observed when applying transcutaneous systems?

    _____

9. IPPB refers to _____.

Select the correct needle for the purpose. Needle size may be used for more than one purpose.

	Purpose		Needle
10.	Subcutaneous injection	**a.**	21 gauge, 1½ inch
11.	Intravenous injection	**b.**	25 gauge, ⅝ inch
12.	Allergy testing	**c.**	18 gauge
13.	Intramuscular injection	**d.**	27 gauge, ⅜ inch

14. What are the two purposes of the tuberculin syringe?

    _____

    _____

15. The insulin syringe is calibrated in _____, and 1 ml is equal to _____ in an insulin syringe.

16. On a *standard* insulin syringe, each calibration represents _____ unit/s.

On a *Lo-Dose* insulin syringe, each calibration represents _____ unit/s.

Match the injection with the proper technique:

Injection		Technique	
17. _____	Intramuscular	**a.**	Needle 45-degree angle, skin pinched up
18. _____	Subcutaneous	**b.**	Needle flat, bevel up, skin taut
19. _____	Intradermal	**c.**	Needle 90-degree angle, skin taut

20. List the five sites for intramuscular injections and when each is used.

_____

_____

_____

_____

_____

21. Why is the Z-track method used? _____

Describe Z-track administration. _____

_____

_____

22. Define local effects. _____

_____

List four areas to administer medication for local effects.

_____ _____

_____ _____

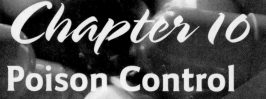

Chapter 10
Poison Control

Objectives

Upon completion of this chapter, the learner should be able to

1. Define the Key Terms
2. Identify four routes by which poisons may be taken into the body
3. List five conditions in which vomiting, after the ingestion of poisons, could be injurious to the patient
4. Describe the first step to take in the event of any poisoning and the procedure to follow
5. Explain the purpose of activated charcoal and when it is given
6. Name three clinical procedures required when caring for patients who have been poisoned
7. Describe appropriate therapy for poisoning by inhalation, external poison, and insect sting
8. Identify two groups of people at risk for poisoning
9. List 10 recommendations for patient education to help prevent poisoning

Key Terms

Antidotes

Emetic

Ingestion

Poison

A **poison** is a substance taken into the body by ingestion, inhalation, injection, or absorption that interferes with normal physiological functions. In some cases, only a small amount of a substance can cause severe tissue damage directly (e.g., corrosives). In other cases, the substance can be beneficial in small amounts, but lethal in excessive amounts (e.g., overdose of medication).

In a case of suspected poisoning, the best policy is to contact a Poison Control Center directly, or through an emergency care facility. Instructions can then be given by phone for appropriate emergency treatment based on the type of poison and the patient's condition, age, and size.

POISONING BY INGESTION

The most common type of poisoning is by **ingestion,** or swallowing. Children between the ages of one and five are most at risk for poisoning. Before 2004 it was recommended that children who had ingested poisons be given the **emetic** ipecac syrup to induce vomiting. However, extensive research conducted through The American Association of Poison Control Centers, Toxic Exposure Surveillance System, identified several concerns regarding ipecac.

1. Outcomes failed to justify its effectiveness.

2. Adverse effects, such as persistent vomiting could interfere with other treatment.

3. There has been evidence of widespread abuse of ipecac by people with anorexia and bulimia.

Therefore, in early 2004, The American Academy of Pediatrics (AAP) issued a policy statement on poison treatment in the home. The AAP recommended against keeping ipecac in the home and further recommended that ipecac presently in the home be disposed of safely.

The first step to take in any poisoning is to contact your local Poison Control Center. This number can be obtained by calling the national toll-free Poison Control number: **1-800-222-1222.** Callers should be prepared to give details regarding the poison and the age, weight, and health status of the individual who took the poison. Mention allergies and asthma if present.

Under the following conditions vomiting could be injurious to the patient and should be avoided if possible:

1. Ingestion of corrosive substances such as mineral acids or caustic alkalis (e.g., carbolic acid, ammonia, drain cleaners, oven cleaners, dishwasher detergent, and lye). Check also for burns around or in the mouth. Vomiting can cause additional tissue damage.

2. Ingestion of volatile petroleum products (e.g., gasoline, kerosene, lighter fluid, and benzene). Vomiting can cause aspiration and/or asphyxiation.

3. Ingestion of convulsants (e.g., strychnine or iodine). Vomiting can precipitate seizures.

4. If patient is semiconscious, severely inebriated, in shock, convulsing, or has no gag reflex. Vomiting could cause choking, aspiration, and/or asphyxiation.

5. If patient is less than one year old.

6. In patients with cardiac or vascular disease, vomiting can increase blood pressure and precipitate a stroke, cardiac arrhythmias, or atrioventricular block.

If any of the above-mentioned conditions exist, the patient should be transported *immediately* to an emergency care facility. Trained personnel can remove the stomach contents by gastric lavage, if appropriate, and administer appropriate antidotes as indicated. **Antidotes,** such as CNS (central nervous system) stimulants and/or CPR (cardiopulmonary resuscitation), may be required in poisoning with CNS depressants. Gastric lavage is *not* used in patients who have ingested corrosives, because of the danger of perforating the damaged tissue of the esophagus. If perforation exists, surgery is required. Observation is required in an acute care facility.

Sometimes a substance such as activated charcoal is administered to minimize systemic absorption of the ingested poison. However, activated charcoal is given *only after* emesis or gastric lavage, or if antidotes are *not* to be given via the gastric route; charcoal would interfere with absorption of any drugs in the stomach.

Personnel caring for poisoning victims should observe the following cautions:

- *Be sure to save emesis.* It may be necessary to send it to a laboratory to determine the type of poison. If there is doubt about the poison, the doctor may also order urine and blood tests for toxicology.
- Closely monitor the vital signs of patients who have taken poison of any kind.
- Observe closely for possible confusion, tremors, convulsions, visual disturbances, loss of consciousness, respiratory distress, or cardiac arrhythmias.

POISONING BY INHALATION

Poisoning by inhalation requires symptomatic treatment: fresh air, oxygen, and CPR if indicated. Inhaling insect spray may require administration of an antidote.

EXTERNAL POISONING OF SKIN OR EYES

External poisons should be flushed from the skin or eyes with a continuous stream of water for at least 15 min. The patient should then be transported to an emergency care facility for further treatment as required. Systemic absorption of poisons through the skin may require administration of an antidote.

POISONING BY STING AND SNAKEBITE

Poisoning by insect sting (e.g., bee, wasp, scorpion, or fire ant) should be treated with immediate application of household ammonia to the site or with a paste made of bicarbonate of soda and water, after removing the stinger of a bee or wasp. An ice pack can also be applied to the site of the sting. If the patient is allergic, watch closely for possible anaphylactic reaction. CPR and administration of adrenalin and corticosteroids may be required. Transport the patient to an emergency care facility immediately if indicated. Some allergic persons carry a kit with medication prescribed by their doctor (e.g., antihistamine and Isuprel SL to be self-administered if stung, or epinephrine for self-injection or injection by someone else).

After emergency care is completed, aftercare to lessen the pain, discomfort, and redness associated with stings, can include application of topical corticosteroid ointment. (See Topical Corticosteroids in Table 12-1.)

Do not apply ice or a tourniquet to a snakebite. Venom is very irritating and may cause sloughing of the tissues. Keep the patient quiet in order to slow circulation, and transport the patient, lying down, to an emergency care facility for *antivenom injections.* If possible, take the snake along, in a closed container, for identification purposes. It may be nonpoisonous.

PEOPLE AT RISK

Poisonings are the leading cause of health emergencies for children in the nation and a major cause of death among young children because of their natural curiosity and active lifestyle. The danger is particularly great with flavored medications, such as aspirin or iron tablets. Great care must be taken to prevent poisoning of young children. The child between the ages of one and five years old is most **at risk.**

Keep all chemicals in a locked cupboard. Keep infrequently used drugs, for example, pain medications, in a locked box, such as a tackle box or file box with a lock. Be sure that medications taken daily by adults are always in childproof containers. Be particularly vigilant when visiting with elderly friends or relatives who may not have childproof containers for their pills.

The Food and Drug Administration (FDA) reports that iron pills are the leading cause of poisoning deaths in children under six. Although iron supplements have been sold in bottles with child-resistant caps, in the last decade more than 110,000 children were poisoned by eating adult iron pills and at least 33 have died. Therefore, in 1994 the FDA proposed requiring iron supplements to be sold in special "blister packs."

The health care worker can play a major role in reducing the number of accidental poisonings in children by stressing preventive measures to parents. One educational program teaches the child to stay away from dangerous products by labeling them with a "Mr. Yuk" sticker. Figure 10-1

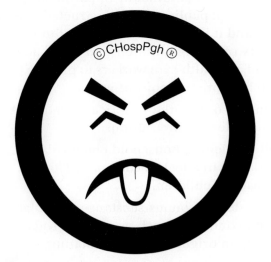

Figure 10-1 Mr. Yuk and similar stickers may be obtained from many Poison Control Centers throughout the United States. The telephone number of the nearest Poison Control Center is frequently printed on these stickers. (Permission to reproduce Mr. Yuk has been granted by Children's Hospital of Pittsburgh.)

(Mr. Yuk says "No!") is a warning label for children who cannot read. These stickers are available from many poison information centers throughout the United States.

Another group at risk for poisoning is older adults. Overdoses of medication can result in toxicity, with symptoms of confusion, dizziness, weakness, lethargy, ataxia, tremors, or cardiac irregularities. *Toxic reactions* from medications taken by older adults can possibly result from

1. Slower metabolism, impaired circulation, and decreased excretion, causing medication to remain in the body longer and build up to dangerous levels

2. Wrong dosage caused by impaired vision or poor memory (patients may forget that they have taken medicine and take a double dose)

3. Interactions when many different medications are taken and over-the-counter medications, or herbal remedies are self-administered with inadequate medical supervision

4. Medical conditions affecting absorption

(See Chapter 27: Drugs and Older Adults.)

Many medicines and common household products resemble candy or food. Children may be attracted to the unique shapes and bright colors used in packaging. Impaired vision may contribute to mistakes by adults, especially older adults. It is important to keep medicines and dangerous chemicals in an area separate from food and medicines. Don't be fooled by look-alikes (Figure 10-2).

Patient Education

Poisons

Public education is of paramount importance in preventing poisoning. The general public must be instructed in precautions with medications, and it is especially important to inform the parents and caretakers of young children and older adults. It is the responsibility of all health care workers to provide the necessary information to help prevent poisoning.

To prevent poisoning, the American Medical Association recommends the following precautions:

1. Keep all medicines, household chemicals, cleaning supplies, and pesticides in a locked cupboard. There is no place that is "out of reach of children."

2. Never transfer poisonous substances to unlabeled containers or to food containers such as milk or soda bottles or cereal boxes. Keep in original labeled container.

3. Never store poisonous substances in the same area with food. Confusion could be fatal.

4. Never reuse containers of chemical products.

5. When discarding medication, always flush down the toilet. Never discard it in a wastebasket.

6. Do not give or take medications in the dark.

7. Never leave medications on a bedside stand. Confusion while a person is sleepy could result in a fatal overdose.

8. Always read the label before taking any medication or pouring any solution for ingestion.

9. Never tell children the medicine you are giving them is candy.

10. When preparing a baby's formula, taste the ingredients. Never store boric acid, salt, or talcum near the formula ingredients.

11. Never give or take any medication that is discolored, has a strange odor, or is outdated.

12. Don't take medicine in front of children.

13. Keep pocketbooks, purses, and pillboxes out of reach of children.

14. Rinse out containers thoroughly before disposing of them.

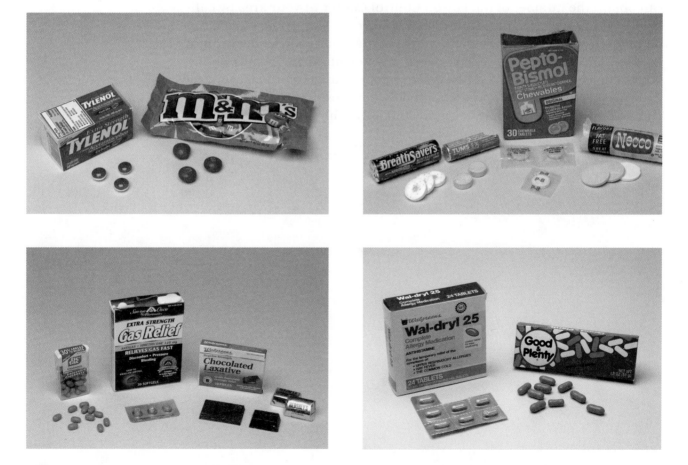

Figure 10-2   Look-alikes: Don't be fooled! Many common household products and medicines resemble candy or food. Keep these products in separate areas. The compared products are chosen for illustration purposes only. The manufacturers do not intend any misuse of their products.

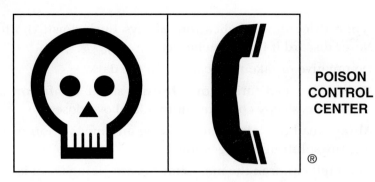

POISON
CONTROL
CENTER

®

Figure 10-3 Obtain the number of your nearest Poison
Control Center and place it near or on your telephone.
(Permission to reproduce Poison Control Center logo has been
granted by the American Association of Poison Control Centers,
Inc., Washington DC.)

Obtain the number of your nearest Poison Control Center (Figure 10-3) and place it on or near your telephone. There are more than 70 Poison Control Centers throughout the United States and Canada with computerized data to give you the latest information about poisons. Remember, *the wrong treatment is often more dangerous than none.* You can obtain the number of the Poison Control Center in your area by calling 1-800-222-1222, or the nearest emergency care facility, or by logging on to the Webite (http://www.aapcc.org) of the American Association of Poison Control Centers, or check the emergency numbers in your phone book. The Poison Control Center is also a good source of information regarding poisonous plants, insects, snakes, reptiles, and poisonous marine organisms, for example, stingray and jellyfish.

CHAPTER REVIEW QUIZ

Complete the statements by filling in the blanks:

1. Poisons can be taken into the body in four different ways:

   _____

   _____

   _____

   _____

2. In cases of poison ingestion, vomiting is to be avoided under the following five conditions:

   _____

   _____

   _____

   _____

   _____

3. Gastric lavage is contraindicated when a patient has ingested what type of substance?

   _____

4. When is activated charcoal administered?

   _____

5. Why are gastric contents saved after emesis or gastric lavage?

   _____

6. What is the treatment for poisons that contact skin or eyes?

   _____

7. What two groups of people are most at risk for poisoning?

   _____

   _____

8. Name four conditions that may lead to toxic medication reactions in older adults.

   _____

   _____

   _____

   _____

9. What is the leading cause of poisoning deaths in children under six years of age?

_____

10. What is the number of the National Poison Control Center?

_____

Note: A *Comprehensive Review Exam* for Part I can be found at the end of the text following the Summary.

Answers to this comprehensive exam are available in the Instructor's Guide.

PART II
Drug Classifications

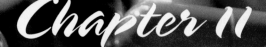

Chapter 11
Vitamins, Minerals, and Herbs

Objectives

Upon completion of this chapter, the learner should be able to

1. Categorize vitamins as water-soluble or fat-soluble
2. List vitamins and their sources, function, signs of deficiency, and symptoms of overdose if known
3. Identify vitamins by name as well as letter
4. List minerals and their sources, function, and signs of deficiency
5. Identify the chemical symbol for each mineral
6. Describe conditions that may require vitamin and/or mineral supplements
7. Explain the role of antioxidants in nutrition therapy
8. Describe why and how consumers should be more vigilant in the use of herbal products
9. Define the Key Terms

The National Academy of Sciences and the National Research Council of the Food and Nutrition Board have listed U.S. Recommended Dietary Allowances (U.S. RDA) of vitamins and minerals necessary for maintenance of good nutrition in the average healthy adult under normal living conditions in the United States. This information was published by the National Academy of Sciences, Washington, DC. A major revision is currently under way to replace the RDA. The revised recommendations are called Dietary Reference Intakes (DRI) and reflect the collaborative efforts of both the United States and Canada. Until 1997, the RDA were the only standards available, and they will continue to serve health professionals until DRI can be established for all nutrients. For this reason, both the 1989 RDA and the 1997

DRI for selected nutrients are presented here. Research is ongoing in this area. The National Academies issue periodic reports, such as those released in April 2000, urging caution with megadoses of antioxidant supplements that can cause adverse side effects.

Under special circumstances, vitamin and mineral **supplements** are required for optimal function and health. *Indications for vitamin and mineral supplements include:*

Inadequate diet. Due to anorexia, weight reduction or other special diets, illness, alcoholism, or poor eating habits

Malabsorption syndromes. Chronic gastrointestinal disorders or surgery that result in chronic diarrhea

Increased need for certain nutrients. As in pregnancy and lactation (especially iron and calcium), infants under one year of age, adolescence, debilitation, illness, unusual physical activity, postmenopausal women (calcium)

Deficiency due to medication interactions. For example, potassium deficiency with diuretic use

Nutrients function in groups or teams. Therefore, if diet supplementation is warranted, it is likely that both vitamins and some additional minerals are needed. An example of this teamwork is bone growth, development, and strength, which depend on calcium, magnesium, vitamin A, vitamin D, and several other nutrients (fluoride, etc.). However, patients should be advised to avoid self-medication with large doses of vitamins or minerals, which may not be indicated if the diet is well balanced and the individual is in good health. **Overdoses** of some vitamins, especially A and D, and some minerals, for example, iron, can be injurious to health. A need or **deficiency** should be established by a physician's diagnosis or blood test before exceeding Recommended Dietary Allowances (RDA). Supplementary (prophylactic) multivitamin preparations may reasonably contain 50%–150% of the RDA of vitamins (except the amount of vitamins A and D and folic acid should not exceed the RDA). Combination vitamin preparations containing iron should not be used unless a deficiency has been established with a blood test or physician's diagnosis.

It is important to differentiate between water-soluble and fat-soluble vitamins in order to avoid build-up in the body with possible symptoms of overdose. Megadoses of vitamins (more than the RDA) should be taken only if prescribed by a physician and/or approved by the FDA. *Remember, the RDA includes the amount from foods you eat as well as supplements.* Research reports have indicated a possibility of damage to tissues with large quantities of vitamins (above RDA), especially those stored in the fat cells of the body.

The Recommended Dietary Allowances listed on the following pages are established for average, normal, healthy adults. Larger amounts are required with certain conditions (e.g., *pregnancy, lactation, and some illnesses*). Larger amounts are required for males than females. The RDAs on the following pages show the amount required for females first, with the amount for males afterward. Smaller amounts are required for children (consult references). However, megadoses should *never* be taken except under the direct supervision of a physician.

FAT-SOLUBLE VITAMINS

The **fat-soluble** vitamins are A, D, E, and K.

Vitamin A (Retinol, Retinal, Beta Carotene)

Vitamin A is processed in the body from the carotene of plants, especially yellow-orange and dark-green leafy vegetables, fruits, oily saltwater fish, dairy products, and eggs (RDA 800–1,000 units/day/DRI 700–3,000 mcg/day). Beta carotene is an antioxidant. (See Antioxidants, later in this chapter.)

Necessary for:

Resistance to infection

Proper visual function at night

Normal growth and development of bones and soft tissue, and maintaining healthy epithelial tissue (skin and mucous membranes)

Healing of wounds (sometimes prescribed for acne)

Possible connection to reproduction

Deficiencies may result from:

Malabsorption of fats or diarrhea

Obstruction of bile

Presence of mineral oil in the intestines

Overcooking of vegetables in an open container (heat and air cause oxidation)

Prolonged infection or fever

Signs of deficiency include:

Night blindness

Slow growth, anorexia, weight loss, bone and teeth deformities

Dry eyes and skin, pruritus (itching)

Supplements of vitamin A (e.g., Aquasol A) may be necessary for:

Infants fed unfortified skim milk or mild-substitute formulas

Those with prolonged infection or fever

Diabetes or hypothyroidism

Liver disease

Vitamin A has been used as a screening test for fat absorption

Some dermatological disorders, for example, psoriasis, are being treated investigationally with retinoids (synthetic vitamin A products). A retinoid product, *Accutane,* is prescribed for severe acne. This product can cause fetal abnormalities and is therefore contraindicated in pregnancy. *Accutane* has also caused increased intracranial pressure, possible liver changes, and other adverse side effects associated with hypervitaminosis A. (See Chapter 12 Skin Medications.)

Symptoms of overdose (hypervitaminosis A) from greater than 50,000 units (15,000 mcg of retinol) in adults and 20,000 units (6,000 mcg of retinol in infants and children) include:

* Irritability and psychiatric symptoms
  Fatigue, lethargy
  Headache, insomnia
* Brittle nails, dry skin and hair
* Anorexia, nausea, diarrhea, and jaundice
  Acute toxicity with increased intracranial pressure, vertigo, coma
* Joint pain, myalgia
  Stunted growth, fetal malformations

Caution should be used with kidney or liver problems or diabetes.

* Long-term use of large doses of vitamin A is *contraindicated* for women who are, or may become, pregnant. *Fetal malformations* have been reported following maternal ingestion of large doses of vitamin A, either before or during pregnancy.

Vitamin D (Calciferol, Cholecalciferol, Ergocalciferol)

Vitamin D is synthesized in the body through the action of sunlight on the skin. Other sources include fish oils and food products fortified with vitamin D, such as milk and cereals (RDA 400 units/day/DRI 5–15 mcg).

Necessary for:

Maintenance of normal nerves and muscles

Regulating the absorption and metabolism of calcium and phosphorus for healthy bones and teeth

Pregnancy and lactation, when it is especially important

Signs of deficiency include:

Poor tooth and bone structure (rickets)

Skeletal deformities

Osteoporosis, osteomalacia

Tetany (muscle spasms)

Vitamin D supplements are prescribed as calcifediol, calcitriol, or ergocalciferol to prevent or treat rickets or osteomalacia and to manage hypocalcemia in cases of parathyroid malfunction. The difference between therapeutic dosage and that causing hypercalcemia is very small and dosage must be carefully regulated and monitored.

Symptoms of vitamin D overdose and toxicity include:

Nausea, anorexia, weight loss
* Muscle and/or bone pain
* Kidney damage and kidney stone

* Hypercalcemia and convulsions, calcium deposits in soft tissues
* Fetal disorders

Caution not to exceed the RDA of vitamin D especially with:

> Cardiovascular disorders
> Kidney diseases
> Pregnancy (possible fetal malformations or mental retardation)
> Lactation

Interactions (overdose may antagonize) with:

> Digitalis
> Thiazide diuretics
> Mineral oil may interfere with intestinal absorption of vitamin D.

Vitamin E (Tocopherol)

Vitamin E is abundant in nature, found especially in cereals, wheat germ, seeds, nuts, vegetable oils, eggs, meat, and poultry (RDA 30 units/day/DRI 15–1,000 mg/day). Vitamin E has antioxidant properties (see Antioxidants later in this chapter).

Necessary for:

> Normal metabolism
> Protection of tissues of the eyes, skin, liver, breast, muscles, and lungs
> Protecting red blood cells (RBCs) from damage
> Decreasing platelet clumping

Research is ongoing in the use and benefits of vitamin E supplements as one of the treatment protocols for management of early Alzheimer's disease and for possibly slowing the progress of such symptoms as memory loss. However, such supplements will neither cure nor prevent the disease.

Deficiencies are found in those with:

> Alcohol abuse
> Malabsorption syndromes, for example, celiac disease, sprue, cystic fibrosis
> Pathological conditions of liver and pancreas
> Sickle-cell anemia
> Also found in premature infants or low-birth-weight neonates

Signs of deficiency are not firmly established. Premature infants may show irritability, edema, or hemolytic anemia. Deficient adults may show muscle weakness and some abnormal laboratory values, such as low RBC count.

 Vitamin E overdose (1200 units) can result in prolonged clotting times.

Note: Vitamin E supplements should be discontinued ten days prior to surgery because of the danger of prolonged bleeding time. Vitamin E supplements should not be taken while on anticoagulant therapy because of increased risk of bleeding.

Interactions: Excessive use of mineral oil may decrease the absorption of vitamin E.

Vitamin K (Phytonadione)

Vitamin K is found in green or leafy vegetables, cabbage, vegetable oils, cheese, eggs, and liver and is absorbed in the small intestine in the presence of bile salts (RDA 60–80 mg/day/DRI 90–120 mcg/day).

Necessary for blood clotting.

Deficiencies may result from reduced prothrombin in the blood due to:

Insufficient clotting factors in the newborn

Malabsorption syndromes, ulcerative colitis, prolonged diarrhea

Coumarin overdose

Prolonged use of salicylates, quinine, and broad-spectrum or long-term hyperalimentation antibiotics

Signs of deficiency include:

Increased clotting time

Petechiae and bruising

Blood in the urine (hematuria)

Blood in the stool (melena)

Vitamin K is usually prescribed as phytonadione (Mephyton tabs or Aqua-Mephyton IM or SubQ). Vitamin K is sometimes administered as an antidote for bleeding complications during coumarin therapy. Vitamin K is only effective for bleeding disorders due to low concentrations of prothrombin in the blood. It is not effective for bleeding from other causes such as heparin overdose.

The American Academy of Pediatrics recommends that vitamin K (phytonadione) be routinely administered to infants at birth to prevent hemorrhagic disease of the newborn. Some state regulations currently require this prophylaxis.

Adverse effects are rare, but hypersensitivity reactions have occurred with IV injections. **Toxicity** in infants can cause jaundice or hemolytic anemia.

Note: Patients receiving anticoagulant therapy should be consistent in the amount of vitamin K–rich foods they eat daily in order to keep prothrombin levels stable. Large amounts of vitamin K–rich foods can counteract the anticoagulant therapy. See Chapter 25, Cardiovascular Drugs, for more information regarding anticoagulant therapy.

WATER-SOLUBLE VITAMINS

The water-soluble vitamins include the B-complex vitamins and vitamin C.

Vitamin B₁ (Thiamine)

Vitamin B_1 is a coenzyme utilized for carbohydrate metabolism. It is found in whole grains, wheat germ, peas, beans, nuts, yeast, meat, especially pork and organ meats, oysters, collard greens, oranges, and enriched cereals (RDA 1–1.5 mg/day).

Necessary for normal function of the nervous and cardiovascular systems.

Deficiencies in the United States may be due to:

> Chronic alcoholism
>
> Malabsorption

Signs of deficiency (beriberi; symptoms sometimes vague) include:

> Anorexia and constipation, GI upset, nausea
>
> Neuritis, pain, tingling in extremities, loss of reflexes
>
> Muscle weakness, fatigue, ataxia
>
> Mental depression, memory loss, confusion
>
> Cardiovascular problems
>
> Hypersensitivity reactions have occurred mainly following repeated IV administration of the drug.

Vitamin B₂ (Riboflavin)

Vitamin B_2 is a coenzyme utilized in the metabolism of glucose, fats, and amino acids. It is found in milk; eggs; nuts; meats, especially liver; yeast; enriched bread; and green leafy vegetables (RDA 1.3–1.8 mg/day).

Necessary for cell growth and metabolism with release of energy from carbohydrates, protein, and fat in food. Also functions to regulate certain hormones and in formation of RBCs.

Deficiencies of vitamin B_2 in the United States may be due to:

> Chronic alcoholism
>
> Poor diet
>
> Medications such as probenecid

Signs of deficiency include:

> Glossitis (inflammation of the tongue)
>
> Cheilosis (cracking at corners of mouth)
>
> Dermatitis, photophobia, vision loss, burning or itching eyes

Vitamin B₆ (Pyridoxine)

Vitamin B_6 is a coenzyme utilized in the metabolism of carbohydrates, fats, protein, and amino acids. It is found in meats, fish, poultry, legumes, peanuts, soybeans, wheat germ, whole-grain cereals, and bananas (RDA 1.6–2 mg/day). There is significant loss of B_6 when foods are frozen.

Deficiencies may be due to:

Chronic alcoholism

Drug interactions with isoniazid, other antitubercular drugs, oral contraceptives

Cirrhosis

Malabsorption syndromes

Signs of deficiency include:

Seizure activity in infants

Neuritis, dermatitis, nausea, vomiting, and depression in adults

Caution: Overdose in pregnant women may result in newborns with seizures who have developed a need for greater than normal amounts of pyridoxine.

Patient Education

Patients taking levodopa alone (not combined with carbidopa) should be instructed not to take vitamin B_6 supplement because it antagonizes the action of levodopa.

Vitamin B₁₂ (Cobalamin, Cyanocobalamin)

Vitamin B_{12} is found in meats (especially organ meats), poultry, fish and shellfish, milk, cheese, and eggs. Absorption of vitamin B_{12} depends on intrinsic factor, which is normally present in the gastric juice of humans. Absence of this factor leads to vitamin B_{12} deficiency and pernicious anemia (RDA 2 mcg/day).

The National Academy of Sciences now suggests that all Americans over the age of 50 begin taking a low-dose vitamin B_{12} supplement (6 mcg per day) or regularly eat breakfast cereals that are fortified with the vitamin. The problem is that as many as 30% of adults over 50 have diminished gastric acid production, and therefore they lack intrinsic factor, which is necessary for absorption of vitamin B_{12}. This is especially true for those taking medications that reduce gastric acid, for example, cimetidine (Tagamet).

Necessary for maturation of red blood cells and maintenance of the nervous system.

Deficiencies can be associated with:

Vegetarian diets without meat, eggs, or milk products

Gastrectomy or intestinal resections

Malabsorption syndromes

Pernicious anemia, megaloblastic (macrocytic) anemia

Signs of deficiency include:

Anemia and weakness first symptoms of clinical deficiency

Poor muscle coordination

Numbness of hands and feet (paresthesia)

Mental confusion, disorientation, memory loss, and irritability

Treatment for pernicious anemia consists of vitamin B_{12}, cyanocobalamin (Betalin 12 or Rubramin), 100–1,000 mcg IM monthly for life to prevent neurological damage.

Side effects include:

Transient diarrhea

Itching and urticaria

Anaphylaxis (rare)

Interactions may occur (decreased absorption of B_{12}) with:

Aminoglycoside antibiotics

Anticonvulsants

Slow-release potassium and colchicine

Patient Education

Patients should avoid taking large doses of vitamin B_{12} without confirmed deficiency, as megadoses may mask symptoms of folic acid deficiency or cause complications in those with cardiac or gout conditions.

Folic Acid (Folacin)

Folic acid is a vitamin included in the B-complex group and is found in leafy and green vegetables (broccoli), avocado, beets, orange juice, kidney beans, and organ meats (RDA 400 mcg/day). Folic acid is lost with overcooking and reheating.

Necessary for protein synthesis, production of RBCs, cell division, and normal growth and maintenance of all cells. Deficiency during pregnancy can result in neural tube defects, such as spina bifida, in the newborn.

Deficiencies can be associated with:

Improper diet

Chronic alcoholism

Liver pathology

Intestinal obstruction

Megaloblastic and macrocytic anemia

Malabsorption syndromes, malnutrition

Renal dialysis or prolonged use of some medicines (listed below)

Signs of deficiency include:

Anorexia, weight loss, weakness

Irritability, behavior disorders

Caution: Folic acid (Folvite) *should not be given to anyone with undiagnosed anemia,* since it may mask the diagnosis of pernicious anemia. OTC vitamin supplements should contain no more than 0.4 mg; however, 1-mg doses are available by prescription.

Interactions of folic acid, over RDA, could interfere with action of the following drugs:

Phenytoin (Dilantin)

Estrogen (oral contraceptives)

Barbiturates, or nitrofurantoin

Patient Education

Patients should avoid taking folic acid supplements without consulting a physician first.

Niacin (Nicotinic Acid, Niacinamide)

Niacin is a vitamin included in the B-complex group and is found in meat, chicken, milk, eggs, fish, green vegetables, cooked dried beans and peas, soybeans, nuts, peanut butter, and enriched cereal products (RDA 15–19 mg/day).

Necessary for lipid metabolism and nerve functioning, especially in circulation and maintenance of all cells.

Deficiency results in pellagra, a severe skin and mucous membrane disorder progressing to systemic and central nervous system disorders.

Signs of niacin deficiency include:

Peripheral vascular insufficiency

Dermatitis and varicose ulcers

Diarrhea

Dementia, hallucinations, depression

Mouth sores

Lethargy, weakness, anorexia, indigestion

Niacin is used primarily to prevent and treat pellagra. Other treatment indications (usually as an adjunct with other medications) include:

Many vascular disorders (e.g., vascular spasm, arteriosclerosis, Raynaud's disease, angina, and varicose and pressure ulcers)

Circulatory disturbances of the inner ear, Ménière's syndrome

Lower blood lipid levels (see Chapter 25)

Daily doses of up to 1,000 mg appear to be safe.

Side effects of niacin, especially over 1,000 mg daily, can include:

* Headache, flushing, and burning sensations of face, neck, and chest
* Postural hypotension

Jaundice

Nausea, diarrhea, vomiting

* Increased blood glucose and uric acid

Caution for patients with liver disease, gallbladder disease, gout, or diabetes

Patient Education

Patients should be instructed regarding possible side effects, especially flushing and a burning sensation, and should be cautioned to rise slowly from a reclining position. They should be told that the flushing usually resolves within two weeks. Taking niacin in divided doses, or extended-release products, can sometimes lessen this effect. Sometimes aspirin is prescribed to counteract flushing.

Vitamin C (Ascorbic Acid)

Vitamin C is a water-soluble vitamin found in fresh fruits and vegetables, especially citrus fruits, cantaloupe, tomatoes, cabbage, green peppers, and broccoli. It is unstable when exposed to heat or air or combined with alkaline compounds (e.g., antacids). Adding baking soda to vegetables for color retention destroys vitamin C (RDA 75–90 mg/day).

Necessary for formation of intracellular substances (collagen), and for normal teeth, gums, and bones. Also required for iron absorption. Vitamin C is considered an antioxidant. (See Antioxidants later in this chapter.) Also promotes healing of wounds and bone fractures.

Deficiencies are associated with:

Diet lacking fresh fruit and vegetables

Alcoholism, infections

Smoking

Signs of the vitamin C deficiency disease (scurvy) include:

Muscle weakness and cramping

Sore and bleeding mouth and gums, loose teeth

Capillary fragility (bruising); dry, scaly skin

Poor healing

Supplements of ascorbic acid are available in capsules, tablets (extended-release), solution, chewables, or injection form. They are indicated for:

Treatment of scurvy (adults 100–250 mg bid, children 100–300 mg/day divided doses)

Hemodialysis patients (100–200 mg daily)

Infants beginning at two to four weeks of age (20–50 mg/day)

Prevention or treatment of the common cold (1–2 g/day)

Dosages larger than that recommended are to be avoided because of the potential for side effects. In addition, since ascorbic acid is water soluble, more than 50% of the dose is excreted in the urine of normal subjects. Excretion of less than 20% of the dose over 24 h suggests vitamin C deficiency.

Side effects of large doses of vitamin C, more than RDA, can include:

✳ Heartburn, abdominal cramps, nausea, vomiting, and diarrhea

✳ Increased uric acid levels; may precipitate gouty arthritis

✳ Increased urinary calcium; may precipitate kidney stone formation

✳ Scurvy in neonates following large amounts during pregnancy

False negative for colon cancer test

Interactions may occur with:

Aspirin, causing elevated blood levels of aspirin

Barbiturates, tetracyclines, estrogens, oral contraceptives, which may increase requirements for vitamin C

Alcohol and smoking, which may decrease vitamin C level

Patient Education

Patients should be given the following information concerning vitamin C:

Vitamin C is destroyed by heat and air; therefore, raw fresh fruits and vegetables are best.

Large quantities of supplemental vitamin C are to be avoided, unless prescribed by a doctor, because of potential side effects, such as gastric irritation, increased uric acid, and kidney stones.

Antacids should not be taken at the same time as vitamin C supplements because the alkaline compound neutralizes the ascorbic acid.

Megadoses of vitamin C taken during pregnancy may cause the newborn to require larger than average amounts of ascorbic acid.

See Table 11-1 for a summary of water- and fat-soluble vitamins.

Table 11-1 Summary of Fat-Soluble and Water-Soluble Vitamins

NAME (FAT SOLUBLE)	FOOD SOURCES	FUNCTIONS	DEFICIENCY/TOXICITY

Vitamin A (retinol, beta carotene)	Animal
	   Oily saltwater fish
	   Dairy products
	   Eggs
	Plants
	   Dark-green leafy vegetables
	   Deep yellow or orange fruit and vegetables
		Dim light vision
		Maintenance of mucous membranes
		Growth and development of bones
		Healing of wounds
		Resistance to infection
		Beta carotene is an antioxidant
			Deficiency
			Retarded growth
			Faulty bone and tooth development
			Night blindness
			Dry skin
			Xerophthalmia (dry eyes)
			Toxicity
			(hypervitaminosis A)
			Irritability, lethargy, headache
			Joint pain, myalgia
			Stunted growth, fetal malformations
			Jaundice, nausea, diarrhea
			Dry skin and hair

Vitamin D (cholecalciferol)	Animal
	   Fish oils
	   Fortified milk
	Plants
	   Fortified cereals
		Healthy bones and teeth
		Muscle function
		Enables absorption of calcium
			Deficiency
			Softening bones:
			   Rickets (in children)
			   Osteomalacia (in adults)
			Poorly developed teeth
			Muscle spasms
			Toxicity
			(Hypercalcemia), convulsions
			Kidney stones, kidney damage
			Muscle/bone pain
			Nausea, anorexia
			Fetal disorders

Vitamin E (tocopherol)	Plants
	   Vegetable oils
	   Seeds, nuts
	   Wheat germ, cereals
		Antioxidant
		Decreases platelet clumping
		Normal metabolism and tissue protection
			Deficiency
			Destruction of RBCs, muscle weakness
			Toxicity
			Prolonged bleeding time

Vitamin K (phytonadione)	Animal
	   Egg yolk, cheese
	   Liver
	Plants
	   Vegetable oil
	   Green leafy vegetables
	   Cabbage, broccoli
		Blood clotting	**Deficiency**
			Prolonged blood clotting time
			Blood in urine and stool
			Toxicity
			Jaundice in infants

(continued)

Table 11-1 Summary of Fat-Soluble and Water-Soluble Vitamins—*continued*

NAME (WATER SOLUBLE)	FOOD SOURCES	FUNCTIONS	DEFICIENCY/TOXICITY

Vitamin B_1 (thiamine)	Animal
	  Pork, beef, liver
	  Oysters
	Plants
	  Yeast
	  Whole and enriched grains, wheat germ
	  Beans, peas, collard greens, nuts, asparagus
	  Oranges
		Normal nervous and cardiovascular systems	**Deficiency**
			GI upset, constipation
			Neuritis, mental disturbance
			Cardiovascular problems
			Muscle weakness, fatigue
			Toxicity
			None known

Vitamin B_2 (riboflavin)	Animal
	  Milk
	  Meat, liver
	Plants
	  Green vegetables
	  Cereals
	  Enriched bread
	  Yeast
		Aids in energy metabolism of glucose, fats, and amino acids	**Deficiency**
			Cheilosis
			Glossitis
			Photophobia, vision problems, itching eyes
			Dermatitis, rough skin
			Toxicity
			None

Vitamin B_6 (pyridoxine)	Animal
	  Pork, beef, chicken, tuna, salmon
	Plants
	  Whole-grain cereals, wheat germ
	  Legumes, peanuts, soybeans
	  Bananas
		Synthesis of amino acids
		Antibody production
		Maintenance of blood glucose level
			Deficiency
			Anorexia, nausea, vomiting
			Dermatitis
			Neuritis, depression
			Toxicity
			Seizures in newborn

Vitamin B_{12} (cyanocobalamin)	Animal
	  Seafood/shellfish
	  Meat, poultry, liver
	  Eggs
	  Milk, cheese
	Plants
	  None
		Synthesis of RBCs
		Maintenance of nervous system
			Deficiency
			Nerve, muscle, mental problems
			Pernicious anemia
			Toxicity
			None

Niacin (nicotinic acid)	Animal
	  Milk
	  Eggs
	  Fish
	  Poultry
	Plants
	  Legumes, nuts
	  Green vegetables
		Lipid metabolism
		Nerve functioning
			Deficiency
			Pellagra
			Toxicity
			Headache, flushing
			Increased blood glucose and uric acid

Table 11-1 Summary of Fat-Soluble and Water-Soluble Vitamins—*continued*

NAME (WATER SOLUBLE)	FOOD SOURCES	FUNCTIONS	DEFICIENCY/TOXICITY

Folacin (folic acid)	Animal
	  Organ meats
	Plants
	  Green leafy vegetables
	  Avocado, beets
	  Broccoli, kidney beans
	  Orange juice
		Synthesis of RBCs, leukocytes, DNA and RNA
		Needed for normal growth and reproduction
			Deficiency
			Increased risk of neural tube defects
			Macrocytic anemia
			Irritability, behavior disorders
			Toxicity
			None

Vitamin C (ascorbic acid)	Fruits
	  All citrus, cantaloupe
	Plants
	  Broccoli
	  Tomatoes
	  Brussel sprouts
	  Cabbage
	  Green peppers
		Normal teeth, gums, and bone
		Prevention of scurvy
		Formation of collagen
		Healing of wounds
		Absorption of iron
		Antioxidant
			Deficiency
			Scurvy
			Poor healing
			Muscle cramps/ weakness
			Ulcerated gums/mouth, loose teeth
			Capillary fragility (bruising)
			Toxicity
			Raise uric acid level, gout
			GI distress
			Kidney stones
			Rebound scurvy in neonates

MINERALS

Minerals are chemical elements occurring in nature and in body fluids. The correct balance of each is required for maintenance of health. Minerals dissolved in the body fluids are called *electrolytes* because they carry positive or negative electrical charges required for body activities, such as conduction of nerve impulses, beating of the heart, skeletal muscle contraction, absorption of nutrients from the GI tract, protein synthesis, energy production, blood formation, and many other body processes.

Necessary for:

Homeostasis (body balance).

The correct ratio of fluids to electrolytes must be maintained for normal functioning of the body. Fluids and minerals are excreted daily and must be replaced with fluid and food intake.

The principal minerals in the body and their chemical symbols are sodium (Na), chloride (Cl), potassium (K), calcium (Ca), and iron (Fe).

Sodium and Chloride

Sodium and chloride are the principal minerals in the extracellular body fluids. Blood contains approximately 0.9% sodium chloride. The best source of sodium and chloride is table salt (NaCl).

Deficiencies of sodium and chloride are associated with:

Excessive fluid loss: bleeding, diarrhea, vomiting, or excessive perspiration

Insufficient oral intake (starvation or extended fasting)

Alkalosis (chloride deficiency)

Treatment consists of intravenous therapy with sodium chloride (NaCl) according to needs:

Normal saline solution (0.9% sodium chloride)

Half-normal saline solution (0.45% sodium chloride)

Quarter-normal saline solution (0.2% sodium chloride)

Sometimes other minerals are required and are also added to the intravenous fluids.

Potassium (K)

Potassium is another of the principal minerals within cells. Natural sources of potassium include citrus, bananas, tomatoes, potato skin, cantaloupe, avocadoes, dried fruits, cooked dried beans, and peas.

Necessary for:

Acid-base and fluid balance

Normal muscular irritability (heartbeat regulation)

Deficiencies are associated with:

Insufficient oral intake due to surgery, anorexia, or weight-reduction diets

Diarrhea or vomiting

Diabetic ketoacidosis

Diaphoresis (excessive perspiration)

Diuretic use, especially thiazides and furosemide

Digitalis toxicity

Long-term use of corticosteroids or long-term use of laxatives

Kidney disease

Signs of deficiency include:

Muscular weakness, paralysis

Cardiac arrhythmias

Lethargy and fatigue, mental apathy and confusion

Treatment consists of:

KCL given IV postoperatively or for severe dehydration (diluted according to directions)

One of the numerous oral products available, usually in effervescent tablet or powder form, to be dissolved in water or juice and taken after meals (e.g., K-Lyte 50–100 mEq daily), or capsules to be swallowed (e.g., Micro-K), extended-release tablets (e.g., K-Dur, or Slow-K), or oral liquid preparations (e.g., Kaochlor).

Side effects of potassium overdose can include:

Nausea, vomiting, or diarrhea

GI bleeding, or abdominal pain

Pain at the injection site or phlebitis may occur during IV administration of solutions containing 30 mEq or more potassium per liter. IV solutions containing potassium should always be run at a slow rate to prevent pain or hyperkalemia.

Hyperkalemia (excessive potassium in the blood) is not likely to result from oral administration, except in the case of severe renal impairment. Care must be taken when adding potassium to IV solutions that the dilute solution is thoroughly mixed, inverted, and agitated, before the solution is hung for administration. Never add potassium to hanging IV solution.

Symptoms of potassium overdosage can include:

Confusion

Weakness or paralysis of extremities

Fall in the blood pressure and/or *cardiac arrhythmias* from hyperkalemia

Caution with use of potassium in the following conditions:

Cardiac disease

Renal impairment

Gastric or intestinal ulcers (extended-release products contraindicated)

Mental confusion (unable to follow directions properly)

Patient Education

Patients taking potassium should be instructed regarding:

Natural sources of potassium-rich foods

Conditions requiring potassium supplements

Directions for taking potassium supplements with or after meals to avoid GI distress and following directions on package carefully

The importance of *dissolving* the tablet in at least four to eight oz of water *completely* before taking it and *never* holding the tablet in the mouth or swallowing the tablet whole

Notifying a doctor immediately of any side effects

Calcium (Ca)

Calcium is a mineral component of bones and teeth. It is absorbed in the small intestine with the help of vitamin D. Natural sources include milk and dairy products (RDA 1,000–1,200 mg/day). In postmenopausal women not receiving estrogen therapy, the RDA is about 1,500 mg/day. Those who are lactose intolerant (unable to take milk) should include dark-green leafy vegetables (except spinach), broccoli, and canned fish with the bones. (DRI 1,000–1,300 mg/day, with the higher figure recommended for adolescents of both sexes and postmenopausal women.)

Necessary for:

Strong bones and teeth

Contraction of cardiac, smooth, and skeletal muscles

Nerve conduction

Blood coagulation, capillary permeability, and normal blood pressure

The balance between calcium and magnesium is important in the prevention of heart disease

Deficiencies (supplements required) are associated with:

Pregnancy and lactation

Postmenopausal women (or those with estrogen deficiency)

Hypoparathyroidism

Long-term use of corticosteroids, some diuretics, or anticonvulsants

Chronic diarrhea, pancreatitis, renal failure

Lack of weight-bearing exercise

Signs of deficiency may include:

Osteoporosis, or osteomalacia (softening of bones), including frequent fractures, especially in the elderly

Rickets in children (softening of bones)

Muscle pathology, including cardiac myopathy or tetany (muscle spasm) and leg cramps

Increased clotting time

Treatment consists of calcium supplements 400–600 mg daily PO. A higher-dosage supplement is required for those not including calcium-rich foods in the diet, (e.g., without dairy products). The RDA, *including foods,* are 1,200 mg/day for adults and 1,500 mg/day for postmenopausal women not taking estrogen. Many products and combinations are available including calcium gluconate, calcium carbonate, or calcium lactate. Of these three, calcium carbonate delivers the highest amount of elemental calcium per tablet.

Adding vitamin D for calcium metabolism may be necessary without exposure to sunlight (see Vitamin D).

Side effects of calcium salts can include:

Constipation from oral products

Tissue irritation from IV products

✴ When injected IV, calcium salts should be administered *very slowly* to prevent tissue necrosis or *cardiac arrhythmias*

Caution: Calcium should be used cautiously, if at all, with:

Cardiac disease

Renal disease

Respiratory conditions (e.g., sarcoidosis)

Administration: Most oral calcium supplements should be administered 1–1.5 h after meals, unless specified otherwise on the label.

Interactions may occur with:

Digitalis, resulting in potentiation (may cause arrhythmias)

Tetracycline, resulting in antagonism (inactivates the antibiotic)

Patient Education

Patients taking calcium should be instructed regarding:

Calcium-rich diet, especially dairy products and vitamin D–fortified milk, which can be low-fat

Necessity for calcium supplements, usually recommended for women beginning at age 35, and especially for postmenopausal women not on estrogen therapy

Importance of upright exercise, for example, walking at least three to four times per week to preserve bone mass

Importance of outdoor activity because sunlight helps create vitamin D necessary for calcium metabolism

Taking calcium supplements 1–1½ h after meals, unless specified otherwise on the label

Not taking calcium at the same time as other medicines

Iron (Fe)

Iron is the oxygen-carrying component of blood. Iron is a mineral found in meat (especially liver), egg yolk, beans, spinach, enriched cereals, dried fruits, prune juice, and poultry.

Necessary for hemoglobin formation.

Deficiencies (supplements recommended) with:

Hemorrhage and excessive menstrual flow

Internal bleeding, ulcers, and GI tumors

Pregnancy

Infancy

Puberty at time of growth spurt

Patients undergoing hemodialysis

Signs of deficiency may include:

Paleness of the skin and/or mucous membranes

Lethargy and weakness

Vertigo

Air hunger

Decline in mental skills

Irregular heartbeat and function

Cravings for nonfood items, for example, ice, clay, or starch (called pica)

Treatment of anemia due to iron deficiency consists of administration of iron preparations:

Oral iron products. Ferrous sulfate (Feosol, Fer-in-Sol, and others). Adults 50–100 mg tid after meals (not with milk, coffee, or tea), infants and children 4–6 mg/kg daily in three divided doses in juice or with meals (not with milk).

Injectable iron. Iron dextran (INFeD) 50–100 mg *deep* IM by the *Z-track method only.* Extreme caution is urged to prevent solution contacting the subcutaneous tissue because of its irritating effect. A fresh 2-inch needle is recommended at the time of administration. Iron dextran also can be given IV *slowly* after testing for sensitivity with a small trial dose.

Side effects of taking iron preparations can include:

 Black stools

Nausea and vomiting (GI effects can be minimized by taking iron after or with meals, *but not with coffee, tea, or milk*)

Constipation or diarrhea

Anaphylactic reactions or phlebitis with IV administration of iron dextran

Contraindicated in patients with peptic ulcer, regional enteritis, or ulcerative colitis

Parenteral iron should *not* be administered concomitantly with oral iron therapy.

Iron should *not* be administered without confirming a diagnosis of deficiency with a blood test and determining cause of deficiency.

Interactions may occur with:

Vitamin C or orange juice, taken at same time, which *enhances* iron absorption

Coffee or tea taken within two hours of iron, which reduces iron absorption by as much as 50%

Tetracycline, absorption of which is inhibited by oral iron preparations when taken within two hours

Antacids, which decrease iron absorption (should not be given at same time)

Symptoms of acute overdose of iron may occur within minutes or days and include:

Lethargy

Shock

Vomiting and diarrhea

Erosion of GI tract/hemochromatosis

Liver or kidney damage

Patient Education

Patients taking iron supplements should be instructed regarding:

Avoidance of self-medication without established need (blood test) and without medical supervision to determine why hemoglobin is low. Taking iron when not prescribed could mask the symptoms of internal bleeding or GI malignancy.

Black stools to be expected

Taking iron at meals to minimize GI distress and with orange juice for better absorption

Interactions (i.e., avoidance of coffee, tea, milk, or antacids at same time)

Caution with flavored children's tablets (overdosage can be dangerous, even fatal)

Taking liquid iron preparations with drinking straw to avoid temporary stain of dental enamel

The iron in meats is called heme iron and is better absorbed than nonheme iron in vegetables and fruits

Nonheme iron is absorbed better if consumed with a rich source of vitamin C (e. g., orange juice)

Zinc

Zinc is a component of numerous enzymes and is an essential element in metabolism. It is usually found in adequate amounts in a well-balanced diet. Rich sources include lean meat, organ meats, oysters, poultry, fish, and whole grain breads and cereals (RDA 8–11 mg/d). Zinc is an antioxidant.

Necessary for:

Wound healing

Mineralization of bone

Insulin glucose regulation

Normal taste

Deficiencies (supplements recommended) with:

>   Inadequate or vegetarian diet

>   Chronic, nonhealing wounds

>   Major surgery or trauma

Deficiency symptoms can include:

>   Poor wound healing

>   Reduced taste perception

>   Poor alcohol tolerance, glucose intolerance

>   Anemia, slowed growth, sterility

>   Dermatitis and hair loss

Toxicity (more than 2 g/day) may cause:

>   Nausea, GI distress, vomiting

>   Copper deficiency with extended use of high levels of zinc

Treatment consists of tablets or capsules administered with meals tid to minimize gastric distress. Standard supplement of zinc is no more than 50 mg/24 h. If a zinc supplement is required for more than 90 days, blood levels should be monitored. Chronic consumption of high levels of zinc may cause copper deficiency.

Many combinations of various vitamins and minerals are available in OTC products with various strengths and forms.

Patient Education

Vitamins and Minerals

Patients should be instructed regarding:

Well-balanced diets and natural sources of vitamins and minerals

Food preparation to avoid loss of vitamins

Information regarding signs of deficiency and overdose/toxicity

Caution taking supplements without established need or without medical supervision, especially megadoses, fat-soluble vitamins, and iron

Proper administration to minimize side effects

See Table 11-2 for summary of major minerals.

Table 11-2 Summary of Major Minerals

NAME	FOOD SOURCES	FUNCTIONS	DEFICIENCY/TOXICITY
Calcium (Ca)	Milk, cheese, yogurt Sardines Salmon Green vegetables except spinach	Development of bones and teeth Contraction of cardiac, smooth and skeletal muscles Nerve conduction Blood clotting	**Deficiency** Osteoporosis, osteomalacia Rickets (in children) Muscle pathology Heart disease Increased clotting time **Toxicity** None known
Potassium (K)	Oranges, bananas Dried fruits Tomatoes	Contraction of muscles Heartbeat regulation Transmission of nerve impulses Maintaining fluid balance	**Deficiency** (Hypokalemia) Muscle weakness Cardiac arrhythmias Lethargy, mental confusion **Toxicity** (Hyperkalemia) Confusion Weakness Cardiac arrhythmias
Sodium (Na)	Table salt Beef, eggs Milk, cheese	Maintaining fluid balance in blood Transmission of nerve impulses	**Deficiency** Hyponatremia **Toxicity** Increase in blood pressure
Chloride (Cl)	Table salt	Gastric acidity Regulation of osmotic pressure Activation of salivary amylase	**Deficiency** Imbalance in gastric acidity Imbalance in blood pH **Toxicity** Diarrhea
Magnesium (Mg) (DRI 320–420 mg)	Green vegetables Whole grains	Synthesis of ATP (adenosine triphosphate) Transmission of nerve impulses Relaxation of skeletal muscles	**Deficiency** (seldom) Imbalance Weakness **Toxicity** Diarrhea
Iron (Fe)	Meat Liver Eggs Poultry Spinach Dried fruits Dried beans Prune juice	Hemoglobin formation	**Deficiency** (anemia) Pale Weak Lethargy Vertigo Air hunger Irregular heartbeat **Toxicity** Lethargy, shock Vomiting, diarrhea Erosion of GI tract Liver or kidney damage

(continued)

Table 11-2 Summary of Major Minerals—*continued*

NAME	FOOD SOURCES	FUNCTIONS	DEFICIENCY/TOXICITY
Iodine (I)	Freshwater shellfish and seafood Iodized salt	Major component of thyroid hormones Regulating rate of metabolism Growth, reproduction Nerve and muscle function Skin and hair growth	**Deficiency** Goiter Hypothyroidism **Toxicity** "Iodine goiter" Hyperactive, enlarged goiter
Zinc (Zn)	Meat Liver Oysters Poultry Fish Whole-grain bread and cereal	Wound healing Mineralization of bone Insulin glucose regulation Normal taste Antioxidant	**Deficiency** Poor wound healing Reduced taste perception Alcohol/glucose intolerance **Toxicity** GI distress Copper deficiency with extended use of high levels of zinc

ANTIOXIDANTS

No discussion of nutrition would be complete without an explanation of the antioxidants, as we know them. **Antioxidants,** sometimes referred to as "anticancer foods," or "natural drugs," inhibit cell destruction in damaged or aging tissues. Nucleic acids, which make up the genetic code within the cell, usually act to regulate normal cell function and the growth and repair of damaged or aging tissues.

Free radicals attack the cells, causing damage, which prevents the transport of nutrients, oxygen, and water into the cell and the removal of waste products. This damage affects the nucleic acids in their function of growth and repair of tissue. Free radical damage is associated with several age-related diseases. For example, damage to the nucleic acids might initiate growth of abnormal cells, the first step in cancer development. Also, free radical attack to the cell membranes of the tissues lining the blood vessels can lead to cholesterol accumulation in the damaged arteries, the initial state of atherosclerosis and heart disease. Additionally, free radicals are associated with inflammation, drug-induced organ damage, immunosuppression, and possibly other disorders as well.

The body has developed an antioxidant system response to defend itself from free radicals. An antioxidant is defined as any compound that fights against the destructive effects of free radical oxidants. This system is comprised of enzymes, vitamins, and minerals. Antioxidants function in the prevention of free radical formation by binding to, and neutralizing, destructive substances before they damage cells and tissues.

The antioxidant vitamins—vitamin C, vitamin E, and beta carotene—can function independently of enzymes. Antioxidant minerals include copper, manganese, selenium, and zinc. These minerals work with antioxidant enzymes and are essential to proper enzyme function. If the diet is inadequate in these minerals, the enzyme is not produced, or is ineffective.

Research on antioxidants is ongoing. However, statistical findings at this time indicate that "natural" antioxidants in foods are much more effective than synthetic products.

A report issued in April 2000 by the National Academies stated that, "insufficient evidence exists to support claims that taking megadoses of antioxidants can prevent chronic diseases." They also state that extremely large doses may lead to health problems, rather than confer benefits.

The pharmaceutical magazine, *Drug Topics,* January 2000, provides a caution that taking antioxidants while undergoing chemotherapy or radiation treatments could be contraindicated. Chemotherapy and radiation generate free radicals, and they need an oxidative process to actually kill tumor cells. By giving antioxidants concurrently with chemotherapy or radiation, you actually can increase the tumor cell's life. It is recommended that patients stop taking antioxidants two days before chemotherapy or radiation, and avoid them during the treatment and for two days after completion of the treatment.

Patient Education

Patients asking about antioxidants should be instructed regarding:

Foods that provide antioxidant action

Natural antioxidants in certain foods, which are more effective than synthetic products

ALTERNATIVE MEDICINES
Herbs and Other Dietary Supplements

As a provider of health care, you will be asked about dietary supplements and, in particular, about **herbal** remedies. It is important for you to be able to answer these questions effectively and refer your patients to reliable sources of information. There are many books on the market and articles on the Internet describing the use of herbal remedies. In assessing the value of these resources, question the source, the credentials of the author, the research involved in collecting the data, and the reliability and validity of the statistics. Be sure that the information is based on fact, not opinion. You have a responsibility to caution your patients regarding the dangers of taking remedies not approved by the FDA, and especially the risk of possible interactions between "natural products" and prescription drugs.

The FDA has published a report entitled *A FDA Guide to Dietary Supplements,* which answers many questions on this subject. The following information was taken from that report and from the *FDA Talk Paper* of January 2000: *FDA Finalizes Rules for Claims on Dietary Supplements.*

Congress passed the Dietary Supplement Health and Education Act of 1994 (DSHEA), which amended the Food, Drug, and Cosmetic Act to recognize dietary supplements as distinct from food additives and drugs, which are monitored and regulated by the FDA. *Food supplements are not subject to the same scrutiny and restrictions,* so consumers and manufacturers have the responsibility for checking the safety of dietary supplements and determining the truthfulness of label claims.

Dietary Supplements

Dietary supplements have traditionally referred to products made of one or more of the essential nutrients, such as vitamins, minerals, and protein. DSHEA broadens the definition to include, with some exceptions, any product intended for ingestion as a supplement to the diet. This includes vitamins, minerals, herbs, botanicals, other plant-derived substances, amino acids (the individual building blocks of protein), and concentrates, metabolites, constituents, and extracts of these substances.

It is easy to spot a supplement because DSHEA requires manufacturers to include the words "dietary supplement" on product labels. Also, since March 1999, a "Supplement Facts" panel is required on the labels of most dietary supplements. The supplement manufacturers are required to document substantiation of their claims. They must also include a disclaimer on their labels that the dietary supplements *are not drugs and receive no FDA premarket approval.* The rule, published in the January 6, 2000, *Federal Register,* also prohibits "structure/function" claims (claims that the products affect the structure or function of the body) without prior FDA review. Supplement labels also *may not, without prior FDA review, bear a claim that they can prevent, treat, cure, mitigate, or diagnose disease.*

Drugs used as traditional medicines are sometimes derived from plants. However, before marketing, they must undergo extensive clinical studies to determine their effectiveness, safety, possible interactions, and appropriate dosages before FDA approval. *The FDA does not authorize or test dietary supplements.*

Dietary supplements come in many forms, including tablets, capsules, powders, softgels, gelcaps, and liquids. Though commonly associated with health food stores, dietary supplements also are sold in grocery, drug, and national discount chain stores, as well as through mail-order catalogs, TV programs, the Internet, and direct sales.

Under DSHEA, once a dietary supplement is marketed, FDA has the responsibility for showing that a dietary supplement is *unsafe* before it can take action to restrict the product's use. This was the case when, in June 1997, the FDA proposed, among other things, to limit the amount of ephedrine alkaloids in dietary supplements (marketed as ephedra, Ma huang, and epitonin, for example) and provide warnings to consumers about hazards associated with use of dietary supplements containing the ingredients. The hazards ranged from nervousness, dizziness, and changes in blood pressure and heart rate, to chest pain, heart attack, hepatitis, stroke, seizures, psychosis, and death. The proposal stemmed from the FDA's review of adverse event reports it had received, scientific literature, and public comments. Finally, in 2004, the FDA announced a ban on the weight-loss aid ephedra. However, there are numerous other dangerous supplements still on the market. In May 2004, *Consumer Reports* identified a dozen supplements that according to government warnings and adverse-event reports were too dangerous to be on the market. However, the following unsafe supplements were still available at that time in retail stores or by shopping online: *Aristolochia* (linked to kidney failure and cancer), *yohimbe* (linked to heart and respiratory problems), *bitter orange* (linked to high blood pressure, heart attacks and stroke), and *chapparal, comfrey, germander,* and *kava* (linked to liver failure). These products and others listed in *Consumer Reports'* "dirty dozen" (*Dangerous Supplements*), can have many other trade names. For details, consult *Natural Medicines Comprehensive Database.*

Fraudulent Products

Consumers need to be on the lookout for fraudulent products. These are products that don't do what they say they can or don't contain what they say they contain. At the very least, they waste consumers' money, and they may cause physical harm. Fraudulent products often can be identified by the types of claims made in their labeling, advertising, and promotional literature. Some possible indicators of fraud, says Stephen Barrett, M.D., a board member of the National Council Against Health Fraud, are

- Claims that the product is a secret cure and use of such terms as "breakthrough," "magical," "miracle cure," and "new discovery." "If the product were a cure for a serious disease, it would be widely reported in the media and used by health care professionals," he says.

- Claims that a product is backed by scientific studies, but with no list of references or references that are inadequate. For instance, if a list of references is provided, the citations cannot be traced, or if they are traceable, the studies are out-of-date, irrelevant, or poorly designed.

Quality Products

The growing market for supplements, with fewer regulations, creates the potential for quality-control problems. For example, the FDA has identified several manufacturers that were buying herbs, plants, and other ingredients without first adequately testing them to determine whether the product they ordered was actually what they received, whether the ingredients were free from contaminants, and were of the strength stated.

To help protect themselves, consumers should:

- Look for ingredients in products with the U.S.P. notation, which indicates that the manufacturer followed standards established by the U.S. Pharmacopoeia.

- Realize that the label term "natural" doesn't guarantee that a product is safe. "Think of poisonous mushrooms," says Elizabeth Yetley,

Ph.D., Director of FDA's Office of Special Nutritionals. "They're natural."

- Consider the name of the manufacturer or distributor. Supplements made by a nationally known food and drug manufacturer, for example, have likely been made under tight controls because these companies already have in place manufacturing standards for their other products.

- Write to the supplement manufacturer for more information. Ask the company about the conditions under which its products were made.

- Avoid products sold for considerably less money than competing brands.

Reading and Reporting

Consumers who use dietary supplements should always read product labels, follow directions, and heed all warnings.

Supplement users who suffer a serious harmful effect or illness that they think is related to supplement use should call a doctor or other health care provider. He or she, in turn, can report it to FDA MedWatch by calling 1-800-FDA-1088 or going to http://www.fda.gov/medwatch/report/hcp.htm on the MedWatch website. Patients' names are kept confidential.

Much remains unknown about many dietary supplements regarding their health benefits and potential risks. Therefore, consumers who decide to take advantage of the expanding market should do so with care, making sure to have the necessary information and consulting with their doctors regarding any health conditions that could be compromised or any medications they are taking that may interact adversely with the herbs. "The majority of supplement manufacturers are responsible and careful," FDA's Yetley says. "But, as with all products on the market, consumers need to be discriminating. FDA and industry have important roles to play, but consumers must take responsibility, too."

Your responsibility as a health care provider includes warning your clients, and others who may seek your advice, regarding the dangers of taking products not approved by the FDA and not adequately tested. You must also caution them about the possibility of fraudulent products and lack of quality control. Most importantly, you must warn them about possible interactions with the medicines they are taking and the potential for serious adverse reactions. Issue special warnings to diabetics and those taking cardiac drugs or anticoagulants because of the increased risk of very serious interactions and problems.

All of the herbal remedies on the market are too numerous to mention in this book. However, you will find some of the more popular ones, along with cautions or interactions known at this time, listed in Table 11-3. Stay informed. Some sources of current information are listed at the end of the chapter. See Table 11-3 for a list of some herbs, possible uses, cautions, and interactions.

Table 11-3 Herbs

HERBS[a]	POSSIBLE USES[b]	POSSIBLE SIDE EFFECTS, CAUTIONS, INTERACTIONS
Aloe vera	Topical use for minor burns, shallow wound healing	Not for deep, surgical wounds
Black cohosh	Phytoestrogen for menopausal symptoms and premenstrual syndrome (PMS)	Can cause bradycardia Do not take with estrogen or with history of breast cancer
Capsaicin	Topical pain reliever, anti-inflammatory for arthritis For post-herpetic neuralgia and neuropathy	Local burning sensation, may fade with time
Chamomile	Sedative tea, insomnia, nausea	Those allergic to pollens; e.g., ragweed, may be allergic to it
Chondroitin Sulfate	Anti-inflammatory for arthritis	Occasional mild GI effects Reliability of content varies Shark cartilage or cattle cartilage may be contaminated
Echinacea	Proven *ineffective* in 2005 studies for prevention and treatment of colds	Can cause allergies and rashes Contraindicated in those with autoimmune disease; e.g., HIV, MS, or lupus, and chronic use, longer than eight weeks
Ephedra	Banned by the FDA in 2004 due to danger of heart problems and stroke	
Flaxseed oil	For constipation Source of omega-3 fatty acids Possibly anti-inflammatory	May interact with anticoagulants to cause bleeding Diarrhea possible
Feverfew	Migraine headaches, prevention and treatment	No toxic reactions known Sensitive individuals may develop dermatitis from external contact
Garlic	To lower blood pressure and cholesterol Anti-infective, immune enhancing	Risk of bleeding with anticoagulants Nausea, vomiting, diarrhea, heartburn, flatulence
Ginger	Nausea, motion sickness	Doses higher than 6 g can cause gastric irritation
Gingko (GBE)	Improve mental function and memory in elderly and Alzheimer's patients Antidepressant, anxiolytic, antioxidant	May interact with anticoagulants to cause bleeding and strokes Rare GI upset, headache
Ginseng	Antistress, antifatigue	Not for long-term use May cause hypertension, nausea, vomiting, diarrhea, nervousness, mental changes Contraindicated in pregnancy

(continued)

Table 11-3 Herbs—*continued*

HERBS[a]	POSSIBLE USES[b]	POSSIBLE SIDE EFFECTS, CAUTIONS, INTERACTIONS
Glucosamine	Anti-inflammatory for arthritis	Elevated cholesterol Insulin resistance, higher blood glucose
Kava	FDA warning March 2002 Banned in Canada, Germany, So. Africa and Switzerland	Possible liver damage, often irreversible; deaths reported
Licorice	Anti-infective, for cough, anti-inflammatory, menopausal symptoms, PMS, peptic ulcer—deglycyrrhizinated licorice (DGL)	Hypertension, fluid retention Do not take with diuretics
Melatonin	For insomnia, improves sleep cycle, especially with older adults and for jet lag Boosts immune system Antioxidant protection	Side effects rare, nightmares Contraindicated in pregnancy
SAM-e	Anti-inflammatory for osteoarthritis and fibromyalgia Antidepressant	Not to be taken with other antidepressants Not for severe depression or bipolar disorder Package should be airtight and lightproof; not stable
Saw palmetto	For benign prostatic hypertrophy (BPH) Antiandrogen	Rare GI upset See a physician for diagnosis and treatment
Soy	Menopause symptoms Phytoestrogen Cancer-preventing qualities	No known side effects Counteracts thyroid medicine Do not take together
St. John's wort	Mild to moderate depression Not for severe depression or bipolar disorder	Photosensitivity—may cause hives Insomnia, irritability, headache Do not combine with other antidepressants or alcohol Interacts with warfarin, oral contraceptives, anticonvulsants, digoxin, theophylline, and other drugs
Valerian	For anxiety, insomnia	Morning-after drowsiness Avoid during pregnancy Short-term use only

[a]The listing of these herbs does not constitute a recommendation for their use. This is only a representative list of some of the more popular herbs and those that could be problematic. There are many others on the market. Always check current, reliable references for the most up-to-date information regarding dosage, adverse effects, and interactions.

[b]Although some of the herbs listed here have been tested for use with the conditions mentioned, *they are not approved by the FDA. There is no guarantee that they will help the condition. There is always the possibility of adverse effects. Use with caution and at your own risk.*

Patient Education

Dietary Supplements

Patients should be instructed regarding:

- Consulting a physician or pharmacist before taking any "herbal remedies." Some herbs may be contraindicated with certain diagnoses.

- Taking a list of all products you are using, including herbal remedies, vitamins and minerals, OTC (nonprescription) medicines, and prescription drugs to a physician or pharmacist. Many of these products can interact, with dangerous, even life-threatening results. Physician consult is important before starting any "alternative medicines." Do not mix prescription drugs and herbal remedies for the same condition.

- The fact that "natural" does not mean "safe."

- Not taking more than the recommended amount listed on the label. Even vitamins and minerals in excess of the RDA can cause serious problems. Herbs that may be safe in small doses could be harmful at larger doses or over a prolonged period of time. Products without dosage recommendations should be avoided.

- All products should carry a lot number, expiration date, and manufacturer's name, address, and phone number. Products should be *avoided* that lack this information, or that claim an effect on the body's structure or function, or claim to be able to cure a disease or condition.

- Herbal products should be stored away from young children and pets.

- Herbal products should not be used for children without the approval of a pediatrician.

- Herbal remedies should not be used if you are pregnant, trying to become pregnant, or nursing.

- These products should not be taken with alcohol without first determining the safety of such a combination.

- These products should not be used as a substitute for proper rest and nutrition. A balanced diet is necessary for good health.

Following are some of the references used in preparing the Alternative Medicine section of this book. You may find these resources useful in researching information for your patients and yourself. The most current information can frequently be found on the Internet; several Web sites are also listed.

REFERENCES

Burgess, Leslie (March 2000). Exploring herbal medicine's risks and benefits. *Caring for the ages,* Vol. 1, No. 3, 1–18. American Medical Directors Assoc., New York, New York: Lippincott.

Cupp, Melanie Johns (1999). *Herbal remedies: Adverse effects and drug interactions*. Shawnee Mission, KS: The American Academy of Family Physicians.

Foster, Steven (1998). *101 medicinal herbs*. Loveland, CO: Interweave Press.

Foster, Steven, & Tyler, Varro E. (1999). *Tyler's honest herbal*. 4th ed. New York: Haworth Herbal Press.

Graedon, Joe, & Graedon, Teresa (1999). *The people's pharmacy guide to home and herbal remedies*. New York: Martin's Press.

Krinsky, Norman I. (2000). *Antioxidants' role in chronic disease prevention still uncertain, huge doses considered risky*. Washington, DC: National Academies News.

McCaleb, Rob (2000). *The encyclopedia of popular herbs*. Boulder, CO: Prima Publishing.

PDR for herbal medicines. 2nd ed. (2000). Montvale, NJ: Medical Economics Company.

ONLINE REFERENCES

American Society of Health System Pharmacists (2000). *Alternative medicines: Playing it safe*. Available: *www.safemedication.com/meds/altmeds.html*

FDA Consumer (1998). *Dietary supplements associated with illnesses and injuries*. Available: *http://www.cfsan.fda.gov/dms/supplmnt*

HerbMed (2001). A free online database of herbs providing scientific data behind the use of herbs for health. Available: *www.herbmed.org*

McCaleb, Rob, President Herb Research Foundation (2000). *Controversial products in the natural foods market*. Available: *www.ibiblio.org/herbs/controv.html*

WORKSHEET 1 FOR CHAPTER 11
FAT-SOLUBLE VITAMINS

Complete all columns. To complete the Symptoms of Overdose column, refer to the *side effect icon* in the chapter (✹).

Vitamin	Sources	Cause of Deficiencies	Signs of Deficiencies	Symptoms of Overdose and Side Effects	Interactions and Cautions
A					
D					
E					
K					

WORKSHEET 2 FOR CHAPTER 11
WATER-SOLUBLE VITAMINS

Complete all columns.

Vitamin	Sources	Cause of Deficiencies	Signs of Deficiencies	Symptoms of Overdose and Side Effects	Interactions and Cautions
B$_1$					
B$_2$					
B$_6$					
B$_{12}$					
Folic acid					
Niacin					

WORKSHEET 3 FOR CHAPTER 11
VITAMINS AND MINERALS

Complete all columns.

Vitamins and Minerals	Sources	Cause of Deficiencies	Signs of Deficiencies	Symptoms of Overdose and Side Effects	Interactions and Cautions
C					
Potassium					
Calcium					
Iron					

A. Case Study (Vitamins and Minerals)

Miss I. M. Puny, a 30-year-old secretary, calls the physician's office asking for a prescription for iron because she feels tired and weak. The patient should be given the following information:

1. No iron medication should be taken before first taking all the following steps EXCEPT

    a. Checking hemoglobin   c. Trying multivitamins

    b. Assessing all symptoms   d. Determining cause of deficiency

2. Symptoms of iron deficiency may include all of the following EXCEPT

    a. Nausea and diarrhea   c. Air hunger

    b. Pale skin   d. Dizziness

3. Iron is found in all of the following foods EXCEPT

    a. Liver   c. Milk

    b. Spinach   d. Red meat

4. Oral iron products can cause all of the following EXCEPT

    a. Constipation   c. Black stools

    b. Diarrhea   d. Nervousness

5. Iron products should be taken with which one of the following?

    a. Coffee   c. Orange juice

    b. Tea   d. Milk

B. Case Study (Vitamins and Minerals)

Mr. M. I. Grate, a 40-year-old physical education instructor, comes to the health fair to get the latest advice on vitamin C supplements to prevent colds, cancer, and premature aging. He should receive the following advice:

1. Vitamin C can be found naturally in all of the following foods EXCEPT

    a. Citrus   c. Cabbage

    b. Broccoli   d. Cheese

2. All of the following *decrease* vitamin C levels EXCEPT

    a. Smoking   c. Raw vegetables

    b. Alcohol   d. Slow cooking

3. Megadoses of vitamin C can cause all of the following EXCEPT

    a. Constipation   c. Kidney stones

    b. Gouty arthritis   d. GI distress

4. Functions of vitamin C include all of the following EXCEPT

    a. Healing of wounds   c. Prevention of liver disease

    b. Absorption of iron   d. Prevention of scurvy

5. Vitamin C interacts with all of the following drugs EXCEPT

    a. Tetracycline   c. Aspirin

    b. Estrogen   d. Tylenol

CHAPTER REVIEW QUIZ

Multiple Choice

1. Which is *not* true of antioxidants?
   a. Inhibit cell breakdown in damaged tissue
   b. Consist of enzymes, vitamins, and minerals
   c. Only found in synthetic products
   d. Fight free radicals

2. Free radical damage can be associated with all of the following conditions EXCEPT:
   a. Stunted growth
   b. Inflammatory conditions
   c. Heart disease
   d. Immunosuppression

3. Which is *not* an antioxidant vitamin?
   a. Ascorbic acid
   b. Beta carotene
   c. Vitamin B
   d. Vitamin E

4. Which is *not* an antioxidant mineral?
   a. Copper
   b. Selenium
   c. Zinc
   d. Iron

5. Which of the following statements is true?
   a. Patients should stop taking antioxidants during chemotherapy.
   b. Patients should continue antioxidants during radiation therapy.

6. When buying dietary supplements, you should look for which term on the label?
   a. Natural
   b. FDA
   c. U.S.P.
   d. New discovery

7. All of the following herbs can interact with anticoagulants to cause bleeding EXCEPT:
   a. Flaxseed oil
   b. Garlic
   c. Gingko
   d. Ginseng

8. Which is *not* true of glucosamine?
   a. Always combined with chondroitin
   b. Can elevate cholesterol
   c. Anti-inflammatory
   d. Can raise blood glucose

9. Which is *not* true of soy products?
   a. For menopause symptoms
   b. Phytoestrogens
   c. Counteract thyroid meds
   d. Can cause bradycardia

10. Which is *not* true of St. John's wort?
    a. Interacts with oral contraceptives
    b. Can be combined with SSRI's
    c. Causes photosensitivity
    d. For moderate depression

Chapter 12
Skin Medications

Key Terms

Antifungals

Antipruritics

Antiseptics

Antiviral

Bactericidal

Demulcents

Emollients

Keratolytic

Objectives

Upon completion of this chapter, the learner should be able to

1. Define the Key Terms

2. Describe application procedures for various skin medications

3. Identify side effects of the seven major categories of skin medications and contraindications when appropriate

4. Compare and contrast scabicides and pediculicides

5. Explain the factors that influence the absorption of skin medications

6. Classify drugs according to their action: antipruritic, emollient, keratolytic, antifungal, anti-infective, or agents to treat acne

7. List five possible side effects of long-term topical corticosteroid therapy

8. List five contraindications for topical corticosteroid therapy

9. Describe special contraindications and cautions with Accutane therapy for acne

10. Describe important patient education for all skin medications in this chapter

The skin is the largest organ of the body. Since such a great area is involved, many conditions can affect the skin, causing annoyance and discomfort. Skin ailments can range from minor ones, such as pruritus (itching), to major ones, such as severe burns. Treatment is usually topical or local (applied to the affected area), but skin conditions are sometimes treated internally with oral medications or injections for their systemic effects.

This chapter primarily explains *topical* medications. Medications given parenterally or orally to relieve inflammation or itching, such as corticosteroids and antihistamines, are discussed more extensively in other chapters.

Topical skin preparations can be classified *according to action* in seven principal categories

1. Antipruritics relieve itching.

2. Emollients and demulcents soothe irritation.

3. Keratolytic agents loosen epithelial scales.

4. Scabicides and pediculicides treat scabies or lice.

5. Antifungals control fungus conditions.

6. Local anti-infectives prevent and treat infection.

7. Agents to treat acne.

Factors that influence the rate of absorption of medication include condition and location of the skin, heat, and moisture. If the skin is thick and callused, absorption will be slower. If the skin is moist, macerated (raw), or warm, absorption will be more rapid. Sometimes the physician will order that the skin be premoistened or plastic wrap be applied over the ointment to aid absorption; in other cases, the skin must be left exposed to the air to slow absorption and reduce systemic effects. At times, the length of time for the medication to remain on the skin is very important. Complete understanding of appropriate directions for each topical medication is vital *before administration.*

ANTIPRURITICS

Antipruritics are used short term to relieve discomfort from dermatitis (rashes) associated with allergic reactions, poison ivy, hives, and insect bites. They relieve itching by use of products singly or in combination containing:

Local anesthetics (e.g., the "-caines," such as benzocaine)

Drying agents (e.g., calamine)

Anti-inflammatory agents (e.g., corticosteroids) applied locally or given PO for systemic effect. Topical agents are preferred because of fewer adverse effects.

Antihistamines administered PO for systemic effect (antihistamines applied topically can cause hypersensitivity reactions—use only a few days)

See Chapter 26 for further information on antihistamines.

Side effects of antipruritics can include:

 Skin irritation, rash

Stinging and a burning sensation

 Allergic reactions (especially with the "-caines")

 Sedation from antihistamines PO or paradoxical agitation in children

Patient Education

Patients being treated with antipruritics should be instructed to:

Clean area thoroughly before application

Rub in gently until medication vanishes

Use caution if they have allergies

Avoid contact with eyes or mucous membranes

Avoid covering with dressings unless directed by physician

Avoid prolonged use (not longer than one week)

Discontinue if condition worsens or irritation develops

Trim children's fingernails to reduce possibility of infection from scratching

Contraindications for antipruritics include:

On open wounds for corticosteroids—healing delayed

For prolonged use (especially corticosteroids)

The "-caines" for allergic persons

CORTICOSTEROIDS

The corticosteroids are used *both topically and systemically* to treat dermatological disorders associated with allergic reactions. Topical corticosteroids are also used to treat psoriasis and seborrheic dermatitis. (See Table 12-1.) See Chapter 23, Endocrine System Drugs, for more in-depth information regarding corticosteroids.

Side effects of corticosteroid ointments and creams, especially used long term (e.g., psoriasis), can include:

 Epidermal thinning, with frequent skin tears and increased risk of infection

 Increased fragility of cutaneous blood vessels

Irritation, burning, or stinging

Ulceration, especially with occlusive dressings

 Activation of latent infections and slow healing

Hyperglycemia, glycosuria, and Cushing's syndrome, with *prolonged use* of *high-potency* products

Contraindications with corticosteroids include:

Skin infections, bacterial or fungal, and cutaneous or systemic viral infections

Open wounds

Immunosuppressed, for example, HIV (human immunodeficiency virus) infections

Those receiving chemotherapy

Table 12-1 Topical Medications for the Skin: Antipruritics, Emollients, Demulcents, and Keratolytics

GENERIC NAME	TRADE NAME	AVAILABLE	COMMENTS
Antipruritics			
benzocaine	Americaine, Solarcaine, Orajel	Ointment, spray, gel, lotion	Can cause hypersensitivity reaction
diphenhydramine	Benadryl, Caladryl	Lotion, cream, gel, spray	Antihistamine
corticosteroid	Cortaid, Topicort, Valisone, Aristocort, Synalar, others	Ointment, cream, lotion, solution	Also used for psoriasis and seborrhea
dibucaine	Nupercainal	Ointment, cream	Potential for hypersensitivity
Emollients and Demulcents			
vitamins A and D	A & D	Ointment	
	Desitin (with zinc oxide)	Ointment	
Keratolytic			
coal tar	Zetar, Tegrin, Neutrogena	Shampoo, oil, cream	For dandruff, seborrheic dermatitis, or psoriasis
podophyllin	Podophyllin	Liquid	For anogenital warts; systemic toxicity possible
salicylic acid	Clearasil, Neutrogena	Cream, liquid, gel	For dandruff, psoriasis, acne, warts, corns, calluses (stains clothing)
sulfur	Many combinations with other kerolytics	Cream, lotion, shampoo	For acne, scabies, seborrheic dermatitis

Note: This table lists only typical medications and does not include all of those on the market.

Children

Pregnancy or lactation

Acne, rosacea, or perioral dermatitis

EMOLLIENTS AND DEMULCENTS

Emollients and **demulcents** are used topically to protect or soothe minor dermatological conditions, such as diaper rash, abrasions, and minor burns.

KERATOLYTICS

Keratolytic agents, for example, salicylic acid, are used to control conditions of abnormal scaling of the skin, such as dandruff, seborrhea, and psoriasis or to promote peeling of the skin in conditions such as acne, hard corns, calluses, and warts. Antifungals are also used at times for seborrheic dermatitis and dandruff (see Table 12-1).

Side effects can include:

✳ Severe skin irritation, pruritus, or stinging

✳ Irritation to eyes or mucous membranes

✳ Photosensitivity

Systemic effects in allergic individuals (e.g., headache and GI symptoms)

Note: When podophyllum is used for genital warts, it should be removed 1–4 hours after application.

Contraindications include:

Open areas of skin

Pregnancy and lactation

Small children

For prolonged periods of time

Patient Education

Keratolytics

Patients should be instructed to:

Use only as directed, and for entire treatment period, even if improved

Avoid contact with eyes and mucous membranes

Avoid prolonged use

Discontinue and seek medical aid if irritation occurs

Avoid contact with surrounding tissues when applied as a caustic to corns or calluses

---

SCABICIDES AND PEDICULICIDES

Scabies is caused by an itch mite that burrows under the skin. Pediculosis is caused by infestation of lice on the hairs of the scalp, pubic area, and trunk. Both are easily transmitted from one person to another by direct contact or through contact with contaminated clothing or bed linens. Effective treatment includes laundering in hot water or dry cleaning all clothing and bedding. Sometimes concurrent treatment of close contacts is recommended.

Scabicides (permethrin or lindane) must be applied *according to directions* on the package insert, left in place the required period of time, and then rinsed thoroughly.

Pediculicides, for example, lindane (Kwell), are used in topical treatment of lice infestations. Pyrethrins (e.g., RID), are considered safer for pediculosis.

Side effects, rare when applied topically according to directions, may include:

> Slight local irritation, rash, or conjunctivitis

> Dermatitis with frequent application

However, with excessive or prolonged use, or with oral ingestion, or inhalation of vapors, CNS symptoms and hepatic or renal toxicity may occur. Anemia and seizures have been reported, especially with lindane. Therefore, lindane should be used only in patients who cannot tolerate or have failed first-line treatment with safer medications for the treatment of lice.

Contraindications include:

> Acutely inflamed, raw, or weeping surfaces

> Since lindane (Kwell) can be absorbed systemically following topical application, it should be avoided during pregnancy, lactation, or with infants, children, older adults, and those who weigh less than 110 lb.

However, permethrin is a safer alternative under these conditions for scabies. Pyrethrins (e.g., RID) are a safer alternative than lindane for pediculosis.

Due to the toxicity of lindane, the oral antiparasitic agent ivermectin (Stromectol), has been used successfully as an alternative (off-label) to mass treat scabies in an institutional setting and to treat head lice resistant to standard therapies. It is given orally as a single dose (weight-based), with a repeat dose 10–14 days later.

Patient Education

Patients being treated with scabicides or pediculicides should be instructed to:

Follow directions carefully (read and understand the medication guide dispensed with the lindane prescription); itching may still occur after the successful killing of lice and is not necessarily an indication for retreatment with lindane shampoo

Thoroughly launder clothing and bedding

Use caution to prevent accidental oral ingestion

Use caution with infants who might suck their thumbs

Inform sexual partner if condition is present in pubic area

Alert school if head lice infestation occurs

ANTIFUNGALS

Antifungals, for example, nystatin (Mycostatin), are useful in the treatment of monilial infections (candidiasis), such as thrush, diaper rash, vaginitis, athlete's foot, and jock itch.

Effective treatment includes topical administration according to directions on the package insert and good hygiene practices, including washing, drying, and exposure to air when possible.

For the treatment of candidiasis of the oral cavity, an oral suspension or oral lozenges should be administered four times daily for 14 days. For infants, administer after the feeding, which is followed by water to rinse mouth *before therapy.* Place one-half dose in each side of the mouth. For adults, apply *after meals* and *after rinsing* of mouth. Then the entire dose should be used to thoroughly coat inside the mouth, holding for as long as possible (e.g., several minutes), before swallowing. In both cases, the patient should be NPO for at least one hour after treatment.

With inadequate response to treatment, cultures should be obtained to confirm the diagnosis and assist in the selection of the most appropriate medication.

Side effects, although rare, may include:

Contact dermatitis

Itching, burning, and irritation

Contraindication or caution applies to the use of vaginal preparations during pregnancy. Use only under medical supervision. Some products can cause fetal abnormalities.

See Table 12-2 for a summary of the antifungals, scabicides, and pediculicides.

Patient Education

Patients being treated with antifungals should be instructed to:

Carefully wash and *dry* affected areas

Expose to air whenever possible

With genital fungus, avoid tight undergarments, pantyhose, and wet bathing suits

With athlete's foot, use open sandals instead of sneakers

Follow application instructions carefully. Use for entire time, even if asymptomatic

Remove any stains with soap and warm water

Continue prescribed vaginal treatment even during menstruation, or if symptomatic relief occurs, until entire regimen is completed

Consult doctor before vaginal preparations are used during pregnancy

For oral suspensions or lozenges, apply after meals and after thorough rinsing of mouth. No food or liquids for at least 1 h after treatment.

For vaginal infections, refrain from intercourse until treatment is complete

Consider treating partner if reinfection occurs

Table 12-2 Medications for the Skin: Scabicides, Pediculicides, Antifungals, Antiseptics, Burn Medications, and Acne Medications

GENERIC NAME	TRADE NAME	AVAILABLE	COMMENTS
Scabicides and Pediculicides			
permethrin	Acticin, Elimite	Cream	Apply from head to feet, wash off after 8–14 h
	Nix	Liquid	Apply to hair, to remain 10 min
lindane	Kwell	Lotion, shampoo	Treat all hairy areas Toxic potential
pyrethrins	RID, A-200	Gel, shampoo, solution	For lice only
Antifungals[a]			
terbinafine	Lamisil	Cream, gel, spray, solution, tabs	Very effective for onychomycosis
clotrimazole	Mycelex, Lotrimin	Lozenges, cream, lotion, sol, vaginal cream, tabs	For oral, topical, or vaginal application
ketoconazole	Nizoral	Cream, shampoo	Topical antifungal, shampoo for dandruff
nystatin	Mycostatin	Oral suspension, lozenges, cream, lotion, ointment, vaginal tab, powder	Apply oral suspension or lozenges PC, then NPO 1 h
tolnaftate	Tinactin	Aerosol spray, cream, powder, solution	Avoid inhaling spray or powder
zinc undecylenate	Cruex, Desenex	Powder, soap, cream	Avoid inhaling powder
Antiviral			
acyclovir[a]	Zovirax	Ointment, orally	See Chapter 17 for dosage
valacyclovir	Valtrex	Orally	
Topical Anti-infectives and Antiseptics			
chlorhexidene	Hibiclens	Solution, liquid, foam	Antimicrobial skin cleanser, surgical scrub; rinse thoroughly
povidone-iodine	Betadine	Aqueous solution, oint., liquid scrub	Bactericidal, antiseptic, surgical scrub; watch for allergies
Burn Medications			
nitrofurazone	Furacin	Cream, powder for sol	Watch for allergies
silver sulfadiazine	Silvadene	Cream	Watch for allergies
mafenide	Sulfamylon	Cream, 5% topical solution	Watch for allergies
Acne Medications			
benzoyl peroxide	Benzac, Oxy-10, Panoxyl-5 and 10	Bar, cream, gel, liquid, lotion	Antibacterial activity Drying actions, for type 1
isotretinoin	Accutane, Sotret	10, 20, 30, 40 mg caps	Absolutely contraindicated in pregnancy, for type 4
salicylic acid	Clearasil, Neutrogena	Cream, liquid, gel Cream, lotion	For type 1 For type 1
sulfur	Many combinations with other kerolytics		

[a]Oral preparations are discussed in Chapter 17.

Note: Other preparations are available. This is a representative list.

195

ANTIVIRALS

Acyclovir has an **antiviral** effect on herpes simplex (cold sores or genital herpes), herpes zoster (shingles), and varicella zoster (chickenpox) viruses. Acyclovir (Zovirax) is available in oral and parenteral preparations (see Chapter 17), or in ointment applied topically. Topical therapy is substantially less effective than systemic therapy (parenteral or oral). Topical acyclovir therapy is *not a cure,* and does not reduce the frequency or delay the appearance of new lesions. However, topical therapy generally decreases the duration of viral shedding, the duration of pain and itching, and the time required for crusting and healing of lesions. It is effective in first episode genital herpes infection, but recurrent infections have shown little, if any, therapeutic benefit from topical therapy. The ointment should be applied as soon as possible following onset of signs and symptoms of infections. Take care not to get the ointment in the eyes. It is *not effective in preventing infections.*

For more effective treatment of herpes zoster (shingles), acyclovir (Zovirax) is available orally. Valacyclovir (Valtrex) is a derivative of acyclovir, which can be dosed less frequently, improving patient compliance. Both of these oral antivirals need to be started within 72 h of rash onset and are most effective if started within the first 48 hours of onset.

LOCAL ANTI-INFECTIVES

Antiseptics

Antiseptics are substances that inhibit the growth of bacteria (bacteriostatic). The term is used most frequently to describe chemicals applied to body tissues, especially the skin. *Disinfectants* are included in this category, but chemicals that kill bacteria (**bactericidal**) are frequently too strong to be applied to body tissues and are *usually* applied to inanimate objects, such as furniture, floors, and instruments. Sometimes a chemical can be used as an antiseptic on skin and also as a disinfectant on inanimate objects by increasing the strength.

The two major antiseptics in use today are chlorhexidene and povidone-iodine, used for surgical scrubs and as bacteriostatic skin cleansers. Some iodine preparations are also bactericidal and are used in the treatment of superficial skin wounds and to disinfect the skin preoperatively. Chlorhexidene (Hibiclens) should not be used on wounds involving more than the superficial layers of skin. It is important to rinse thoroughly after use.

Side effects of chlorhexidene can include:

* Dermatitis and irritation
  Photosensitivity
* Allergic reactions, especially in the genital area

Side effects of povidone-iodine (Betadine) can include:

* Skin irritation or burns
* Allergic reactions

Contraindications or extreme cautions for chlorhexidene include:

> Pregnancy, lactation
>
> Not for frequent use for total body bathing
>
> Not for use in eyes and ears

Povidone-iodine contraindications include:

> Not for those allergic to iodine
>
> Not for use on open wounds
>
> Not for use in newborns (risk of iodine absorption)

Patient Education

Patients being treated with local anti-infectives should be instructed to:

Rinse chlorhexidene *thoroughly*

Avoid chlorhexidene for total body bathing or frequent use

Avoid use of chlorhexidene on open skin lesions, mucous membranes, and genital areas

Take care to avoid chlorhexidene or povidone-iodine in the eyes or ears; flush thoroughly

Use caution with povidone-iodine in anyone with allergies

Burn Medications

Burn treatments include topical application of medications to prevent or treat infections. The two most commonly used agents for this purpose are silver sulfadiazine (Silvadene) and mafenide (Sulfamylon). Apply with a sterile-gloved hand. Nitrofurazone (Furacin) is used for those allergic to sulfa.

Side effects of burn medications can include:

* Pain, burning, and itching
* Allergic reactions
* Staining of the skin temporarily

Contraindications or extreme caution applies to newborns or to patients with:

> Impaired kidney or liver function (cumulative effects)
>
> History of allergy, especially to sulfa drugs

Patient Education

Patients using burn medications should be instructed to:

Use aseptic technique to prevent infection

Watch for allergic reactions

Keep careful intake and output record

Keep area covered at all times with cream and sterile dressing

Antibacterial Agents

There are many prescription and over-the-counter (OTC) topical antibacterial agents on the market, including ointments, creams, and solutions too numerous to mention here. These products have the potential for adverse side effects, including local, hypersensitivity, and systemic reactions. For further information regarding antibacterial agents, see Chapter 17, Anti-infective Drugs.

Patient Education

Patients using any topical antibacterial agent should be instructed to:

Read and follow carefully all directions on the package

Check all ingredients carefully for possible allergies

If there is no improvement, the condition worsens, or there are other untoward reactions (e.g., inflammation, itching, rash, or swelling), stop the medication and consult a physician.

See Table 12-2 for a summary of scabicides, pediculicides, antifungals, antivirals, antiseptics, burn medications, and acne medications.

AGENTS USED TO TREAT ACNE

Acne is a common condition of the skin that affects almost everyone to some degree during the teenage years and even some people into adulthood. Acne is most commonly seen on the face, scalp, neck, chest, back, and shoulders. *Acne is graded depending upon the degree of severity from type 1 (least) to type 4 (most).*

Patients with *type 1* acne may choose from several relatively mild *nonprescription topical* medications such as sulfur, salicylic acid, and benzoyl peroxide. A patient with *type 2* acne might be *prescribed topical antibiotics,* such as, tetracycline or erythromycin. For *Type 3* acne, a course of *oral antibiotics* (tetracyclines or erythromycin—see Chapter 17) may be prescribed in addition to topical products. *Type 4 acne does not respond to topical therapy;* rather *systemic hormones ("birth control pills")* or retinoids (e.g., Accutane) may be prescribed.

Accutane is *absolutely contraindicated* in pregnancy (Food and Drug Administration [FDA] risk category X). There is an extremely high risk that birth defects can occur if pregnancy occurs while taking Accutane in any amount even for a short period of time. To prevent Accutane exposure during pregnancy, the SMART Program has been developed. This program requires prescribers, pharmacists, and patients to comply with certain conditions before prescribing, dispensing, or receiving Accutane.

Accutane therapy *should not be initiated* in females of childbearing potential, regardless of whether or not they are sexually active, *until neg-*

ative results from two urine or serum pregnancy tests are confirmed and the patient or her guardian completes the consent form. Monthly pregnancy tests during Accutane therapy are also required. Women who are, or might become, sexually active with a male partner must also select and use two forms of effective contraception simultaneously for at least one month before beginning, during, and for one month following discontinuation of therapy. *They must also sign a patient information/consent form about Accutane and birth defects.*

Side effects of benzoyl peroxide can include:

* Skin irritation, mild stinging, redness, dry skin

Contraindications for benzoyl peroxide include:

Pregnancy, breast-feeding

Use in patients with skin diseases (dermatitis, eczema, sunburn, etc.) may increase risk of skin irritation

Benzoic acid or paraben hypersensitivity

Avoid exposure to the eyes or mucus membranes, can cause severe irritation

Side effects of Accutane can include:

* Mucotaneous effects (inflammation of lips, dry skin, dry mouth, nose-bleed, peeling, itching, photosensitivity)

Alterations in lipid profiles; decreases in hemoglobin/hematocrit

* Musculoskeletal pain, back pain, arthralgia, myalgia

GI effects (anorexia, colitis, increased appetite, nausea/vomiting, thirst)

* CNS effects (dizziness, drowsiness, fatigue, headache, lethargy, malaise, weakness)

* Depression, emotional lability, psychosis, aggression, violent behavior (rarely, suicidal ideation)

Decreased tolerance to contact lenses

Contraindications for Accutane include:

Pregnancy (see discussion above), breast-feeding

Use in children <12 years of age

Retinoid (i.e., vitamin A)/paraben hypersensitivity

Prolonged exposure to sunlight (UV)—use sunscreen and protective clothing

Driving or operating machinery at night due to *decreased* night vision and other visual disturbances

Use cautiously in patients with psychiatric disorders

Osteoporosis or other bone disorders

Patient Education

Patients being treated with acne agents should be instructed to:

Use preparations every day as directed; often takes several weeks to be effective (your acne may actually get worse during the first few weeks of treatment, then start to improve)

Do not use benzoyl peroxide with other topical acne products or retinoids

Avoid prolonged exposure to sunlight (UV)—use sunscreen and protective clothing; avoid drugs such as sulfas that make you more sensitive to the sun

Avoid cosmetic procedures to smooth your skin, including waxing, dermabrasion, or laser therapy, during and for at least six months after Accutane therapy, due to the possibility of scarring

Avoid multivitamins or nutritional supplements that contain vitamin A, tetracycline antibiotics, certain antacids (aluminum hydroxide), and certain birth control pills (progestin-only) while taking Accutane

Make sure you receive, read, and understand the *Isotretinoin Medication Guide* every time you get a prescription or refill

Accutane can cause birth defects; do not get pregnant while taking this drug!

CAUTIONS FOR TOPICAL MEDICATIONS

Skin medications by prescription or OTC are too numerous to mention. Many patients use products without adequate instruction in administration, side effects, or precautions. The health care worker has a responsibility to advise patients whenever possible to use great caution with self-medication to avoid ineffective or dangerous treatment. Both the health care worker and the lay person should *read instructions completely* before administration of any medication.

Patient Education

Patients using topical medications should be instructed regarding:

Never taking by mouth

Keeping out of reach of children

Being sure labels are not obscured and are read completely

Discontinuing at once with any side effects and seeking medical advice

Not taking beyond time limit listed on medication container

If allergies are known, avoiding self-medication without medical advice

WORKSHEET FOR CHAPTER 12
DRUGS FOR THE SKIN

List the drugs according to category and complete all columns. To complete the Side Effects column, refer to the side effects icon in the chapter (✷).

Classifications and Drugs	Purpose	Side Effects	Contraindications or Cautions	Patient Education
Antipruritics 1. 2. 3.				
Emollients and Demulcents 1.				
Kerolytics 1. 2. 3. 4.				
Scabicides and Pediculicides 1. 2. 3.				

WORKSHEET FOR CHAPTER 12
DRUGS FOR THE SKIN

List the drugs according to category and complete all columns. To complete the Side Effects column, refer to the side effects icon in the chapter (✸).

Classifications and Drugs	Purpose	Side Effects	Contraindications or Cautions	Patient Education
Antifungals 1. 2. 3.				
Antivirals 1. 2. Oral for Shingles				
Antiseptics 1. 2.				
Burn Medications 1. 2.				

Classifications and Drugs	Purpose	Side Effects	Contraindications or Cautions	Patient Education
Acne Medications Type I *Topical* 1. sulfur 2. salicylic acid 3. benzoyl peroxide				
Type 2 *Topical* Antibiotics 1. tetracycline 2. erythromycin				
Type 3 *Oral* Antibiotics 1. tetracycline 2. erythromycin				
Type 4 Oral 1. contraceptives 2. retinoids (Accutane)				

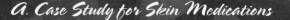

A. Case Study for Skin Medications

Jay Skalin, a 35-year-old male, comes to the dermatologist's office with a request for corticosteroid cream for an outbreak of psoriasis on his hands. He asks if he will be able to use the same medicine for his jock itch and athlete's foot and for an abrasion on his son's knee. He will need the following information.

1. Topical corticosteroids are *contraindicated* for many conditions. The *only* appropriate use listed below is for
   a. Open wounds   c. Fungal conditions
   b. Viral infections   d. Allergic reaction

2. Topical corticosteroids are *contraindicated* in many circumstances. Which circumstance would allow its use?
   a. With immunosuppression   c. With psoriasis
   b. With children's rash   d. With chemotherapy

3. Corticosteroid cream can be used for all of the following EXCEPT
   a. Jock itch   c. Hives
   b. Poison ivy   d. Insect bites

4. Side effects of prolonged use of corticosteroid cream can include all of the following EXCEPT
   a. Easy bruising   c. Thin skin
   b. Thick scabs   d. Irritation

5. Other medications to treat psoriasis include kerolytics listed below EXCEPT
   a. Zetar   c. Salicylic acid
   b. Tegrin   d. Lindane

B. Case Study for Skin Medications

Melody Lane goes to the physician for her 6-week postpartum check. She complains of vaginal itching and says that her baby has "white spots in his mouth." The following information would be helpful:

1. Fungal infections (candidiasis) can cause all of the following EXCEPT
   a. Thrush   c. Diaper rash
   b. Acne   d. Vaginitis

2. Oral candidiasis can be treated with all of the following EXCEPT
   a. Lozenges   c. Extended-release capsules
   b. Suspension   d. Topical application

3. Treatment for oral candidiasis includes all of the following instructions EXCEPT
   a. Treat ac   c. NPO after
   b. Rinse first   d. Swallow solution

4. Customary treatment of monilial vaginal infections can include all the following EXCEPT
   a. Cream   c. NPO after
   b. Lotion   d. Tablets

5. Treatment for vaginal monilial infections includes all of the following instructions EXCEPT
   a. Avoid tight undergarments   c. Discontinue when better
   b. Continue during menstruation   d. Consult M.D. if pregnant

CHAPTER REVIEW QUIZ

Multiple Choice

1. For the treatment of scabies in an extended care facility, which is the safest treatment?
   - a. Lindane
   - b. Ivermectin
   - c. Ketoconazole
   - d. Nystatin

2. Treatment for type I acne could include any of the following medicines EXCEPT:
   - a. Salicylic acid
   - b. Sulfur
   - c. Accutane
   - d. Benzoyl peroxide

3. The most effective treatment for shingles includes all of the following EXCEPT:
   - a. Start within 72 h
   - b. Zovirax
   - c. Valacyclovir caps
   - d. Acyclovir ointment

4. Contraindications for Accutane therapy include all of the following EXCEPT:
   - a. Pregnancy
   - b. Sunlight exposure
   - c. Adolescence
   - d. Psychiatric disorder

5. Side effects of Accutane therapy can include all of the following EXCEPT:
   - a. Muscle pain
   - b. Low night vision
   - c. Depression
   - d. Increased salivation

6. Which antipruritic could cause a hypersensitivity reaction?
   - a. Caladryl
   - b. Benzocaine
   - c. Cortaid
   - d. Benadryl

7. Which keratolytic is used to treat genital warts?
   - a. Coal tar
   - b. Salicylic acid
   - c. Podophyllum
   - d. Sulfur

8. Kwell, used to treat lice infestations, is contraindicated in all of the following conditions EXCEPT:
   - a. Infancy
   - b. Older adult
   - c. Pregnancy
   - d. Obesity

9. Which burn medicine would be more likely to be used with someone allergic to sulfa?
   - a. Silvadene
   - b. Sulfamylon
   - c. Furacin

10. Which statement is NOT true with chlorhexidine (Hibiclens)?
    - a. Used with deep wounds
    - b. Can cause photosensitivity
    - c. Rinse after use
    - d. Can cause dermatitis

Chapter 13
Autonomic Nervous System Drugs

Objectives

Upon completion of this chapter, the learner should be able to

1. Define the Key Terms
2. Compare and contrast characteristics of the four categories of autonomic nervous system drugs
3. List the most frequently used (key) drugs in each of the four categories and the purpose of administration
4. Describe the possible side effects of each of the key drugs

Key Terms

Adrenergic

Anticholinergics

Autonomic

Beta-blockers

Cholinergic drugs

The autonomic nervous system (ANS) can be thought of as being *automatic, self-governing,* or *involuntary.* That is to say, we have no control over the action of the autonomic nervous system. Chemical substances called *neurotransmitters* are released at the nerve endings to transmit the nerve impulses from nerve to nerve at the synapses or from nerve to muscle at the myoneural junctions.

The autonomic nervous system is divided into the *sympathetic* and the *parasympathetic* divisions. Drugs that affect the function of the autonomic nervous system are divided into four categories:

1. Adrenergics (sympathomimetics)
2. Adrenergic blockers (alpha- and beta-blockers)
3. Cholinergics (parasympathomimetics)
4. Cholinergic blockers (anticholinergics)

ADRENERGICS

The sympathetic nervous system can be thought of as the emergency system used to mobilize the body for quick response and action. Key words to illustrate this action are *fright, fight,* and *flight*. If someone is startled in a dark place by a sudden motion, the body automatically mobilizes the sympathetic nerves to prepare the body to handle the fright by flight or a fight. The blood pressure, pulse, and respiration increase. The peripheral blood vessels constrict, sending more blood inward to the vital organs and skeletal muscles and speeding up the heart action. The bronchioles dilate to allow for a greater oxygen supply. The pupils dilate.

The chemical substances (neurotransmitters) released at the sympathetic nerve endings are called catecholamines and include epinephrine *(adrenalin),* norepinephrine, and dopamine. Drugs that mimic the action of the sympathetic nervous system are called sympathomimetic or **adrenergic**, e.g. isoproterenol.

Actions of the adrenergics include:

> Cardiac stimulation
>
> Increased blood flow to skeletal muscles
>
> Peripheral vasoconstriction
>
> Bronchodilation
>
> Dilation of pupils (mydriatic action)

Uses for the adrenergics include:

> Restoring rhythm in cardiac arrest
>
> Elevating blood pressure in shock of all kinds
>
> Constricting capillaries (e.g., applied topically to relieve nosebleed or nasal congestion or combined with local anesthetics for minor surgery)
>
> Dilating bronchioles in acute asthmatic attacks, bronchospasm, or anaphylactic reaction
>
> Ophthalmic procedures (mydriatic agent)

Side effects of the adrenergics may include:

* Palpitations
* Nervousness or tremor
* Tachycardia
* Cardiac arrhythmias
  Anginal pain
* Hypertension
  Tissue necrosis (when applied to laceration of periphery, for example, nose, fingers, and toes)
* Hyperglycemia
  Headache and insomnia

Contraindications or extreme caution with adrenergics applies to:

Angina

Coronary insufficiency

Hypertension

Cardiac arrhythmias

Angle-closure glaucoma

Organic brain damage

Hyperthyroidism

Caution for adrenergics also with administration; check dosage carefully (small amounts only). Give subcutaneous, IM (deltoid), or IV.

Interactions of adrenergics may occur with:

CNS drugs (e.g., alcohol, monoamine oxidase inhibitors [MAOIs], and antidepressants)

Propranolol (Inderal) or other beta-adrenergic blockers

Terazosin (Hytrin) or other alpha-adrenergic blockers

See Table 13-1 for a summary of the adrenergics.

Table 13-1 Adrenergics

GENERIC NAME	TRADE NAME	DOSAGE	COMMENTS
epinephrine	Adrenalin	0.1–0.5 ml 1:1,000 sol SubQ or IMª (deltoid) 5–10 ml 1:10,000 sol IV	For bronchospasm, asthma, cardiac arrest, anaphylaxis
ephedrine	Ephedrine	25–50 mg IM or SubQ	To raise blood pressure
dopamine	Intropin	2–5 mcg/kg/min IV	To raise blood pressure, cardiotonic
isoproterenol	Isuprel	10–15 mg SL q6–8h or inhalations 4×/d, 0.02–0.2 mg IV or IM	For asthma or bronchospasm; for heartblock or ventricular arrhythmias
metaraminol	Aramine	0.5–5 mg IV	To raise blood pressure in shock
norepinephrine	Levophed	2–4 mcg/min IV	For severe shock

ªUse caution with dosage. This caution applies to both dosages.

ADRENERGIC BLOCKERS

Drugs that block the action of the sympathetic nervous system are called adrenergic blockers. The most commonly used drugs in this category are beta-adrenergic blockers, or **beta-blockers,** such as propranolol (Inderal) (Table 13-2).

Table 13-2 Adrenergic Blockers

GENERIC NAME	TRADE NAME	DOSAGE	COMMENTS
propranolol[a]	Inderal	PO 160–480 mg daily divided doses	Begin with smaller dose and increase gradually to optimum dose for blood pressure control
		PO 10–20 mg 4×/d (initial dose)	For angina
		PO 10–30 mg 4×/d IV 1–3 mg slowly Use extreme caution	For arrhythmias
		PO 80 mg initial dose, increase to 160–240 mg daily divided doses	For migraine

[a]A beta-adrenergic blocker or beta-blocker. Others available and vary with condition.

Uses of the beta-blockers include treatment of the following:

> Hypertension
>
> Cardiac arrhythmias
>
> Angina pectoris
>
> Migraine headache

Side effects of beta-blockers may include:

* Hypotension
* Bradycardia
* Fatigue or lethargy
> Nausea and vomiting
>
> Hypoglycemia
* Confusion

Contraindications or extreme caution applies to use of beta-blockers with:

> Congestive heart failure or atrioventricular block
>
> Hypotension
>
> Asthma
>
> Diabetes

Interactions of beta-blockers may occur with:

> Digitalis
>
> Insulin or oral antidiabetic agents
>
> Theophylline

MAOIs and tricyclic antidepressants

Epinephrine

Alcohol

See Chapter 15 for a discussion of alpha-adrenergic blockers.

Patient Education

Patients taking beta-blockers, frequently given for cardiovascular disease, should be instructed regarding:

Rising slowly from reclining position to avoid postural hypotension

Possible slow heartbeat and reporting dizziness, difficulty breathing, or excessive weakness to the physician

Avoiding alcohol, antihistamines, muscle relaxants, tranquilizers, and sedatives because they potentiate CNS depression and sedation

Reporting sexual dysfunction or depression to the physician for possible dosage regulation or change to different medication

Not discontinuing the medication abruptly, except on advice of physician

Consulting physician before using over-the-counter (OTC) cold preparations

CHOLINERGICS

The parasympathetic nerve fibers synthesize and liberate *acetylcholine* as the mediator. Drugs that mimic the action of the parasympathetic nervous system are called parasympathomimetic or **cholinergic drugs** (e.g., bethanechol, neostigmine, and pilocarpine).

Actions of the cholinergics include:

Increased gastrointestinal (GI) peristalsis

Increased contraction of the urinary bladder

Increased secretions (sweat, saliva, and gastric juices)

Increased skeletal muscle strength

Lowered intraocular pressure

Constriction of pupils

Slowing of the heart

Uses for the cholinergics include treatment of:

Nonobstructive urinary retention (bethanechol)

Abdominal distention (neostigmine)

Myasthenia gravis (neostigmine)

Open-angle glaucoma (pilocarpine)

Side effects of the cholinergics may include:

* Nausea, vomiting, and diarrhea
* Muscle cramps and weakness
* Slowing of the heart, hypotension
* Sweating, excessive salivation, lacrimation, and flushing
* Respiratory depression, bronchospasm

Acute toxicity or cholinergic crisis is treated with atropine sulfate IV.

Contraindications or extreme caution with the cholinergics applies to:

Benign prostatic hypertrophy (BPH)

GI disorders (e.g., ulcer and obstruction)

Asthma

Cardiac disorders

Hyperthyroidism

Interactions of cholinergics occur with:

Procainamide

Quinidine

See Table 13-3 for a summary of the cholinergics.

Table 13-3 Cholinergics

GENERIC NAME	TRADE NAME	DOSAGE	COMMENTS
bethanechol	Urecholine	10–50 mg PO 4×/d, or 2.5–5 mg SubQ	For postpartum or postoperative urinary retention, **not** with benign prostatic hypertrophy
edrophonium	Tensilon	1–2 mg IV, then 8 mg if no response	Test for myasthenia gravis
neostigmine	Prostigmin	45–150 mg PO in divided doses daily 0.5–2 mg IM or IV q1–3h	Treatment for myasthenia gravis Neuromuscular blockade reversal
pilocarpine	Isopto Carpine	Ophthalmic gtt, dose varies	To lower intraocular pressure with glaucoma

Patient Education

Patients taking cholinergic drugs, or exposed to insecticides containing cholinergic agents (e.g., malathion), should be instructed regarding:

Reporting immediately to physician or emergency room any symptoms of prolonged GI distress (e.g., nausea, vomiting, and diarrhea), excessive perspiration, slow heartbeat, or depressed respiration

Avoiding combination of cholinergic medications with heart medications or antibiotics

CHOLINERGIC BLOCKERS

Cholinergic blockers, or **anticholinergics**, are drugs that block the action of the parasympathetic nervous system. Therefore, they are also called parasympatholytic. Atropine is the classic example of a cholinergic blocker.

Anticholinergics most commonly used as preoperative medications include atropine and glycopyrrolate (Robinul). They reduce the secretions of the mouth, pharynx, bronchi, and GI tract and reduce gastric activity. Anticholinergics, as preoperative medication, also are used to prevent cholinergic effects during surgery, such as hypotension or bradycardia and some cardiac arrhythmias associated with general anesthetics or vagal stimulation. However, only *atropine* acts as a bronchodilator and reduces the incidence of laryngospasm that can occur during general anesthesia. (See Table 13-4 for anticholinergics.)

Actions include:

Drying (all secretions decreased)

Decreased GI and genitourinary (GU) motility

Dilation of pupils

Uses of anticholinergics:

Antispasmodic and antisecretory for GI or GU hypermotility

Preoperative and preanesthetic uses

Neuromuscular block and other spastic disorders

Antidote for insecticide poisoning, cholinergic crisis, or mushroom poisoning

Emergency treatment of bradycardia and atrioventricular heart block with hypotension

Dilation of pupils (mydriatic)

Prevention and treatment of bronchospasm (bronchodilator, e.g., Atrovent inhaler)

Side effects of anticholinergics may include:

Fever or flushing

Blurred vision, headache

✳ Dry mouth, constipation, and urinary retention

✳ Confusion and/or excitement, especially older adults

✳ Palpitations and tachycardia

Interactions with potentiation of sedation and drying occur with antihistamines (e.g., diphenhydramine).

Contraindications or extreme caution applies to use of atropine with:

Asthma and other chronic obstructive pulmonary disease (COPD)—atropine *inhalations* recommended rather than oral or parenteral administration, which can reduce bronchial secretions and obstruct airflow.

Angle-closure glaucoma

GI or GU obstruction

Cardiac arrhythmias

Hypertension

Hypothyroidism, hepatic, or renal disease

Patient Education

Patients receiving cholinergic blockers should be instructed regarding:

Dried secretions (e.g., dry mouth)

Possible blurring of vision

Reporting fast heartbeat or palpitations

Avoiding oral anticholinergics with chronic obstructive lung disease and asthma, using inhalants only as prescribed, never OTC

See Table 13-4 for a summary of the anticholinergics.

Table 13-4 Cholinergic Blockers

GENERIC NAME	TRADE NAME	DOSAGE[a]	COMMENTS
atropine	Atropine[b]	0.4–0.6 mg IM	Preoperative
		2 mg IM or IV qh	For insecticide or mushroom poisoning
		0.6–1 mg IV	For bradycardia or atrioventricular block
glycopyrrolate	Robinul	0.1–0.2 mg IM or IV	Preoperative
propantheline	Pro-Banthine	15 mg PO AC and 30 mg at bedtime	For bladder spasm
scopolamine	Transderm Scop	72-h patch	Prevent motion sickness
homatropine[b]	Isopto Homatropine	Ophthalmic gtt	Mydriatic

[a]Use caution to give correct dosage.

[b]Other anticholinergics used in ophthalmic conditions are discussed in Chapter 18.

See Figure 13-1 for a summary of the autonomic nervous system drugs.

The Autonomic Nervous System

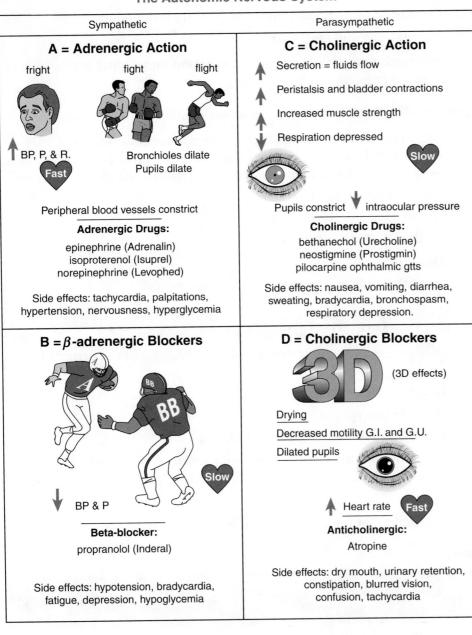

Figure 13-1 The autonomic nervous system drugs can be as simple as A, B, C, D.

WORKSHEET FOR CHAPTER 13
AUTONOMIC NERVOUS SYSTEM DRUGS

List the drugs according to category and complete all columns. To complete the Side Effects column, refer to the side effects icon in the chapter (✴). Learn generic or trade names as specified by instructor.

Classifications and Drugs	Purpose	Side Effects	Contraindications or Cautions	Patient Education
Adrenergics 1. 2. 3. 4. 5.				
Adrenergic Blocker 1.				
Cholinergics 1. 2.				
Cholinergic Blockers 1. 2. 3. 4.				

A. Case Study for Autonomic Nervous System Drugs

Arlie Woods, a 33-year-old, receives epinephrine (Adrenalin) in the emergency room for a severe asthma attack. Health care personnel should have the following information.

1. Adrenalin has all of the following actions EXCEPT
   a. Peripheral vasodilator   c. Bronchodilator
   b. Dilation of pupils   d. Cardiac stimulant

2. All of the following doses of Adrenalin are appropriate EXCEPT
   a. 0.4 ml IM (deltoid)   c. 5 ml SubQ
   b. 0.3 ml SubQ   d. 1 ml IV

3. Epinephrine is also used to treat all of the following conditions EXCEPT
   a. Nosebleed   c. Anaphylaxis
   b. Hypertension   d. Cardiac arrest

4. Side effects can include all of the following EXCEPT
   a. Tremors   c. Tachycardia
   b. Hypoglycemia   d. Insomnia

5. She should be told all of the following about epinephrine EXCEPT
   a. May cause sedation   c. May cause headaches
   b. Avoid alcohol   d. Palpitations possible

B. Case Study for Cholinergic Blockers

Milton Noteworthy was brought into the emergency room with complaints of nausea, diarrhea, and sweating. He says that he "ate mushrooms found in the woods." The following information would be helpful.

1. Mushroom poisoning mimics parasympathetic nervous system (cholinergic) action with all of the following symptoms EXCEPT
   a. Increased peristalsis   c. Salivation
   b. Urinary retention   d. Bradycardia

2. Treatment includes cholinergic blockers. Which of the following is *not* a cholinergic blocker?
   a. Urecholine   c. Atropine
   b. Banthine   d. Scopolamine

3. Which is the drug of choice to treat cholinergic toxicity (e.g., mushroom or insecticide poisoning)?
   a. Urecholine   c. Atropine
   b. Banthine   d. Scopolamine

4. Side effects of cholinergic blockers include all of the following EXCEPT
   a. Dry mouth   c. Urinary retention
   b. Diarrhea   d. Dilated pupils

5. Other side effects of cholinergic blockers can include all of the following EXCEPT
   a. Flushing   c. Blurred vision
   b. Confusion   d. Bradycardia

CHAPTER REVIEW QUIZ

Match the type of drug with the action.

Action	ANS drugs
1. _____ Increases muscle strength	**a.** Adrenergic
2. _____ Drying	**c.** Adrenergic blocker
3. _____ Increases blood pressure	**c.** Cholinergic
4. _____ Increases peristalsis	**d.** Anticholinergic
5. _____ Lowers intraocular pressure	
6. _____ Antispasmodic	
7. _____ Bronchodilator	
8. _____ Lowers blood pressure	
9. _____ Constricts pupils	
10. _____ Antiarrhythmic	

Match the type of drug with possible side effects.

Side Effects	ANS Drugs
11. _____ Bronchospasm	**a.** Adrenergic
12. _____ Hyperglycemia	**b.** Adrenergic blocker
13. _____ Diarrhea	**c.** Cholinergic
14. _____ Flushing	**d.** Anticholinergic
15. _____ Lethargy	
16. _____ Hypoglycemia	
17. _____ Constipation	
18. _____ Nervousness	
19. _____ Confusion	

20. Is the autonomic nervous system voluntary or involuntary?

Chapter 14
Antineoplastic Drugs

Objectives

Upon completion of this chapter, the learner should be able to

1. Define the Key Terms
2. Name three characteristics associated with administration of antineoplastic drugs
3. Name the eight major groups of antineoplastic agents
4. List the side effects common to most of the antineoplastic agents
5. Describe appropriate interventions in caring for patients receiving antineoplastic agents
6. Explain precautions in caring for those receiving radioactive isotopes
7. Describe the responsibilities of those caring for patients receiving chemotherapy
8. Explain appropriate education for patient and family when antineoplastic agents are administered
9. List safety factors for those who care for patients receiving cytotoxic drugs

Key Terms

Antineoplastic

Chemotherapy

Cytotoxic

Immunosuppressive

Palliative

Proliferating

Antineoplastic (against new tissue formation) refers to an agent that counteracts the development, growth, or spread of malignant cells. Cancer therapy frequently includes a combination of surgery, radiation, and/or chemotherapy.

Chemotherapy is a constantly growing field in which many old and new drugs and drug combinations are used for **palliative** effects (alleviation of symptoms) or for long-term or complete remissions in early treatment of cancer. Antineoplastic drugs are **cytotoxic** (destructive to cells), especially to cells that are **proliferating** (reproducing rapidly). Unfortunately, the toxic effects of the antineoplastic drugs are not confined to malignant cells alone, but also affect other proliferating tissue, such as bone marrow, gastrointestinal epithelium, skin, hair follicles, and epithelium of the gonads, resulting in numerous adverse side effects.

One of the most significant developments in cancer treatment today is the use of targeted therapies. Many of these newer antineoplastics are *monoclonal antibodies* that are designed to target only cancer cells, thereby sparing normal tissues. This reduces host toxicity while simultaneously increasing toxicity to cancer cells and improving survival rates in cancer patients.

Many antineoplastic agents also possess **immunosuppressive** properties, which decrease the production of antibodies and phagocytes, and reduce the inflammatory reaction. Suppression of the immune response results in increased susceptibility of the patient to infection.

Antineoplastic drugs are frequently administered in high doses on an *intermittent* schedule. Because most normal tissues have a greater capacity for repair than do most malignant tissues, normal cells may recover during the drug-free period.

Chemotherapy is *individualized* and frequently modified according to the patient's response to treatment. A *combination of several drugs* is frequently prescribed to delay the emergence of resistance, with the choice of agents based on the type of malignancy, areas involved, extent of the cancer, physical condition of the patient, and other factors. Careful planning is required to maximize the effectiveness of therapy and to minimize the side effects and discomfort for the patient. Understanding of the treatment program and possible side effects is essential for all concerned: the nurse, the patient, and the family. Preplanning includes provision for symptomatic relief, such as antiemetics, as well as reassurance and availability of support staff to answer questions, explore feelings, and allay fears. The treatment of cancer is highly complex. Only health care workers on oncology units, in cancer treatment centers, or in oncologist's offices would be expected to know the names of the numerous drugs. However, anyone who is in contact with patients on antineoplastic therapy should be aware of the frequent possible side effects to expect and appropriate interventions for the comfort of the patient. Patient education and support are extremely important.

Antineoplastic agents can be generally classified into eight major groups: antimetabolites, alkylating agents, plant alkaloids, antibiotic antineoplastics, steroid hormones, antiestrogen, antiandrogen, and biological response modifiers. Another category is radiation oncology, in which radioactive isotopes are used to treat certain types of cancer.

ANTIMETABOLITES

Antimetabolites are used in the treatment of leukemia, osteogenic sarcoma, squamous cell carcinoma, breast cancer, and other malignancies, especially those involving the genital areas. Some antimetabolites include methotrexate, fluorouracil, cytarabine, and 6-mercaptopurine.

Methotrexate has also been used for severe, resistant cases of psoriasis, rheumatoid arthritis, and lupus.

Side effects of antimetabolites can include:

 Anorexia, nausea, vomiting, and diarrhea

Ulceration and bleeding of the oral mucosa and gastrointestinal (GI) tract

Bone marrow suppression, including leukopenia with infection, anemia, and thrombocytopenia with hemorrhage

Rash, itching, photosensitivity, and scaling

Alopecia (regrowth of hair may take several months)

> *Note:* Leucovorin (a reduced form of folic acid) is sometimes used as a "rescue agent" following methotrexate administration to reduce methotrexate-induced hematological and GI toxicity.

Contraindications or extreme caution with antimetabolites applies to:

Renal and hepatic disorders

Pregnancy

GI ulcers

ALKYLATING AGENTS

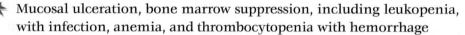Alkylating agents are used in the treatment of a wide range of cancers, including brain tumors, sarcomas, lymphomas, and leukemias. Some alkylating agents include carmustine, cisplatin, and thiotepa, used for metastatic ovarian, testicular, and bladder cancer and sometimes in palliative treatment of other cancers.

Side effects of alkylating agents can include:

Nausea, vomiting, and diarrhea

Mucosal ulceration, bone marrow suppression, including leukopenia, with infection, anemia, and thrombocytopenia with hemorrhage

Neurotoxicity, including headache, vertigo, and seizures

Rash and alopecia

Loss of reproduction capacity

Pulmonary fibrosis

Hemorrhagic cystitis (with ifosfamide and cyclophosphamide; Mesna—a chemoprotectant—is given prior to chemotherapy with ifosfamide to prevent this toxicity

Contraindications or extreme caution with alkylating agents applies to:

Debilitated patients

Pregnancy

Renal disease (with cisplatin and carboplatin)

PLANT ALKALOIDS

Plant alkaloids, for example, vinblastine or vincristine, are used in combination with other chemotherapeutic agents in the treatment of leukemias, Hodgkin's disease, lymphomas, sarcomas, and other malignancies.

Side effects of plant alkaloids can include:

* Neurotoxicity, including numbness; tingling; ataxia; foot drop; pain in the jaw, head, or extremities; and visual disturbances (less common with vinblastine)
* Severe constipation or diarrhea, nausea, and vomiting
* Oral or GI ulceration
* Rash, phototoxicity, and alopecia

  Leukopenia with vinblastine (hematological effects less common with vincristine)

  Necrosis of tissue if intravenous infiltrates into tissue

Contraindications or caution with plant alkaloids applies to:

Pregnancy, hepatic dysfunction, infection

Note: Intrathecal administration of these agents is fatal. This route must not be used. Syringes containing these agents should be labeled, "Warning—For IV use only, fatal if given intrathecally."

Paclitaxel

Paclitaxel (Taxol), another plant alkaloid, was originally extracted from the bark of the Western (Pacific) yew. It is structurally different from other available antineoplastic agents. It is used as second-line or subsequent therapy in patients with metastatic breast or ovarian carcinoma refractory to conventional chemotherapy.

Adverse side effects of Taxol are frequent and include:

* Bone marrow suppression: neutropenia, leukopenia, thrombocytopenia, and anemia
* Hypersensitivity reactions—can be severe, with flushing, rash, dyspnea, chest pain, hypotension, bradycardia
* Peripheral neuropathy
* Nausea, vomiting, diarrhea, mucositis

  Alopecia

Contraindications and cautions with Taxol applies to pregnancy, hepatic dysfunction, infection.

Since paclitaxel (Taxol) is so toxic, the drug is only administered IV under constant supervision of an oncologist, with frequent monitoring of vital signs, and facilities available for emergency interventions if required.

ANTIBIOTIC ANTINEOPLASTICS

Antibiotic antineoplastics are used to treat a wide variety of malignancies, including leukemias, sarcomas, Hodgkin's disease, lymphomas, breast cancer, and tumors of the head, neck, and testicles. Antibiotic antineoplastics include bleomycin, doxorubicin, mitomycin, and others. They are frequently used in combination with other drugs.

Side effects of antibiotic antineoplastics can include:

* Anorexia, nausea, vomiting, and diarrhea
* Bone marrow suppression (especially with bleomycin and mitomycin)
* Cardiotoxicity, including arrhythmias and congestive heart failure (with daunorubicin and doxorubicin)
* Pneumonitis, dyspnea, and rales; pulmonary fibrosis with bleomycin
* Ulceration of mouth or colon
  Alopecia, rash, and scaling

Contraindications or caution with antibiotic antineoplastics applies to:

Pregnancy

Liver disorders

Cardiac disease

HORMONE THERAPY
Corticosteroids

Corticosteroids, such as prednisone, are frequently used in combination with other chemotherapeutic agents in the treatment of leukemias and lymphomas. In addition, large doses of dexamethasone (Decadron) have been found effective in the prevention and treatment of nausea and vomiting associated with many antineoplastic agents, when administered before or with chemotherapy.

Side effects with prolonged use of prednisone (see Chapter 23) include:

* Fluid retention
  Cushingoid features (moon face)
* Fatigue and weakness
* Osteoporosis

Antiestrogen

A *nonsteroidal antiestrogen, tamoxifen,* can be used as primary hormonal therapy for metastatic estrogen receptor–positive breast cancer in both men and postmenopausal women. It is also used in the palliative treatment of advanced metastatic breast cancer or as an adjunct to surgery with positive and negative axillary lymph nodes. Serious adverse side effects are rare and usually dose related, resembling menopausal symptoms. Nausea, vomiting, hot flashes, and night sweats can occur in up to 66% of cases, but usually do not require discontinuation.

Anastrozole (Arimidex), which inhibits the final step in estrogen production, offers an alternative to tamoxifen in postmenopausal women with breast cancer.

Antiandrogen

Antiandrogen drugs include leuprolide acetate (Lupron Depot), a gonadotropin-releasing hormone (GnRH) analog, which is usually administered IM once monthly for prostate cancer. See Chapter 24 for more details.

Bicalutamide (Casodex) is an oral antiandrogen used simultaneously with leuprolide in the treatment of metastatic prostate cancer.

Side effects of antiandrogens can include:

✴ Impotence

✴ Hot flashes, generalized pain, infection, constipation, nausea

Patients should be advised that the drug should be continued even when signs or symptoms of the disease improve.

Sex hormones, including the estrogens, progestins, and androgens, are also used as antineoplastic agents in the treatment of malignancies involving the reproductive system (e.g., cancer of the breast, uterus, or prostate). These hormones are discussed in Chapter 24.

BIOLOGICAL RESPONSE MODIFIERS
Interferons

Interferon alfa is a complex combination of many proteins acting as a biologic response modifier. The action is complex, affecting cell proliferation and other cell functions and immune system response. Its antiviral action is described in Chapter 17. Interferons are used in the treatment of many malignancies, for example, leukemias, sarcomas, and other cancers, especially those resistant to standard treatments. Some interferons are used to treat multiple sclerosis and many other conditions, and research is ongoing.

Adverse side effects of interferons, sometimes severe, are experienced by almost all patients receiving interferon, varying with the dosage and condition. Most common side effects include:

✴ Flulike syndrome—fever, fatigue, headache, muscle aches, and pains

✴ GI symptoms—anorexia, nausea, vomiting, diarrhea, and dry mouth

✴ Nervous system effects—sleep disturbances, mental symptoms

Hematological effects—especially leukopenia

Dyspnea, cough, nasal congestion

Alopecia—transient

MONOCLONAL ANTIBODIES

Monoclonal antibodies (MABs), first developed in the 1970s, were not marketed for cancer treatment until the late 1990s. In the human body, B-cells (a class of white blood cells) produce *endogenous* (within the cell) antibodies in response to foreign stimuli such as bacteria. The antibodies mark the cell for destruction by the immune system, or prevent further cell growth.

MABs are *exogenous* antibodies genetically engineered in the laboratory by combining an antibody-producing B-cell with a cancer cell. This new cell will produce copies or clones of a single antibody, thus the name *monoclonal antibody*. MABs are designed to target only cancer cells, thereby sparing normal tissues (i.e., not *directly* cytotoxic). This reduces host toxicity while simultaneously increasing toxicity to cancer cells.

MABs have fairly specific mechanisms of action that result in fairly specific indications. Bevacizumab (Avastin), in combination with fluorouracil, is indicated for first-line treatment of patients with metastatic carcinoma of the colon or rectum. Rituximab (Rituxan) is used to treat relapsed or refractory (unresponsive to treatment) non-Hodgkin's lymphoma alone or in combination with other antineoplastics. Trastuzumab (Herceptin), combined with paclitaxel, is indicated for first-line treatment of metastatic breast cancer. All MABs are administered intravenously.

Side effects of MABs are common, especially with the first infusion, and can include:

 Fever and chills, headache, dizziness

Nausea and vomiting

Itching, rash, generalized pain

These reactions should occur less frequently with subsequent infusions.

Severe reactions can be minimized by *premedicating* with acetaminophen (Tylenol), diphenhydramine (Benadryl), and/or meperidine (Demerol). Signs of severe reaction can include:

Angioedema, hypotension, dyspnea, bronchospasm (may be necessary to stop infusion)

Hypersensitivity reactions (including anaphylaxis)

Cardiac arrythmias, angina, cardiomyopathy; hypertensive crisis (with Avastin)

Acute renal failure (not with Herceptin)

 Hematological toxicity (i.e., reduced white blood cells [WBCs]); complete blood count (CBC) and platelet count should be monitored frequently

GI perforation, GI bleed; impaired wound healing (all with Avastin)

RADIOACTIVE ISOTOPES

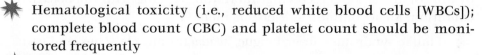

Radioactive isotopes are also used in the treatment of certain types of cancer. Sometimes the radioactive material is injected into the affected site

(e.g., radiogold, injected into the pleural or peritoneal cavity to treat ascites caused by cancer). Radioactive sodium iodine is administered PO or IV to treat thyroid cancer. Radioactive material is sometimes implanted in the body in the form of capsules, needles, or seeds.

The newest targeted therapy provides the added benefit of radiation. Radioimmunotherapy consists of MABs that have radioisotopes attached to them so that whatever the antibody binds to can also be irradiated. Tositumomab (Bexxar) with iodine 131 is indicated for patients with non-Hodgkin's lymphoma that is refractory to rituximab. The primary side effect after radioimmunotherapy is a decreased blood count occurring four to six weeks after treatment. The counts remain low for two to three weeks and then return to normal. The distinct advantage of radioimmunotherapy is that it is usually given one time.

Health care workers caring for patients receiving radioactive isotopes must observe special precautions to prevent unnecessary radiation exposure. Gowns and gloves should be worn when handling excreta. Other isolation procedures, such as handling of linens, will be outlined in the facility's procedure manual. This protocol should be followed with great care by all those who come in contact with patients receiving radioactive materials, for the protection of patients, as well as the health care worker.

CAUTIONS AND RESPONSIBILITIES FOR ANTINEOPLASTIC DRUGS

Health care workers involved in the administration of antineoplastic agents, as well as those who care for these patients, have a number of very important responsibilities.

1. All medications should be given on time and exactly as prescribed to keep the patient as comfortable as possible. Check drug inserts on all new drugs.

2. Intravenous sites must be checked with great care because antineoplastic agents can cause extreme tissue damage and necrosis if infiltration occurs.

3. Intravenous fluids containing antineoplastic agents should not be allowed to get on the skin or into the eyes of the patient or the one administering the medication. Flush skin or eyes copiously if spills occur.

4. Antiemetics should be immediately available and administered as prescribed to minimize nausea and vomiting. Ondansetron (Zofran), dolasetron (Anzemet), and granisetron (Kytril) are examples of antiemetics for this purpose.

5. Careful and frequent oral hygiene is essential to minimize the discomfort and ulceration.

6. Soft foods and cool liquids should be available to the patient as required.

7. Accurate intake and output is important for adequate assessment of hydration.

8. Careful observation and reporting of symptoms and side effects is an essential part of chemotherapy.

9. Aseptic technique is necessary to minimize the chance of infection in patients with reduced resistance to infection.

10. Careful assessment of vital signs is important to identify signs of infection, cardiac irregularities, and dyspnea.

11. The health care worker and family must be informed about all aspects of chemotherapy and answer the patient's questions honestly. Awareness of verbal and nonverbal communication that gives clues to the patient's needs is absolutely necessary.

12. Careful attention to detail, astute observations, appropriate interventions, and compassion are an integral part of care when the patient is receiving chemotherapy.

13. The health care worker should reassure the patient that someone will be available to help at all times. Identify these resources.

Patient Education

Patients being treated with antineoplastic drugs and their families should be instructed regarding:

Side effects to expect, how long they can be expected to continue, and that they are frequently temporary

Comfort measures for coping with unpleasant side effects, (e.g., antiemetics and antidiarrhea agents as prescribed)

Appropriate diet with foods that are more palatable and more likely to be tolerated (e.g., soft foods, bland foods, a variety of liquids, and especially cold foods in frequent, small quantities)

Careful aseptic technique to decrease the chance of infections and reporting any signs of infection (e.g., fever)

Careful oral hygiene with swabs to prevent further trauma to ulcerated mucosa

Observation for bleeding in stools, urine, and gums and for bruises, and reporting this to medical personnel

Reporting of any persistent or unusual side effects, such as dizziness, severe headache, numbness, tingling, difficulty walking, or visual disturbances

Available community resources to assist and support the patient (e.g., Cancer Society, Hospice, or Home Health Services) as required and recommended by the physician

How to obtain information and answers to questions regarding treatment

The right of patients to terminate therapy if they wish

See Table 14-1 for a summary of the antineoplastic agents.

Table 14-1 Antineoplastic Agents

GENERIC NAME	TRADE NAME	GENERIC NAME	TRADE NAME
Antimetabolites		**Antibiotic Antineoplastics**	
cytarabine	Cytosar-U	bleomycin	Blenoxane
fluorouracil	Adrucil	daunorubicin	Cerubidine
methotrexate	Rheumatrex	doxorubicin	Adriamycin
mercaptopurine	Purinethol	mitomycin	Mutamycin
Alkylating Agents		etoposide, VP-16	VePesid
busulfan	Myleran	**Steroid Hormones**	
carboplatin	Paraplatin	dexamethasone	Decadron
carmustine, BCNU	BiCNU, Gliadel	prednisone	Deltasone
chlorambucil	Leukeran	**Antiestrogen**	
cisplatin	Platinol	tamoxifen	Nolvadex
cyclophosphamide	Cytoxan	anastrozole	Arimidex
ifosfamide	IFEX	**Antiandrogen**	
thiotepa	Thioplex	leuprolide	Lupron Depot
Plant Alkaloids		bicalutamide	Casodex
vinblastine	Velban	**Biological Response Modifiers**	
vincristine	Oncovin	interferon	Roferon-A
paclitaxel	Taxol		Intron A
		bevacizumab	Avastin
		rituximab	Rituxan
		tositumomab	Bexxar
		trastuzumab	Herceptin

Note: This listing is not complete but is representative of the most used drugs. Dosage is usually on an intermittent schedule and individualized. New drugs and new combination therapies are under investigation. Research is ongoing.

Cytotoxic Drug Dangers to Health Care Personnel

Anyone who prepares, administers, or cares for patients receiving cytotoxic drugs should be aware of the dangers involved. The American Society of Health-System Pharmacists (ASHP) has published a *Technical Assistance Bulletin (TAB)* that provides detailed advice on recommended policies, procedures, and equipment for safe handling of cytotoxic drugs (see AHFS Drug Information). It is essential that policies and procedures are followed exactly as outlined on the labels provided by the drug company. Guidelines of the individual health care agency must also be followed to the letter for the safety of all concerned.

The danger to health care personnel from handling a hazardous drug stems from a combination of its inherent toxicity and the extent to which workers are exposed in the course of carrying out their duties. This exposure may be from inadvertent ingestion of the drug on foodstuffs, inhalation of drug dust or droplets, or direct skin contact.

Recommended safe handling methods include four broad goals:

1. Protect and secure packages of hazardous drugs. Store separately from nonhazardous drugs.

2. Inform and educate all involved personnel about hazardous drugs and train them in safe handling procedures.

3. Do not let the drugs escape from containers when they are manipulated (i.e., dissolved, transferred, administered, or discarded).

4. Eliminate the possibility of inadvertent ingestion or inhalation and direct skin or eye contact with the drugs.

Specific recommendations for cytotoxic drugs include:

1. When preparing these drugs, wear gloves, long-sleeved gowns, splash goggles, and disposable respirator masks.

2. For administration, wear long-sleeved gowns and gloves. Syringes and IV sets with Luer-Lok fittings should be used and care taken that all fittings are secure.

3. Dispose of syringes, IV tubing and bags, gauze, or any other contaminated material such as linens in a leakproof, puncture-resistant container that is labeled "HAZARD."

4. Wear gloves and gown when handling excreta from patients receiving cytotoxic drugs.

5. Those who are pregnant, breast-feeding, or actively trying to conceive a child should not care for patients receiving cytotoxic drugs.

For more detailed instructions, see *ASHP Technical Assistance Bulletin on Handling Cytotoxic and Hazardous Drugs,* which is reproduced in the AHFS Drug Information book and updated based on information from OSHA (Occupational Safety and Health Administration), National Institutes of Health (NIH), National Study Commission on Cytotoxic Exposure, and the AMA (American Medical Association) Council on Scientific Affairs.

Antineoplastic therapy is complex and changes frequently with ongoing research. Therefore, you are not expected to remember the names of all of the antineoplastic agents. However, you need to know the *common side effects, interventions, cautions, and appropriate patient education.*

A. Case Study for Antineoplastic Drugs

Wanda Woodbirch, a 36-year-old patient with leukemia, has begun chemotherapy at the oncologist's office. She will need the following information.

1. Her therapy will include all of the following EXCEPT
   a. Individualized dosage   c. Radioactive iodine
   b. Intermittent schedule   d. Several drugs

2. All of the following side effects are possible EXCEPT
   a. Nausea   c. Constipation
   b. Alopecia   d. Photosensitivity

3. Many antineoplastic drugs cause bone marrow suppression, which can result in all of the following EXCEPT
    a. Susceptibility to infection   c. Anemia
    b. Increased clotting time   d. Jaundice

4. The following advice is appropriate EXCEPT
    a. Practice good oral hygiene   c. Eat soft foods
    b. Exercise briskly   d. Watch for hematuria

5. The following should be reported to the physician EXCEPT
    a. Fever   c. Blood in stools
    b. Dyspnea   d. Hair loss

B. Case Study for Antineoplastic Drugs

Ila Lake, a 40-year-old patient with metastatic breast cancer, will be followed by the oncologist. The nurse or medical assistant in the office will need the following information.

1. Appropriate treatment might include any of the following drugs EXCEPT
    a. Interferon   c. Tamoxifen
    b. Lupron   d. Taxol

2. The patient will need a supply of all of the following EXCEPT
    a. Analgesics   c. Diuretics
    b. Antiemetics   d. Antidiarrhea drugs

3. Monitoring of the following is necessary EXCEPT
    a. Vital signs   c. Hydration
    b. Neurological signs   d. Blood glucose

4. Patient education includes all of the following EXCEPT
    a. Careful handwashing   c. Brush teeth briskly
    b. Adequate fluids   d. Report air hunger

5. Health care workers who handle cytotoxic drugs should observe the following precautions EXCEPT
    a. Wear gloves   c. Wear long-sleeved gowns
    b. Avoid pregnancy   d. Dispose of waste in dumpster

CHAPTER REVIEW QUIZ

Match the term with the definition:

1. _____ Palliative
2. _____ Cytotoxic
3. _____ Antineoplastic
4. _____ Monoclonal antibodies
5. _____ Proliferating
6. _____ Exogenous antibodies
7. _____ Refractory
8. _____ Immunosuppressive
9. _____ Endogenous antibodies
10. _____ Clone

a. Target only cancer cells
b. Unresponsive to treatment
c. Within the cell
d. Produce a copy
e. Decreases antibody production
f. Alleviation of symptoms
g. Engineered in a laboratory
h. Reproducing rapidly
i. Destructive to cells
j. Counteracts malignant cell growth

Multiple Choice

11. Severe reactions from MABs can be minimized by premedicating with the following drugs EXCEPT
    a. Tylenol
    b. Benadryl
    c. Toradol
    d. Demerol
12. Which is NOT a side effect of many antineoplastic drugs?
    a. Alopecia
    b. Rash
    c. Bone marrow suppression
    d. Constipation
13. Which is NOT a side effect with some antineoplastic drugs?
    a. GI symptoms
    b. Jaundice
    c. Mouth ulcers
    d. Photosensitivity
14. Bone marrow suppression can result in all of the following complications EXCEPT
    a. Anemia
    b. Hemorrhage
    c. Thrombophlebitis
    d. Infection
15. The monoclonal antibodies (MABs) can be administered by which route?
    a. Intramuscular
    b. Intravenous
    c. Oral
    d. Subcutaneous

Chapter 15
Urinary System Drugs

Objectives

Upon completion of this chapter, the learner should be able to

1. Compare and contrast the four types of diuretics for uses, side effects, cautions, and interactions and give examples of each type
2. Define the Key Terms
3. Describe two interactions of other medications with probenecid (Benemid)
4. Identify one medication given for chronic gout that is not uricosuric and one that is
5. Explain the role of certain antispasmodics used to reduce contractions of the urinary bladder
6. Identify the actions of phenazopyridine (Pyridium) and bethanechol (Urecholine)
7. Describe two different treatments for benign prostatic hypertrophy (BPH).
8. Describe appropriate patient education for all medications listed in this chapter

Key Terms

Alpha-blockers

Antispasmodics

Antiandrogens

Benign prostatic hypertrophy (BPH)

Calculus

Cholinergics

Diuretics

Gout

Hyperkalemia

Hypokalemia

Osmotic agents

Uricosuric agents

Urinary analgesic

DIURETICS

The most commonly used drugs influencing function of the urinary tract are the **diuretics,** which increase urine excretion. Diuretics are divided into four categories according to their action: thiazides, loop diuretics, potassium-sparing diuretics, and osmotic agents. The type of diuretic used is determined by the condition being treated. Carbonic anhydrase inhibitors, such as acetazolamide (Diamox), which are diuretics used to lower intraocular pressure, are discussed in Chapter 18, Eye Medications.

Thiazides and Related Diuretics

Thiazides are the most frequently used type of diuretic, increasing excretion of water, sodium, chloride, and potassium. An example is hydrochlorothiazide.

Uses of the thiazides include treatment of:

Edema from many causes (e.g., heart failure and cirrhosis)

Uncomplicated hypertension for most patients, either alone or combined with drugs from other classes (blood pressure is lowered by reducing peripheral vascular resistance as well as by decreasing fluid retention)

Prophylaxis of **calculus** (stone) formation in those with hypercalciuria (excess calcium in the urine)

Electrolyte imbalance from renal dysfunction (metolazone is diuretic of choice)

Side effects of the thiazides may include:

 Hypokalemia (potassium deficiency), may lead to cardiac arrhythmias

Hypochloremia (chloride deficiency), may lead to alkalosis

Muscle weakness or spasm

Gastrointestinal (GI) reactions (e.g., anorexia, nausea, vomiting, diarrhea)

Postural hypotension, vertigo, and headache

Fatigue, weakness, and lethargy

Skin conditions (e.g., rash and photosensitivity; rare)

Hyperglycemia and increased uric acid

Contraindications or caution with thiazides applies to:

Diabetes (may cause hyperglycemia and glycosuria)

History of gout (increased uric acid level)

Severe renal disease

Impaired liver function

Prolonged use (periodic serum electrolyte checks indicated, and potassium supplements recommended to prevent hypokalemia)

Older adults due to greater sensitivity to thiazides (may cause low sodium)

Patients with sulfonamide hypersensitivity

Patient Education

Patients being treated with thiazides should be instructed regarding:

Diet including potassium-rich foods (e.g., citrus fruits and bananas) or potassium supplements (check with the physician first)

If diuretic prescribed for hypertension, a low-sodium diet (may be prescribed by the physician)

Notifying the physician of persistent or severe side effects

Administration with food (to reduce gastric irritation)

Administration in the morning to prevent disruption of sleep cycle

Rising slowly from reclining position to counteract postural hypotension

Limitation of alcohol

Avoiding other medications without consulting physician

Necessity for regular blood test to monitor electrolytes

Interactions with thiazides may occur with:

Nonsteroidal anti-inflammatory agents—risk of renal insufficiency

Corticosteroids to increase potassium loss

Lithium, to cause lithium intoxication

Hypotensive agents, which potentiate blood pressure decrease

Digitalis with increased potential for digitalis toxicity

Probenecid (Benemid) to block uric acid retention

Antidiabetic agents (loss of diabetic control)

Loop Diuretics

These diuretics act directly on the loop of Henle in the kidney to inhibit sodium and chloride reabsorption. Potent diuretics such as furosemide (Lasix), bumetanide (Bumex) and torsemide (Demadex) are not thiazides but act in a similar way to increase excretion of water, sodium, chloride, and potassium. Their action is more rapid and effective than that of thiazides, with a greater diuresis.

Uses of loop diuretics, such as furosemide (Lasix), bumetanide (Bumex), and torsemide (Demadex), include treatment of:

Edema associated with impaired renal function or hepatitic disease

Congestive heart failure

Pulmonary edema

Ascites caused by malignancy or cirrhosis

Hypertension (if thiazides ineffective, loop diuretics sometimes combined with other antihypertensives)

Side effects of loop diuretics may include:

 Fluid and electrolyte imbalance with dehydration, circulatory collapse, chest pain

 Hypokalemia with weakness and vertigo (potassium supplements indicated especially for cardiac patients to prevent arrhythmias)

 Hypotension (close blood pressure checks required)

GI effects, including anorexia, nausea, vomiting, diarrhea, and abdominal pain

 Hyperglycemia and increased uric acid

Blood dyscrasias with prolonged use

Tinnitus, hearing impairment, and blurred vision

Rash, urticaria, pruritus, and photosensitivity

 Allergic reactions to furosemide in those allergic to sulfa, since furosemide and bumetanide are *sulfonamides*

Headache, muscle cramps, mental confusion, dizziness

Contraindications or caution with loop diuretics applies to:

Cirrhosis and other liver disease—careful monitoring required

Kidney impairment

Alkalosis and dehydration

Digitalized patients (cardiac arrhythmias possible unless potassium supplemented)

Those allergic to sulfa

Diabetes

History of gout

Pregnancy and lactation

Children under 18 years of age (Bumex and Demadex)

Note: Torsemide (Demadex) must be given with a potassium-sparing agent to prevent hypokalemia and metabolic acidosis, especially in patients with cirrhosis of the liver.

Interactions of loop diuretics are similar to those of the thiazides:

Corticosteroids—potentiate potassium loss

Lithium—toxicity risk increased

Hypotensive agents—potentiation of effects

Probenecid—may decrease diuretic effects

Digitalis with increased potential for digitalis toxicity and arrhythmias

Additional interactions of loop diuretics may include:

Aminoglycosides increase chance of deafness

Indomethacin decreases diuretic effect

Salicylates with furosemide increase chance of salicylate toxicity

Anticonvulsants (e.g., phenytoin) reduce the diuretic effect of furosemide

Patient Education

Patients being treated with loop diuretics should be instructed regarding the same information as patients taking thiazides:

Dietary or other potassium supplements as prescribed

Notifying the physician of side effects *immediately*

Taking with food before 6 P.M.

Rising slowly from reclining position

Avoiding alcohol

Reporting sudden changes in urinary output, especially decrease

Reporting abrupt or severe weight loss

Limiting exposure to sunlight with furosemide, due to photosensitivity

Not taking any other prescribed or over-the-counter drugs without consulting the physician first

Potassium-Sparing Diuretics

Potassium-sparing diuretics such as spironolactone (Aldactone) and triamterene (Dyrenium), are sometimes administered under conditions in which potassium depletion can be dangerous. Potassium-sparing diuretics also counteract the increased glucose and uric acid levels associated with thiazide diuretic therapy. Spironolactone is the diuretic of choice in patients with cirrhosis. It has also been shown to be very effective in patients with severe heart failure.

Potassium-sparing diuretics are seldom used alone, but are usually combined with thiazide diuretics to increase the diuretic and hypotensive effects and to reduce the danger of **hyperkalemia** (excessive potassium retention). When combination products (e.g., Aldactazide or Dyazide) are given, supplemental potassium is usually *not* indicated, but this varies with individual circumstances and other medications taken concomitantly. *Periodic serum electrolyte checks are indicated.*

Side effects of potassium-saving diuretics are usually mild and respond to withdrawal of the drug, but may include:

* *Hyperkalemia* (especially with potassium supplements), which may lead to *cardiac arrhythmias*

  Dehydration or weakness

  GI symptoms, including nausea, vomiting, and diarrhea

* Fatigue, lethargy, and profound weight loss

* Hypotension

  Gynecomastia with spironolactone

Caution with potassium-sparing diuretics is indicated in patients with:

Renal insufficiency

Cirrhosis and other liver disease

Pregnancy and lactation

Interactions may occur with potassium-sparing diuretics and:

Potassium supplements, angiotensin-converting enzyme (ACE) inhibitors, angiotensin receptor blockers (ARBs), salicylates, and nonsteroidal anti-inflammatory drugs (NSAIDS), to cause hyperkalemia

Lithium to reduce clearance and cause lithium toxicity

Patient Education

Patients being treated with potassium-sparing diuretics should be instructed regarding:

Avoidance of potassium-rich foods and salt substitutes

Reporting signs of excessive dehydration (e.g., dry mouth, drowsiness, lethargy, and fever)

Reporting GI symptoms (e.g., nausea, vomiting, and diarrhea)

Reporting persistent headache and mental confusion

Reporting irregular heartbeat

Monitoring weight and reporting sudden, excessive weight loss

Rising slowly from reclining position

Taking medications after meals

Osmotic Agents

Osmotic agents (e.g., mannitol and urea) are most frequently used to reduce intracranial or intraocular pressure. Mannitol has also been used to prevent and/or treat acute renal failure and during certain cardiovascular surgery. Mannitol is also used alone or with other diuretics to promote excretions of toxins in cases of drug poisoning.

Side effects of osmotic agents can include:

* Fluid and electrolyte imbalance
* CNS symptoms, including headache, vertigo, mental confusion, nausea, and vomiting
* Tachycardia, hypertension, and hypotension
  Allergic reactions
* Severe pulmonary edema

Extreme caution is indicated, and kidney and cardiovascular function should be evaluated before administration of osmotic agents to anyone with:

Kidney failure

Heart failure

Active intracranial bleeding (except during craniotomy)

Severe pulmonary edema

Pregnancy and lactation

Interactions may occur with mannitol to increase urinary excretion of other drugs. Blood levels of drugs, such as lithium, barbiturates, and salicylates, are lowered as a result.

Patient Education

Patients being treated with osmotic agents should be instructed regarding side effects to be reported to the physician immediately. The patient should be reassured that osmotic agents are always given under close medical supervision and serum electrolytes will be monitored frequently by blood tests to detect adverse reactions.

See Table 15-1 for a summary of drugs for diuresis.

Table 15-1 Drugs for Diuresis

GENERIC NAME	TRADE NAME	DOSAGE (VARIES WITH CONDITION)
Thiazide and Related Diuretics (representative list—many others)		
indapamide	Lozol	2.5–5 mg daily PO
hydrochlorothiazide	Esidrix, HydroDIURIL	25–50 mg daily-TID
metolazone	Zaroxolyn	5–20 mg daily
Loop Diuretics		
furosemide	Lasix	20–80 mg daily, PO, IM, or IV
bumetanide	Bumex	0.5–2 mg daily, PO, IM, or IV
torsemide	Demadex	5–20 mg daily, PO; **slow** IV dosage not to exceed 200 mg
Potassium-Sparing Diuretics		
spironolactone	Aldactone	50–100 mg daily
triamterene	Dyrenium	100 mg BID pc
Combination Potassium-Sparing and Thiazide Diuretics		
spironolactone and hydrochlorothiazide	Aldactazide	25–100 mg daily (each component)
triamterene and hydrochlorothiazide	Dyazide, Maxzide	I cap or tab daily
Osmotic Agents		
mannitol	Osmitrol	Parenteral only, dose varies with condition
urea	Ureaphil	Parenteral only, dose varies with condition

MEDICATIONS FOR GOUT

Gout is a form of arthritis in which uric acid crystals are deposited in and around joints, causing inflammation and pain. Joints affected may be at any location but gout usually begins in the knee or foot.

Medications to treat gout include uricosuric agents and allopurinol, which lower uric acid levels.

Uricosuric Agents

Uricosuric agents, such as probenecid (Benemid), act on the kidney by blocking reabsorption and promoting urinary excretion of uric acid. This type of drug is used in the treatment of *chronic* cases of gout and frequent disabling attacks of gouty arthritis. However, the uricosuric agents have no analgesic or anti-inflammatory activity and are therefore *not* effective in the treatment of acute gout. During acute attacks of gout, the probenecid dosage is supplemented with colchicine, which has anti-inflammatory action. (See Chapter 21, Anti-inflammatory Drugs.)

Probenecid is sometimes given with penicillin to potentiate the level of the antibiotic in the blood, for example, with amoxicillin for some gonococcal infections. Probenecid is also given with cefoxitin to treat acute pelvic inflammatory disease.

Side effects of probenecid are rare but may include:

Headache

Nausea and vomiting

Kidney stones and renal colic if large volume of fluids is not maintained

Hypersensitivity reactions, rash, hypotension, and anaphylaxis are rare

Contraindication for probenecid applies to patients with:

History of uric acid kidney stones

History of peptic ulcer

Renal impairment

Blood dyscrasias

Interactions may occur with:

Penicillins and cephalosporins, potentiating therapeutic effect of antibiotics

Oral hypoglycemics, which could cause hypoglycemia through potentiation

Salicylates, which antagonize uricosuric action

NSAIDs (probenecid decreases renal clearance)

Patient Education

Patients being treated with uricosuric agents should be instructed regarding:

Drinking large amounts of fluid

Avoiding taking any aspirin products

Taking other medications at the same time only with physician's order

Taking medications with food

Reporting rash immediately

Allopurinol

Allopurinol (Zyloprim) is another medication, not a uricosuric, used to treat chronic gout. This drug acts by decreasing serum and urine levels of uric acid. It has no analgesic or anti-inflammatory activity and therefore is *not* effective in the treatment of acute gout.

> *Note:* The drug of choice for acute cases of gout or gouty arthritis is *colchicine*, which is discussed in Chapter 21, Anti-inflammatory Drugs.

Allopurinol is also used for the prevention of renal calculi in patients with a history of frequent stone formation and prevention of acute hyperuricemia during radiation of certain tumors or antineoplastic therapy.

Side effects of allopurinol can include:

Rash

Allergic reactions, also fever, chills, nausea, vomiting, diarrhea, drowsiness, and vertigo

Severe hypersensitivity reactions are rare, but increase in patients with renal impairment who receive allopurinol and thiazide diuretics in combination.

Contraindications or caution with allopurinol applies to:

Impaired renal function

History of hypersensitivity reactions

Liver disease

Pregnancy and lactation

Interactions may occur with allopurinol and:

Antineoplastic drugs, potentiating side effects (azathioprine, mercaptopurine)

Alcohol and diuretics, which increase serum urate concentrations

Patient Education

Patients being treated with allopurinol should be instructed regarding:

Drinking large quantities of fluid

Taking medication after meals

Stopping medication and reporting rash to physician immediately

Avoiding alcohol, which increases uric acid

Avoiding other medications unless prescribed by physician

ANTISPASMODICS

Antispasmodics, which are anticholinergic in action (blocking parasympathetic nerve impulses), are used to reduce the strength and frequency of contractions of the urinary bladder (See Chapter 13, Cholinergic Blockers). Antispasmodics, such as propantheline (Pro-Banthine), are used to increase the bladder capacity in patients with neurogenic bladder resulting in incontinence. Another anticholinergic, occasionally used as an antispasmodic, is hyoscyamine (Cytospaz, Levsin) but adverse side effects are common in older adults.

Other chemically similar drugs that exert spasmolytic effects on smooth muscle include tolterodine (Detrol) and oxybutynin (Ditropan). They are used for the relief of symptoms such as urgency, frequency, nocturia, and incontinence. They have similar adverse side effects, especially in older adults.

Tolterodine and oxybutynin XL, or Oxytrol patch, are less than or equally effective as oxybutynin IR (immediate release), but cause significantly fewer anticholinergic adverse effects.

Side effects of antispasmodics are *anticholinergic* in action and can include:

* Drying of all secretions (especially in the eyes and mouth)
* Drowsiness and dizziness—headache
* Urinary retention and constipation
* Blurred vision
* Mental confusion (especially with older adults)
* Tachycardia, palpitations

   Nausea and vomiting

   Rash, urticaria, allergic reactions

Cautions with antispasmodics for:

   Older adults

   Hepatic or renal disease, obstructive uropathy

   Bladder or GI obstruction, or ulcerative colitis

   Cardiovascular disease

Prostatic hypertrophy

Children under five years old—contraindicated

Pregnant or nursing women

Narrow angle glaucoma

Patient Education

Patients being treated with antispasmodics should be instructed regarding:

Reporting side effects that are troublesome for possible dosage adjustment

Reporting effectiveness

Using caution driving or operating machinery

Avoiding alcohol or other sedatives that potentiate drowsiness

CHOLINERGICS

Bethanechol (Urecholine) is a **cholinergic** drug, stimulating parasympathetic nerves, to bring about contraction of the urinary bladder in cases of nonobstructive urinary retention, usually postoperatively or postpartum. It has been called the "pharmacological catheterization." (See Chapter 13, Cholinergics.)

Side effects of bethanechol are cholinergic in action and usually dose related, and can include:

✳ GI cramping, diarrhea, nausea, and vomiting

✳ Sweating and salivation

✳ Headache and bronchial constriction

✳ Slow heartbeat or reflex tachycardia, and orthostatic hypotension

✳ Urinary urgency

Contraindications of bethanecol include:

Obstruction of the GI or urinary tract

Hyperthyroidism

Peptic ulcer, irritable bowel syndrome

Asthma

Cardiovascular disease—bradycardia

Parkinsonism, seizure disorder

Pregnancy and lactation

Interactions may occur with bethanecol and:

Other cholinergic or anticholinesterase agents (e.g., neostigmine) administered concomitantly, which can potentiate effects, with increased possibility of toxicity

Quinidine or procainamide, which antagonize cholinergic effect

Atropine, which antagonizes cholinergic effect (antidote in cases of cholinergic toxicity

ANALGESICS

Phenazopyridine (Pyridium) is an oral **urinary analgesic** or local anesthetic for urinary tract mucosa. It is used to relieve burning, pain, discomfort, and urgency associated with cystitis; with procedures causing irritation to the lower urinary tract, such as cystoscopy and surgery; or with trauma. It should not be taken for more than two days when used with an antibacterial agent.

Phenazopyridine is used *only for symptomatic relief* and is not a substitute for treatment of causative conditions. For treatment of urinary tract infections, anti-infective medication is required (see Chapter 17).

Side effects of Pyridium are rare for the most part but can include:

Headache or vertigo

Mild GI disturbances

Orange-red urine (common)—may stain fabric and contact lenses

Flavoxate (Urispas), an oral urinary antispasmodic agent, also exhibits weak anesthetic and analgesic properties for symptomatic relief, but is not a substitute for antibiotic treatment of urinary tract infections.

Contraindications for urinary analgesics include:

Impaired kidney function, especially in older adults

Severe hepatitis

Phenazopyridine may interfere with various urine, kidney function, or liver function tests.

Patient Education

Patients being treated with phenazopyridine (Pyridium) for urinary tract distress should be instructed regarding color change of urine to orange-red, which may stain fabric, and tears may stain contact lenses.

Phenazopyridine is only temporarily effective against discomfort in the lower urinary tract and is *not* effective against infection. The cause of the discomfort must be determined by examination of urine culture, and appropriate therapy, such as surgery or anti-infective medication, may be given to correct the condition.

TREATMENT OF BENIGN PROSTATIC HYPERTROPHY (BPH)

Antiandrogens

Finasteride (Proscar) and dutasteride (Avodart) are used to reduce prostate size and associated urinary obstruction and manifestations, for example, urgency, nocturia, and urinary hesitancy in patients with **benign prostatic hypertrophy (BPH).** Proscar 5 mg, or Avodart 0.5 mg, is administered daily for a minimum of 6–12 months. This therapy appears to be suppressive rather than curative, and return of the hypertrophy is likely if the drug is withdrawn.

Side effects of **antiandrogens** are infrequent and mild, including impotence, decreased libido, decreased ejaculate, and gynecomastia (including breast tenderness and enlargement).

Cautions: Patients should be screened first for cancer, infection, or other urinary dysfunctions. Liver function abnormalities may be exacerbated. Crushed tablets and soft gelatin capsules should *not be handled by pregnant women* (causes fetal damage).

ALPHA-BLOCKERS

Tamsulosin (Flomax) blocks alpha-1 receptors found in smooth muscle in the bladder neck and prostate, causing them to relax. Consequently, the urine flow rate is improved and the symptoms of BPH are decreased. Other examples of **alpha-blockers** are doxazosin (Cardura) and terazosin (Hytrin), which are used in the treatment of hypertension, as well as for BPH (see Chapter 25, Cardiovascular Drugs).

Side effects of alpha-blockers are infrequent, but can include:

* Dizziness, headache, nasal congestion
* Orthostatic hypotension
  Palpitations (not Flomax)
  Ejaculation dysfunction, decreased libido, impotence

Combination therapy with an antiandrogen (Proscar) and an alpha-blocker (Cardura) in patients with large prostates has recently been shown to significantly reduce the overall clinical progression of BPH and may reduce the need for invasive therapy compared to either agent alone.

See Table 15-2 for a summary of uricosuric agents, antigout medication, antispasmodics, cholinergic agents, analgesic agents, and agents for BPH.

Table 15-2 Other Drugs Affecting the Urinary Tract

GENERIC NAME	TRADE NAME	DOSAGE
Uricosuric Agents		
probenecid	Benemid	250–500 mg BID
probenecid w/colchicine	ColBenemid	1 tab (500 mg/0.5 mg) BID
Antigout Medication		
allopurinol	Zyloprim, Lopurin	200–600 mg daily
Antispasmodic		
propantheline	Pro-Banthine	7.5–30 mg TID on empty stomach
tolterodine	Detrol	1–2mg BID
	Detrol LA	2–4 mg daily
oxybutynin	Ditropan	5 mg BID or TID
		Children over 5, 5 mg BID
	Ditropan XL	5–30 mg daily
	Oxytrol patch	3.9 mg, change q3–4d
hyoscyamine	Cytospaz, Levsin	0.125–0.25 mg PO, SL, 3–4×/d
flavoxate	Urispas	100–200 mg 3–4×/d
Cholinergic[a]		
bethanechol	Urecholine	PO or SubQ, never IM or IV
		Dose according to condition
		Administer PO on empty stomach
Analgesic		
phenazopyridine	Pyridium, Azo Standard	200 mg TID pc
Agents for BPH		
Antiandrogen		
finasteride	Proscar	5 mg daily
dutasteride	Avodart	0.5 mg daily
Alpha-Blockers		
doxazosin	Cardura	1–8 mg at bedtime
tamsulosin	Flomax	0.4–0.8 mg daily pc
terazosin	Hytrin	5–10 mg at bedtime

[a]For bladder contraction.

WORKSHEET FOR CHAPTER 15
URINARY SYSTEM DRUGS

List the drugs according to category and complete all columns.
Learn generic or trade names as specified by instructor.

Classifications and Drugs	Purpose	Side Effects	Contraindications or Cautions	Patient Education
Thiazides 1. 2.				
Loop Diuretics 1. 2. 3.				
Potassium-Sparing Diuretics 1. 2.				
Combination Potassium-Sparing and Thiazide Diuretics 1. 2.				
Osmotic Agents 1. 2.				

(continued)

Classifications and Drugs	Purpose	Side Effects	Contraindications or Cautions	Patient Education
Uricosuric Agents 1. 2.				
Antigout Medication 1.				
Antispasmodic 1. 2. 3.				
Analgesic 1.				
Cholinergic 1.				
BPH Treatment Antiandrogen 1. 2. Alpha-blockers 1. 2. 3.				

A. Case Study for Urinary System Drugs

Phyl Moore, a 60-year-old diabetic with a history of heart disease and hypertension, comes to the clinic complaining of swollen ankles, shortness of breath, weakness, and nausea. He is taking hydrochlorothiazide. You will need to answer his questions with the following information.

1. Hydrochlorothiazide causes increased excretion of all of the following EXCEPT
   a. Sodium
   b. Glucose
   c. Chloride
   d. Potassium

2. Side effects of the thiazides can include all of the following EXCEPT
   a. Fatigue
   b. Nausea
   c. Muscle spasms
   d. Low blood glucose

3. He should be given all of the following advice EXCEPT
   a. Rise slowly
   b. Eat citrus
   c. Take diuretic with meals
   d. Take diuretic at dinner

4. Because of the edema, he will probably be put on a more potent loop diuretic, such as
   a. Dyazide
   b. Osmitrol
   c. Aldactone
   d. Lasix

5. Patients like Mr. Moore taking loop diuretics should be given all of the following advice EXCEPT
   a. Avoid sunlight
   b. Avoid alcohol
   c. Take medicine at bedtime
   d. Check blood glucose

B. Case Study for Urinary System Drugs

Bea Young, an 85-year-old Alzheimer's patient with cardiac arrhythmias is brought to the physician's office by her daughter with a request for medication to decrease her mother's incontinence. She will need the following information:

1. The following medications can reduce bladder contractions EXCEPT
   a. Urecholine
   b. Detrol
   c. Ditropan
   d. Pro-Banthine

2. Side effects of the antispasmodics can include all of the following EXCEPT
   a. Constipation
   b. Drooling
   c. Blurred vision
   d. Mental confusion

3. Other side effects can include all of the following EXCEPT
   a. Nausea
   b. Dizziness
   c. Frequency
   d. Palpitations

4. Which of the following conditions would be treated with antispasmodics?
   a. Renal disease
   b. Kidney stones
   c. Prostatic hypertrophy
   d. Neurogenic bladder

5. Antispasmodics, for example Ditropan, are contraindicated or given with caution in the following conditions EXCEPT
   a. Geriatrics
   b. Renal disease
   c. Neurogenic bladder
   d. Cardiovascular disease

CHAPTER REVIEW QUIZ

Match the medication in the first column with the conditions in the second column that it is used to treat. Conditions may be used more than once.

Medication	Condition
1. _____ Proscar	**a.** Congestive heart failure
2. _____ Benemid	**b.** Gout
3. _____ Hydrochlorothiazide	**c.** Benign prostatic hypertrophy (BPH)
4. _____ Ditropan	**d.** Incontinence
5. _____ Allopurinol	**e.** Edema
6. _____ Lasix	
7. _____ Cardura	
8. _____ Detrol	
9. _____ Bumex	
10. _____ Hydrodiuril	

Choose the correct answer.

11. Patients taking combination potassium-sparing diuretics and thiazides, for example Dyazide, should be given the following instructions EXCEPT:
    a. Avoid salt substitutes
    b. Rise slowly
    c. Take before meals
    d. Report sudden weight loss
12. Osmotic agents, for example mannitol, are used in all of the following conditions EXCEPT:
    a. Hypertension
    b. Intraocular pressure
    c. Drug poisoning
    d. Craniotomy with cerebral pressure
13. The following statements are true of benemid EXCEPT:
    a. Can cause kidney stones
    b. Anti-inflammatory
    c. Used for chronic gout
    d. Interacts with penicillin
14. The following statements are true of urecholine EXCEPT:
    a. Stimulates bladder contractions
    b. For postoperative retention
    c. Cholinergic action
    d. For BPH
15. The following statements are true of Pyridium EXCEPT:
    a. Colors urine orange-red
    b. May interfere with kidney tests
    c. Anti-infective
    d. Analgesic

Chapter 16
Gastrointestinal Drugs

Objectives

Upon completion of this chapter, the learner should be able to

1. Define the Key Terms

2. Describe side effects, contraindications, and interactions of antacids, antiulcer agents, antidiarrhea agents, antiflatulents, cathartics and laxatives, and antiemetics

3. Compare and contrast the five types of laxatives according to use, side effects, contraindications, and interactions

4. Identify examples of drugs from each of the eight categories of gastrointestinal drugs

5. Explain important patient education for each category of gastrointestinal drugs

Key Terms

Antacids

Antidiarrhea

Antiemetics

Antiflatulents

Antiulcer

Gastroesophageal reflux disease (GERD)

Laxatives

Gastrointestinal drugs can be divided into eight categories based on the action: antacids, drugs for treatment of ulcers, antispasmodics, management of inflammatory bowel disease, antidiarrhea agents, antiflatulents, laxatives and cathartics, and antiemetics.

ANTACIDS

Antacids act by partially *neutralizing* gastric hydrochloric acid and are widely available in many over-the-counter (OTC) preparations for the relief of indigestion, heartburn, and sour stomach. Antacids are also prescribed at times (between meals and at hour of sleep) to help relieve pain and promote the healing of gastric and duodenal ulcers. Other antiulcer agents are discussed later in this chapter. Antacids are also used at times in the management of esophageal reflux.

Antacid products may contain aluminum, calcium carbonate, or magnesium, either individually or in combination. Most antacids also contain sodium. Sodium bicarbonate alone is not recommended because of flatulence, metabolic alkalosis, and electrolyte imbalance with prolonged use. Calcium carbonate, for example Tums, may cause constipation.

The choice of a specific antacid preparation depends on palatability, cost, adverse effects, acid neutralizing capacity, the sodium content, and the patient's renal and cardiovascular function. Magnesium and/or aluminum antacids are the most commonly used. Magnesium can cause diarrhea, and aluminum is constipating. Therefore, combinations are frequently used to control the frequency and consistency of bowel movements, for example, Maalox, Gelusil, Mylanta.

Side effects with frequent use of antacids may include:

* Constipation (with aluminum or calcium carbonate antacids)
* Diarrhea (with magnesium antacids)
  Electrolyte imbalance
* Urinary calculi and renal complications
  Osteoporosis (with aluminum antacids)
  Belching and flatulence (with calcium carbonate and sodium bicarbonate)

Contraindications or extreme caution with antacids applies to:

Congestive heart failure

Renal pathology or history of renal calculi

Cirrhosis of the liver or edema

Dehydration or electrolyte imbalance

Interactions of antacids with almost any other drug administered concurrently can alter the effectiveness of the other drugs. Therefore, *antacids should not be taken within two hours of most other drugs.* With the following drugs, antacids may decrease effectiveness of the drug:

Anti-infectives, especially tetracyclines, quinolones, and isoniazid

Digoxin, indomethacin, and iron

Salicylates and thyroid hormones

Antacids with the following drugs may increase action and precipitate side effects:

Diazepam, which increases sedation

Amphetamines and quinidine, which increase cardiac irregularities

Enteric-coated drugs may be released prematurely in the stomach (separate doses from antacids by two hours).

Patient Education

Patients should be instructed regarding:

Avoiding prolonged use (no longer than two weeks) of OTC antacids without medical supervision because of the danger of masking symptoms of gastrointestinal (GI) bleeding or GI malignancy

Avoiding the use of antacids at the same time as any other medication because of many interactions

Avoiding the use of antacids entirely if patient has cardiac, renal, or liver disease or fluid retention

Patients taking medicines in the management of esophageal reflux should also be instructed regarding avoidance of constrictive clothing, treatment of obesity (if appropriate), reducing meal size, avoiding recumbency after meals, and elevating the head of the bed.

AGENTS FOR TREATMENT OF ULCERS AND GASTROESOPHAGEAL REFLUX DISEASE

Some **antiulcer** agents *reduce gastric acid secretion* by acting as *histamine$_2$* blockers. The drugs in this category, cimetidine (Tagamet), famotidine (Pepcid), and ranitidine (Zantac) are used *short term* for the relief of "acid indigestion and heartburn," **gastroesophageal reflux disease (GERD)**, and upper GI bleeding or esophagitis.

Side effects of H$_2$-blockers, usually transient and dose related, can include:

* Diarrhea, dizziness, rash, and headache

    Mild gynecomastia with Tagamet occurs infrequently and is reversible.

* Mental confusion (especially in older adults or debilitated)—rarely with Pepcid

Note: Reduction of gastric juices on a regular basis for extended periods can deplete intrinsic factor, which is necessary for absorption of vitamin B$_{12}$. Especially in individuals over the age of 50, deficiency of this vitamin can possibly lead to conditions such as pernicious anemia, confusion, disorientation, and numbness of extremities. A supplement may be required. (See Chapter 11, Vitamins.)

Contraindications or extreme caution with H$_2$-blockers applies to:

Impaired renal function

Liver dysfunction

Children, pregnancy, and lactation

Interactions with Tagamet may occur with increased blood concentrations of:

Coumarin anticoagulants (also with high doses of Zantac)

Phenytoin

Propranolol

Diazepam

Lidocaine

Theophylline (also with high doses of Zantac)

Tricyclic antidepressants

Antacids may interfere with absorption of Tagamet and Zantac; separate administration by at least one hour.

There is less likelihood for drug interactions with Pepcid.

Misoprostol (Cytotec)

Misoprostol (Cytotec), a synthetic analog of prostaglandin E_1, inhibits gastric acid secretion and protects the mucosa from the irritant effect of certain drugs, for example nonsteroidal anti-inflammatory drugs (NSAIDs—see Chapter 21), especially in those at risk, for example debilitated patients or older adults or those with a history of gastric ulcers. It is not Food and Drug Administration (FDA)-approved for the treatment of gastric or duodenal ulcers.

Side effects of Cytotec can include:

Diarrhea, nausea, and abdominal pain (occurs early in treatment and is usually self-limiting; take with food to minimize)

Menstrual irregularities (begin therapy on the second or third day of next normal menstrual period)

Spontaneous abortion, possibly incomplete, with potentially dangerous uterine bleeding, maternal or fetal death

Contraindications for Cytotec include:

Women of childbearing age

Pregnant women

Children under age 12

Interactions with antacids decrease the rate of absorption. Therefore, it is recommended that antacids should be given at least two hours away and should not be of a magnesium type (which exacerbates diarrhea).

Proton Pump Inhibitors (PPI)

Omeprazole (Prilosec) is a gastric antisecretory agent (proton pump inhibitor), unrelated to the H_2-receptor antagonists. It is used for the short-term (four to eight weeks) symptomatic relief of GERD, for the *short-term* treatment of *confirmed* gastric and duodenal ulcer, and for erosive esophagitis and "heartburn." Other drugs in this category include lanso-prazole (Prevacid), rabeprazole (Aciphex), pantoprazole (Protonix), and esomeprazole (Nexium).

Side effects of proton pump inhibitors can include:

✳ Diarrhea, constipation, nausea, vomiting, abdominal pain

✳ Headache, dizziness

Long-term use on a regular basis of agents that reduce gastric acid can possibly result in vitamin B_{12} deficiency, especially in older adults (see preceding note under antiulcer agents)

Interactions of proton pump inhibitors may occur with:

H_2-blockers (decrease proton pump inhibitor effectiveness)

Sucralfate (delays absorption of most proton pump inhibitors)

Diazepam, phenytoin, warfarin (increased serum levels)

Ampicillin, ketoconazole, iron (results in poor bioavailability)

Food—Nexium, Prevacid, and Prilosec should be given on an empty stomach; Aciphex and Protonix can be given without regard to meals.

Note: **Proton pump inhibitors available as SR tabs should NOT be chewed, broken, or crushed. Proton pump inhibitors available as SR caps may be opened and sprinkled on applesauce or yogurt, given with fruit juices, and swallowed immediately with water (do not chew or crush).**

Sucralfate (Carafate)

Sucralfate (Carafate), an inhibitor of pepsin, is another antiulcer agent that acts in a different way. Sucralfate is *administered on an empty stomach* and then reacts with hydrochloric acid in the stomach to form a paste that adheres to the mucosa, thus protecting the ulcer from irritation. The therapeutic effects of the drug result from local (i.e., at the ulcer site) rather than systemic activity.

Side effects of sucralfate are rare, with constipation occurring occasionally.

Interactions are possible with sucralfate altering absorption and, therefore, other drugs should not be given within two hours of sucralfate. Antacids may decrease binding of sucralfate to mucosa, decreasing effectiveness. Separate administration times by 30 min.

Helicobacter Pylori Treatment

Patients with recurrent or refractory peptic ulcer disease (i.e., resistance to standard antiulcer therapies: antacids, H_2-receptor antagonists, sucralfate), with failure to heal within 12 weeks, or with frequent recurrences, unrelated to NSAIDs, may be suffering from infection with *Helicobacter pylori*. Such infection has been treated successfully with multiple-drug regimens (over 14 days) combining three medications. One such combination package, called Prevpac, contains amoxicillin with clarithromycin and lansoprazole (Prevacid). Another combination, the Helidac pack, contains tetracycline with metronidazole (antibacterial and antiprotozoal), and bismuth salicylate. This treatment and possible side effects are discussed further in Chapter 17, Anti-infective Drugs.

ANTISPASMODICS/ANTICHOLINERGICS
Hyoscyamine

Hyoscyamine (Cystospaz, Levsin, Levsinex) is an anticholinergic/antimuscarinic agent used as adjunct therapy in the management of peptic ulcer disease, hypermotility disorders of the lower urinary or GI tract, and infant colic and as a preoperative medication to control salivation and excessive secretions. GI anticholinergics work by decreasing motility (smooth muscle tone) in the GI tract. As with other antimuscarinic agents, there are no conclusive data from well-controlled studies that indicate that hyoscyamine aids in the healing, decreases the rate of occurrence, or prevents complications of peptic ulcers; more effective agents are available.

Side effects of hyoscyamine, especially in older adults, can include:

* Dry mouth, constipation
* Blurred vision, dizziness, drowsiness
* Urinary retention
  Tachycardia, palpitations
* Confusion (especially in older adults)

Contraindications of hyoscyamine include:

Glaucoma (narrow angle)

Cardiovascular disease

Obstructive GI disease, ulcerative colitis

Obstructive uropathy (BPH, bladder obstruction)

Myasthenia gravis

Pregnancy and lactation

Interactions of hyoscyamine include:

Phenothiazines (decreased antipsychotic effectiveness, increased anticholinergic side effects)

Tricyclic antidepressants (increased anticholinergic side effects)

Opiate agonists (additive depressive effects on GI motility/bladder function)

Patient Education

Patient Education for Those Undergoing Ulcer Therapy

Patients should be instructed regarding:

Cigarette smoking, which seems to decrease the effectiveness of medicines in the healing of duodenal ulcers

Importance of close communication with the physician for possible dosage regulation of other medications taken at the same time

Structuring of environment to reduce stress factors and decrease tension in order to facilitate healing of ulcers and reduce gastric motility and hypersecretion, as an adjunct therapy

Not taking antacids, if ordered, within two hours of taking cimetidine, ranitidine, or any other drug

Taking medications on a regular basis and avoiding abrupt withdrawal, which could lead to rebound hypersecretion of gastric acid

Taking sucralfate (Carafate) one hour before meals, on an empty stomach, and not within two hours of any other medicine

Taking misoprostol (Cytotec) with meals and at bedtime with food, and avoiding magnesium products to lessen incidence of diarrhea

Taking proton pump inhibitors, Nexium, Prevacid, and Prilosec, on an empty stomach; Aciphex and Protonix can be given without regard to meals.

Proton pump inhibitors available as SR tabs should NOT be chewed, broken, or crushed; proton pump inhibitors available as SR caps may be opened and sprinkled on applesauce or yogurt, given with fruit juices, and swallowed immediately with water (do not chew or crush).

Anticholinergic side effects with antispasmodics (e.g., hyoscyamine), especially with older adults

FOR INFLAMMATORY BOWEL DISEASE

Salicylates

Mesalamine (Asacol, Rowasa) and sulfasalazine (Azulfidine) have chemical structures similar to those of aspirin and exhibit anti-inflammatory activity in the GI tract. They are used in the management of Crohn's disease and ulcerative colitis. These salicylates are all designed to reach the ileum and colon, bypassing the stomach and upper intestines. They are safe for long-term use and are well tolerated in most patients.

Side effects of salicylates (often more frequent and severe with sulfasalazine) can include:

✳ Anorexia, nausea, vomiting, diarrhea, abdominal pain, cramps

✳ Headache, weakness, dizziness

Intolerance to sulfasalazine can be minimized by taking the enteric-coated product.

Caution with salicylates applies to:

✳ Allergy to salicylates

✳ Allergy to sulfonamides with sulfasalazine (can cause anaphylaxis or asthma attacks)

✳ Allergy to sulfites (Rowasa enema)

Renal impairment

Hepatic impairment (with sulfasalazine)

Interactions with sulfasalazine include:

Warfarin (increased risk of hemorrhage)

Methotrexate (increased bone marrow suppression)

Cyclosporine (decreased efficacy)

Oral diabetic agents (hypoglycemia)

Glucocorticoids

Glucocorticoids (prednisone, prednisolone, hydrocortisone enema) are used to treat moderate to severe forms of inflammatory bowel disease in patients who are inadequately controlled with salicylates. The oral steroids do not require direct contact with inflamed intestinal tissue to be effective. For a detailed discussion on these agents, see Chapter 23, Endocrine System Drugs.

ANTIDIARRHEA AGENTS

 Antidiarrhea agents act in various ways to reduce the number of loose stools.

Kaolin and Pectin

Kaolin and pectin preparations (e.g., Kapectolin) act as *adsorbents and protectants* to achieve a drying effect (i.e., decrease fluidity of stools).

Side effects are relatively nonexistent, other than transient constipation on occasion.

Interactions are possible, such as impaired absorption, when these agents are administered concurrently with such other medications as:

Digoxin

Contraindicated, without medical supervision, in infants and older adults, and with bowel obstruction.

Patient Education

Patients with diarrhea should be instructed regarding:

Avoiding self-medication for longer than 48 hours or if fever develops without consulting a physician

Diet of a bland nature, excluding roughage, and including foods containing natural pectin (e.g., apple *without* peelings and without sugar added to apple)

Adequate fluid intake (especially tea *without* sugar for its astringent effect) or Gatorade to prevent dehydration

Contacting the physician immediately if complications develop or condition worsens and if observing blood in stool

Taking other medications (e.g., antibiotics or digitalis) two to three hours before or after taking kaolin and pectin products

Diphenoxylate with Atropine and Loperamide

Diphenoxylate with atropine (Lomotil) and loperamide (Imodium) act by slowing *intestinal motility.*

Side effects can include:

✳ With Lomotil, anticholinergic effects (e.g., drying of secretions, blurred vision, urinary retention, lethargy, confusion, or flushing)

✳ With Lomotil or Imodium, abdominal distention, nausea, or vomiting

Contraindications include:

Diarrhea caused by infection or poisoning

Young children and pregnancy

Colitis associated with broad-spectrum antibiotics

Ulcerative colitis

Cirrhosis

Caution with older adults.

Patient Education

Patients taking antidiarrhea agents should be instructed regarding:

Not exceeding the recommended dosage; short-term only

Adequate fluid intake and bland diet

Reporting side effects or complications to the physician immediately, or if symptoms persist

Not taking these medications if diarrhea caused by infection or food poisoning. In this instance kaolin and pectin preparations are preferable.

Lactobacillus Acidophilus

Lactobacillus acidophilus (Lactinex) is an acid-producing bacterium in culture administered orally for simple diarrhea caused by antibiotics, infection, irritable colon, colostomy, or amebiasis. Lactobacillus bacteria help to re-establish normal intestinal flora. The capsules, tablets, or granules may be taken or mixed with cereal, food, juice, or water.

Contraindications for Lactinex apply to:

Anyone with a high fever

Those sensitive to milk products

Long-term use

Patients with prosthetic heart valves/valvular heart disease (risk of bacteremia)

ANTIFLATULENTS

Antiflatulents (e.g., simethicone) are used in the symptomatic treatment of gastric bloating and postoperative gas pains, by helping to break up gas bubbles in the GI tract.

No side effects, contraindications, or drug interactions have been reported.

Contraindications apply only to infant colic because of limited information on safety in children.

Patient Education

Patients should be instructed to avoid gas-forming foods (e.g., onions, cabbage, and beans).

See Table 16-1 for a summary of antacids, antiulcer agents, antidiarrhea agents, antiflatulents, and antispasmodics.

Table 16-1 Antacids, Antiulcer Agents, Antidiarrhea Agents, and Antiflatulents

GENERIC NAME	TRADE NAME	DOSAGE
Antacids (only a sample, many other products available)		
aluminum	Amphojel	Suspension, 320 mg/5 ml
		Tabs, 300–600 mg
calcium carbonate	Tums	Tabs, 500–1,000 mg, also liquid
aluminum-magnesium combinations	Riopan, Maalox, Gelusil, Mylanta	Suspension, tabs (with simethicone); dose varies with product
Agents for Ulcers and GERD		
H₂-Blockers		
cimetidine	Tagamet	200–300 mg q6h PO or IV
	Tagamet HB (OTC)	20 mg daily-BID PO (2 weeks maximum)
famotidine	Pepcid	20–40 mg PO tabs at bedtime
		20 mg IV diluted
	Pepcid AC (OTC)	10 mg daily BID (2 weeks maximum)
ranitidine	Zantac	150 mg tabs BID
		50 mg IV diluted
	Zantac 75 (OTC)	75 mg daily-BID (2 weeks maximum)
Proton Pump Inhibitors		
esomeprazole	Nexium	20–40 mg daily SR caps
lansoprazole	Prevacid	15–30 mg daily SR caps
		SoluTab/susp; 30 mg daily
		IV diluted
omeprazole	Prilosec	20–40 mg qAM ac, SR caps
	Prilosec OTC	20 mg daily AC SR tab (2 weeks maximum)
pantoprazole	Protonix	20–40 mg daily SR tabs; 40 mg daily IV diluted
rabeprazole	Aciphex	20 mg daily SR tab
Gastric Mucosal Agents		
misoprostol	Cytotec	100–200 mcg TID with meals and at bedtime with food
sucralfate	Carafate	1 g 4 ×/d (1 h ac and at bedtime), tabs, susp
Antispasmodic/Anticholinergic		
hyoscyamine	Cytospaz, Levsin, Levsinex	PO 0.125–0.25 mg q4h PRN, elixir, tabs, SL
		ER caps 0.375–0.75 mg q12h
For Inflammatory Bowel Disease		
Salicylates		
mesalamine	Asacol	800 mg PO TID (up to 6 weeks), SR tab
	Rowasa	4 g PR at bedtime (retain 8 h; use 3–6 weeks), enema
sulfasalazine	Azulfidine	500 mg tab or EC tab
		500 mg–1 g 4 ×/d
Antidiarrhea Agents		
diphenoxylate with atropine	Lomotil	Sol or tabs, 2.5–5 mg 4 ×/d
kaolin and pectin	Kapectolin	Susp, 15–30 ml after each BM (max 120 ml/12 h)
loperamide	Imodium	Sol, tabs, caps; 4 mg initially, 2 mg after each loose BM
	Imodium A-D (OTC)	(Rx maximum 16 mg/day; OTC maximum 8 mg/day × 2 days)
Lactobacillus acidophilus	Lactinex, Bacid	2 caps, 4 tabs, or 1 pkg granules 3 or 4 ×/d
Antiflatulent		
simethicone	Mylicon	Suspension, tabs pc and at bedtime
		160–500 mg daily in divided doses

LAXATIVES AND CATHARTICS

Laxatives promote evacuation of the intestine. Included in the laxative category are *cathartics,* or *purgatives,* which promote rapid evacuation of the intestine and alteration of stool consistency. Laxatives can be subdivided into six categories according to their action: bulk-forming laxatives, stool softeners, emollients, saline laxatives, stimulant laxatives, and osmotic laxatives.

Many over-the-counter (OTC) laxatives are self-prescribed and overused by a large portion of the population. Prevention and relief of constipation is better achieved through natural methods (e.g., high-fiber diet, adequate fluid intake, good bowel habits, and exercise). Normal frequency of bowel movements varies from daily to several times weekly. When constipation occurs, the cause should be identified before laxatives are used.

Bulk-Forming Laxatives

Bulk-forming laxatives (e.g., psyllium, cellulose derivatives, polycarbophil, malt soup extract, and bran) are the treatment of choice for simple constipation unrelieved by natural methods. These products are available in powders, flakes, granules, tablets, wafers, or liquids and *must be dissolved and/or diluted* according to manufacturers' directions (note label). The usual procedure is to dissolve the product in one *full glass* of water or juice to be taken orally and followed immediately with another glass of fluid. The proper dosage is administered one to three times per day. Laxative effect is usually apparent within 12–72 h.

Bulk-forming laxatives are the choice for older adults or laxative-dependent patients. Bulk-forming laxatives have been useful in maintaining regularity for patients with diverticulosis. Bulk-forming laxatives have also been used to increase the bulk of stools in patients with chronic, watery diarrhea.

Contraindications apply to patients with acute abdominal pain, partial bowel obstruction, dysphagia, or esophageal obstruction.

Patient Education

Patients should be instructed regarding *dissolving all bulk-forming products completely* in one full glass of liquid and following that with another glass of fluid to prevent obstruction.

Administer immediately when dissolved, before thickening occurs.

Stool Softeners

Stool softeners (e.g., docusate) are another mild form of laxative administered orally. Dosage required to soften stools varies widely depending on the condition and patient response. Stool softeners are the choice for pregnant or nursing women and children with hard, dry stools. Onset of action is usually 12–72 h.

Side effects are rare, with occasional mild, transitory GI cramping or rash.

Contraindications include acute abdominal pain or prolonged use (more than one week) without medical supervision

Caution to avoid stool softeners that also contain stimulant laxatives, for example, Peri-Colace, Correctol.

Patient Education

Patients taking stool softeners should be instructed regarding:

Discontinuance with any signs of diarrhea or abdominal pain

Avoiding use for longer than one week without medical supervision

Interaction with mineral oil, which leads to mucosal irritation

Taking large quantities of fluids to soften stool

Checking package label to be sure no cathartics are included

Emollients

Mineral oil may be administered orally and is usually effective in six to eight hours. Mineral oil is sometimes administered rectally as an oil-retention enema (60–120 ml).

Side effects of emollients may include:

- Seepage of oil from rectum, causing anal irritation
- Malabsorption of vitamins A, D, E, and K only with prolonged oral use

Contraindications for oral mineral oil include:

Children under 5 years old

Bedridden, debilitated, or geriatric patients

Patients with dysphagia, gastric retention, or hiatal hernia

Pregnancy

Prolonged use

Concomitant use of stool softeners

Patient Education

Patients taking mineral oil should be instructed regarding:

Avoiding frequent or prolonged use

Caution with anyone who might have trouble swallowing or who might aspirate the oil

Interaction with docusate (stool softener), which can facilitate absorption of mineral oil, possibly increasing risk of toxicity.

Saline Laxatives

Saline laxatives (e.g., milk of magnesia or citrate of magnesia) should be taken only infrequently in single doses. Saline laxatives should never be taken on a regular or repeated basis. Onset of action is 0.5–3 h.

Side effects of saline laxatives used for prolonged periods or in overdoses can include:

* Electrolyte imbalance
* CNS symptoms, including weakness, sedation, and confusion
* Edema
* Cardiac, renal, and hepatic complications

Contraindications include:

Long-term use

Congestive heart failure or other cardiac disease

Edema, cirrhosis, or renal disorders

Those taking diuretics

Acute abdominal pain

Colostomy

Patient Education

Patients taking saline laxatives should be instructed regarding:

Avoiding saline cathartics with the contraindicated medical conditions

Avoiding frequent or regular use of saline cathartics

Stimulant Laxatives

Stimulant laxatives (e.g., senna, castor oil, and bisacodyl) are cathartic in action, producing strong peristaltic activity, and may also alter intestinal secretions in several ways. Stimulant laxatives are habit-forming, and long-term use may result in laxative dependence and loss of normal bowel function. All stimulant laxatives produce some degree of abdominal discomfort. Their use should be confined to conditions in which rapid, thorough emptying of the bowel is required (e.g., before surgical, proctoscopic, sigmoidoscopic, or radiological examinations, or for emptying the bowel of barium following GI X-rays). Sometimes a combination of oral preparations, suppositories, and/or enemas may be ordered for these purposes. Onset of action is 0.25–8 h.

Side effects of stimulant laxatives are common, especially with frequent use, and can include:

* Abdominal cramps or discomfort and nausea (frequent)

  Rectal and/or colonic irritation with suppositories

✳ Loss of normal bowel function with prolonged use

✳ Electrolyte disturbances with prolonged use

Discoloration of urine with senna and cascara

Contraindications with stimulant laxatives include:

Acute abdominal pain or abdominal cramping—danger of ruptured appendix

Ulcerative colitis

Children, pregnancy, and lactation

Long-term use

Patient Education

Patients taking stimulant laxatives should be given strong warnings against frequent or prolonged use because of danger of laxative dependence and loss of normal bowel function.

Osmotic Laxatives

When administered rectally, glycerin, lactulose, and sorbitol exert an action that draws water from the tissues into the feces and reflexively stimulates evacuation. Lactulose response may take 24–48 h. Glycerin rectal suppositories or enemas usually cause evacuation of the colon within 15–60 min. Only extremely high doses of sorbitol exert laxative action (e.g., 120 ml of a 25%–30% solution rectally or 30–150 ml of a 70% solution orally), resulting in diarrhea. Glycerin may produce rectal irritation or cramping pain.

Polyethylene glycol (Miralax) was the first new prescription laxative to be approved (at that time) in nearly 25 years. Two to four days of therapy may be required to produce a bowel movement.

Patient Education

Patients should be instructed regarding:

High-fiber diet to prevent constipation, including roughage (e.g., bran, whole-grain cereals, and fresh fruits and vegetables)

Adequate fluid intake

Developing good bowel habits (e.g., regular, at an unrushed time of day)

Regular exercise to develop muscle tone

Avoiding any laxative with acute abdominal pain, nausea, vomiting, or fever

Avoiding laxatives if any medical condition is present, unless prescribed by a physician. Bulk-forming laxatives are safest in the long term.

Use of only the mildest laxatives (e.g., stool softeners) on a short-term, infrequent basis

Reporting any prolonged constipation, if above measures are ineffective, to a physician for investigation

ANTIEMETICS

Antiemetics are used in the prevention or treatment of nausea, vomiting, or motion sickness. Many different types of products are available, varying in their actions, the condition treated, and route of administration.

The three antiemetics used most frequently to control nausea and vomiting are Phenergan, Compazine, and Tigan, which are related to the phenothiazine or antihistamines, discussed in Chapters 20 and 26. These drugs are used for symptomatic relief, and their use must be supplemented by restoration of fluid and electrolyte balance, as well as determination of the cause of vomiting.

Prochlorperazine (Compazine) is a phenothiazine that shows a high incidence of extrapyramidal reactions, especially in psychiatric patients receiving phenothiazine long term or in children. It is not recommended for children under age 12. *Caution with older adults. Not for long-term use!*

For *preoperative* preventive antiemetic effect or *postoperative* treatment for nausea and vomiting, a phenothiazine (e.g., Phenergan) is usually the drug of choice. Phenergan can be given *deep* IM, but *never* subcutaneously. Ondansetron (Zofran), granisetron (Kytril), and dolasetron (Anzemet) are also used preoperatively and for nausea *with chemotherapy* and have fewer side effects.

PROPHYLAXIS

For prophylaxis of motion sickness, preventive drugs such as dimenhydrinate (Dramamine) or scopolamine are used. For greatest effectiveness, the Transderm-Scop patch is applied behind the ear 4 h before anticipated exposure to motion and is effective up to 72 h. Dramamine is administered orally 30 min before exposure to motion. Both of these drugs are also available for IM injection in patients who have already developed motion sickness.

Meclizine

Meclizine (Antivert) is an antihistamine used in the prevention and treatment of nausea, vomiting, and/or vertigo associated with motion sickness, and in the symptomatic treatment of vertigo associated with the vestibular system (e.g., Meniere's disease). The onset of action is about 1 h and effects persist 8–24 h after a single oral dose. Although meclizine produces fewer adverse anticholinergic effects than scopolamine, it can cause drowsiness, but to a lesser degree than dimenhydrinate (Dramamine). It is not recommended for children under age 12.

Side effects of the antiemetics vary with the drug and dosage, but the most common include:

* Confusion, anxiety, restlessness (especially with older adults)
* Sedation, drowsiness, vertigo, weakness, depression
* Dry mouth and blurred vision
* Extrapyramidal reactions (involuntary movements), especially in children and older adults with Compazine

  Cardiac arrhythmias with IV administration if too fast

Contraindications or extreme caution with antiemetics applies to:

> Children and adolescents (increased risk of Reye's syndrome)—especially Compazine
>
> Pregnancy and lactation
>
> Debilitated, emaciated, or geriatric patients (require reduced dose)
>
> Angle-closure glaucoma
>
> Prostatic hypertrophy
>
> Cardiac arrhythmias or hypertension
>
> Seizure disorders
>
> COPD and asthma (Phenergan suppresses cough reflex.)

Interactions of antiemetics resulting in potentiation of a sedative effect occur with:

> CNS depressants, including tranquilizers, hypnotics, analgesics, antipsychotics
>
> Alcohol
>
> Muscle relaxants
>
> Metoclopramide (other antiemetics also antagonize the stimulant effects of metoclopramide on the GI tract)

Metoclopramide (Reglan), a dopamine-receptor antagonist, is an antiemetic and a stimulant of upper GI motility. It accelerates gastric emptying and intestinal transit. It is used in a variety of GI motility disorders, especially gastric stasis, *short-term (up to 12 weeks)* treatment of GERD, and for the prevention of cancer chemotherapy–induced emesis.

Side effects of metoclopramide can include:

* Restlessness, drowsiness, fatigue, lassitude
* Depression—*can be severe*
* *Extrapyramidal reactions,* especially in children and young adults, or *irreversible* tardive dyskinesia, especially in older women with long-term therapy

Cautions or contraindications with Reglan include:

> Children or young adults
>
> Older adult patients, *Not for long term!*

Patient Education

Patients taking antiemetics should be instructed regarding:

Taking these medications under medical supervision

Determining the cause of nausea and vomiting

Reporting effectiveness or complications

Administering only as directed

Not combining with any other CNS depressants, alcohol, or muscle relaxants unless prescribed by a physician (e.g., with cancer patients)

See Table 16-2 for a summary of laxatives and antiemetics.

Table 16-2 Laxatives and Antiemetics

GENERIC NAME	TRADE NAME	DOSAGE
Laxatives (only a sample, many other products available)		
Bulk-forming (psyllium)	Metamucil, Konsyl-D, Fiberall, others	Powder, 1 tsp, dissolved in full glass of fluid 1–3 ×/d
Stool softener (docusate)	Surfak, Dialose, Colace, others	Oral caps, liquid 50–300 mg daily
Emollient		
mineral oil	Kondremul, Fleet	5–45 ml PO daily; 60–120 ml PR daily
Saline laxative		
magnesium hydroxide	Milk of Magnesia	Susp, 15–60 ml daily
Stimulant laxatives		
cascara sagrada		5 ml single dose
senna	Senokot	8.6 mg tab, 1–2 BID or 10–15 ml syrup BID
bisacodyl	Dulcolax	5–15 mg tabs
	Correctol	10 mg supp
Osmotic laxatives		
glycerin	Colace suppository	1–2 suppositories PRN
	Enema	5–15 ml PR PRN
lactulose	Cephulac, Enulose	15–60 ml PO daily
polyethylene glycol	Miralax	17–34 g (1–2 capfuls) in 8 oz liquid daily
sorbitol	D-Glucitol	30–150 ml PO of 70% solution
		120 ml PR of 25%–30% solution
Antiemetics		
dimenhydrinate	Dramamine	PO or IM q4–6 PRN for motion sickness (max 400 mg PO, 300 mg IM)
meclizine	Antivert	25–50 mg daily, 1 h before motion (repeat q2h PRN) 25–100 mg in divided doses/Meniere's
metoclopramide	Reglan	PO, IM, IV; dose varies with condition
prochlorperazine	Compazine	5–10 mg PO, IM, IV, 4 ×/d; 25 mg suppository BID
promethazine	Phenergan	Tabs, syrup, deep IM, or suppository 25 mg; (*never* Subq)
scopolamine	Transderm-Scop	0.5 mg patch q72h for motion sickness
trimethobenzamide	Tigan	PO 300 mg, IM 200 mg, suppository 100–200 mg 3-4 ×/d
Antiemetics (Preoperative or with Chemotherapy)		
dolasetron	Anzemet	12.5 mg IV
ondansetron	Zofran	1–4 mg over 2–5 min, 16 mg PO

Note: This is only a representative sample. Others are available. Always read labels carefully, especially with OTC medications.

WORKSHEET FOR CHAPTER 16
GASTROINTESTINAL DRUGS

List the drugs according to category and complete all columns.
Learn generic or trade names as specified by instructor.

Classifications and Drugs	Purpose	Side Effects	Contraindications or Cautions	Patient Education
Antacids 1. aluminum 2. calcium carbonate 3. aluminum/magnesium				
Antiulcer Agents 1. Tagament and Zantac 2. Pepcid and Axid 3. Carafate 4. Cytotec 5. Prilosec, Prevacid. Nexium				
For Inflammatory Bowel Disease Sulfasalazine (Azulfidine) Mesalamine (Rowasa)				
Antidiarrhea Agents 1. Kaopectate 2. Lomotil 3. Imodium 4. Lactinex				
Antiflatulent 1. Simethicone				

(continued)

Classifications and Drugs	Purpose	Side Effects	Contraindications or Cautions	Patient Education
Bulk-forming Laxative 1.				
Stool Softeners 1. 2.				
Saline Laxative 1.				
Stimulant Laxatives 1. 2. 3.				
Antiemetics 1. 2. 3. 4. 5. 6.				
For Vertigo/Meniere's 1.				
Stimulant Upper GI Motility 1.				

A. Case Study for Gastrointestinal Drugs

Homer Hill, a 55-year-old salesman, has been taking antacids for years for recurrent gastric distress. X-ray has confirmed a gastric ulcer. The following information will be helpful.

1. All of the following can result from antacids EXCEPT
   - a. Gastric acid decrease
   - b. Urinary calculi
   - c. Constipation
   - d. Diarrhea

2. All of the following are antiulcer drugs EXCEPT
   - a. Prilosec
   - b. Pepcid
   - c. Azulfidine
   - d. Cytotec

3. All of the following are true of sucralfate (Carafate) EXCEPT
   - a. Take before meals
   - b. Decreases gastric acid
   - c. Coats the stomach
   - d. Action is local

4. The following are true of Tagamet and Zantac EXCEPT
   - a. Reduces gastric acid
   - b. Used long-term for GERD
   - c. Can cause confusion in older adults
   - d. Can cause dizziness

5. Patients with recurrent, resistent peptic ulcers might be treated with a combination of all of the following EXCEPT
   - a. Bismuth salicylate
   - b. Tetracycline
   - c. Metronidazole
   - d. Gentamycin

B. Case Study for Gastrointestinal Drugs

Ila Park, a 70-year-old woman, has been taking cathartics for years, and they are now ineffective. She requests a new one she can take daily. She needs the following information.

1. The only laxative that should be taken daily is
   - a. Dulcolax
   - b. Senokot
   - c. Metamucil
   - d. Milk of Magnesia

2. Stimulant laxatives can cause all of the following EXCEPT
   - a. Electrolyte imbalance
   - b. Reduced peristalsis
   - c. Dependence
   - d. Cramping

3. The following is true of bulk-forming laxatives EXCEPT
   - a. Given with liquids
   - b. Useful for diverticulosis
   - c. Used for chronic diarrhea
   - d. Given only pc

4. The following is true of mineral oil EXCEPT
   - a. Can cause anal irritation
   - b. Used with stool softener
   - c. Can cause vitamin deficiency
   - d. Contraindicated with dysphagia

5. Patient education includes all of the following EXCEPT
   - a. Increase fluids
   - b. High-fiber diet
   - c. Stool softeners used short term
   - d. Milk of magnesia used long term

CHAPTER REVIEW QUIZ

Match the medication in the first column with the condition in the second column that it is used to treat. Conditions may be used more than once.

	Medication		Condition
1. _____	Nexium	**a.**	Diarrhea
2. _____	Antivert	**b.**	Flatulence
3. _____	Rowasa	**c.**	GERD
4. _____	Lactinex	**d.**	Meniere's disease
5. _____	Prevacid	**e.**	Nausea and vomiting
6. _____	Transderm-Scop	**f.**	Constipation
7. _____	Dulcolax	**g.**	Inflammatory bowel disease
8. _____	Simethicone	**h.**	Motion sickness
9. _____	Imodium		
10. _____	Phenergan		

Choose the correct answer.

11. With antacids, which of the following applies to administration?
  a. Before meals
  b. Two hours from other medications
  c. With Tagamet
  d. With milk

12. Misoprostol (Cytotec) can cause all of the following EXCEPT:
  a. Constipation
  b. Menstrual irregularities
  c. Spontaneous abortion
  d. Gastric distress

13. Hyoscyamine (Levsin), an anticholinergic drug, can cause all of the following EXCEPT:
  a. Decreased GI motility
  b. Confusion in older adults
  c. Urinary incontinence
  d. Dry mouth

14. The following statements regarding proton pump inhibitors, for example Prilosec, are true EXCEPT:
  a. Treat GERD
  b. Used long-term
  c. Interact with anticoagulants
  d. GI side effects

15. Compazine, a phenothiazine antiemetic, can cause all of the following EXCEPT:
  a. Confusion
  b. Sedation
  c. Gastric distress
  d. Extrapyramidal reactions

16. The following statements regarding Reglan are true EXCEPT:
  a. Short-term use only
  b. Extrapyramidal effects possible
  c. Can cause depression
  d. Decreases GI motility

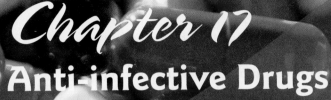

Chapter 17
Anti-infective Drugs

Key Terms

Adverse reactions

Aminoglycosides

Anaphylaxis

Antifungal

Antituberculosis agents

Antiviral

Broad-spectrum

Cephalosporins

Culture and sensitivity
   (C & S) tests

Direct toxicity

Hypersensitivity

Macrolides

Opportunistic infections

Penicillins

Quinolones

Resistance

Sulfonamides

Superinfection

Tetracyclines

Urinary anti-infectives

Objectives

Upon completion of this chapter, the learner should be able to

1. Define the Key Terms

2. Identify side effects, contraindications, and interactions common to each category of anti-infectives

3. Explain the unique features of patient education appropriate for each category of anti-infectives

4. Describe general instructions that should be given to every patient undergoing anti-infective therapy

Treatment of infection is complicated by the great variety of medications available and their differing modes of action (e.g., bacteriostatic versus bactericidal). The first step in treatment is identification of the causative organism and the specific medication to which it is sensitive. **Culture and sensitivity (C & S) tests** will be ordered, based on symptoms (e.g., wound, throat, urine, or blood). It is imperative to obtain the appropriate specimen before administering medication. Results of C & S tests will not be available for 24–48 h. In the meantime, the physician will sometimes order a **broad-spectrum** antibiotic, one that is effective against a large variety of organisms.

Resistance

Sometimes organisms build up **resistance** to drugs that have been used too frequently, and then the drugs are no longer effective. This explains why antibiotics should not be used for the common cold, which is usually caused by viruses and not bacteria. Organisms can also become resistant if infections have been treated incompletely, as when the medication is discontinued before the required number of days to be fully effective.

More than 70% of bacteria that cause nosocomial (hospital-acquired) infections are resistant to at least one of the drugs most commonly used to treat those infections according to the U.S. Centers for Disease Control and Prevention (CDC). Also of concern, infections due to resistant organisms that were seen only in hospital settings are now increasingly being seen in the community. Antimicrobial resistance is rising not only in prevalence but also across all classes of antibiotics.

An example of an organism resistant to most antibiotics is methicillin-resistant *Staphylococcus aureus* (MRSA). Vancomycin IV is one of the very few drugs effective against MRSA, but can cause serious adverse side effects, including ototoxicity and nephrotoxicity. The CDC also reports outbreaks of tuberculosis resistant to standard drug therapy (see Antituberculosis Agents).

Some strains of enterococci have become resistant to most of the antibiotics, including vancomycin. Infections such as bacteremia, endocarditis, or urinary tract infections (UTIs), which are caused by vancomycin-resistant enterococci (*VRE*), can be very difficult to treat. Treatment options are limited and mortality rates are high.

Antimicrobial resistance is caused by many factors. Therefore, the strategies needed to combat the problem are also complex. Effective strategies include better patient and physician *education* on appropriate antibiotic use, accurate diagnosis, and targeted treatment of bacterial infection. Strict adherence to *preventive measures* such as routine handwashing/alcohol wiping between patient visits, and rapid isolation of patients with resistant infections are also extremely important.

Selection of anti-infective drugs is based on several factors:

1. *Status of hepatic and/or renal function.* Lower doses or alternative drugs might be indicated with impairment.

2. *Age of the patient.* Some anti-infectives are more toxic in children or the elderly. Lower doses or alternative drugs might be indicated.

3. *Pregnancy or lactation.* Some anti-infectives can cross the placenta and cause damage to the developing fetus; for example, tetracycline or streptomycin. Others can be carried in breast milk and can cause toxicity to the infant.

4. *Likelihood of organisms developing resistance.* Sometimes a combination of drugs is used to decrease the chance of developing resistance to a single drug. Examples of combination therapy include sulfamethoxazole and trimethoprim combined to treat

urinary tract infections. Another example is the combination of three or more drugs to treat tuberculosis.

5. ***Known allergy to the anti-infective drug.*** In such cases, an alternative should be used.

Adverse Reactions

Adverse reactions to anti-infectives are divided into three categories:

1. ***Allergic hypersensitivity.*** Overresponse of the body to a specific substance. A *mild* reaction with only rash, urticaria (hives), or mild fever is usually treated with corticosteroids or antihistamines, and the medication is *discontinued*. Sometimes severe reactions occur with the first administration of a specific medication (e.g., penicillin), or they may follow a mild reaction. *Severe* reactions may be manifested as **anaphylaxis,** a sudden onset of dyspnea, chest constriction, shock, and collapse. Unless treated promptly with epinephrine, corticosteroids, and CPR (cardiopulmonary resuscitation), death may result.

2. ***Direct toxicity.*** Results in tissue damage, such as ototoxicity (hearing difficulties or dizziness), nephrotoxicity (kidney problems), hepatotoxicity (liver damage), blood dyscrasias (abnormalities in blood components), phlebitis, or phototoxicity. Sometimes the damage can be permanent, or it may be reversible when the medication is discontinued. The health care worker's responsibility involves assessment of physical condition and laboratory reports, and *discontinuance* of medication at the first sign of toxicity.

3. ***Indirect toxicity, or superinfection.*** Manifested as a new infection with different resistant bacteria or fungi as a result of killing the normal flora in the intestines or mucous membranes, especially with broad-spectrum antibiotics. Symptoms of superinfections can include diarrhea, vaginitis, stomatitis, or glossitis. Treatment consists of antifungal medications. Including buttermilk or yogurt in the diet or administering Lactinex (see Chapter 16) helps to restore normal intestinal flora. Probiotics, available OTC in capsule form, are used prophylactically to prevent superinfections, especially severe colitis.

It would be impractical to list all of the anti-infective agents on the market. Therefore, only a few examples of the most frequently used drugs are listed in each category. The antibiotics are divided into therapeutic categories, including aminoglycosides, cephalosporins, macrolides, penicillins, quinolones, and tetracyclines. In addition, antifungals, antituberculosis agents, sulfonamides, and **urinary anti-infectives** are also listed. Miscellaneous anti-infective agents, including some drugs used to treat opportunistic infections associated with AIDS (autoimmune deficiency syndrome), are included. Antiviral drugs, used to treat HIV (human immunodeficiency virus) and other viral infections, are also described.

We have omitted the amebicides, anthelmintics, and antimalarial drugs, as well as vaccines, but urge those in the public health or pediatric fields to investigate these drugs as appropriate to their practice.

VACCINES

Information regarding vaccines and immunizations changes from time to time and requirements may vary by state, territory, or country. Therefore, the most up-to-date information regarding vaccines, immunization recommendations, and requirements can be obtained by contacting the Centers for Disease Control and Prevention (CDC) and the National Immunization Program at http://www.cdc.gov.nip. You can also call the CDC Info Contact Center at 800-232-4636 or the National Immunization Hotline at 800-232-2522 (English) or 800-232-0233 (Spanish).

The CDC has information regarding the latest infection-control measures in place around the world. One recommendation of the CDC regarding influenza vaccine is relevant to your practice. The CDC recommends that all older individuals, and those at any age who are immune compromised or have a serious medical condition, be given the flu vaccine in the last quarter of the year, annually. In addition, all health care workers who have contact with those at risk, as just mentioned, should also receive the flu vaccine. It is your responsibility to stress the importance of this prophylactic measure in helping to prevent serious, possibly fatal, complications from contracting virulent forms of influenza.

AMINOGLYCOSIDES

Aminoglycosides, e.g., gentamycin in combination with other antibiotics, are used to treat many infections caused by *gram-negative* bacteria (e.g., *Escherichia coli, Pseudomonas,* and *Salmonella*) as well as *gram-positive* bacteria (e.g., *Staphylococcus aureus*). Enterococci are generally resistant to aminoglycosides. Aminoglycosides are used in the *short-term* treatment of many serious infections (e.g., septicemia) *only* when other less toxic anti-infectives are ineffective or contraindicated. Examples of aminoglycosides include amikacin, gentamicin, and tobramycin. Because of poor absorption from the gastrointestinal (GI) tract, aminoglycosides are usually administered parenterally, (i.e., IM or IV).

Serum levels (peak and trough) are often drawn to determine optimal dosing and lessen the risk of side effects. These levels measure the amount of drug in the blood at different times, and are used to adjust subsequent doses and/or the frequency between doses. Peak serum levels are drawn 1 hour after the start of the infusion or IM injection of the third dose of aminoglycoside; trough levels are drawn 30 minutes before the next dose.

Serious side effects from aminoglycosides, especially in older adults, dehydrated patients, or those with renal or hearing impairment, can include:

 Nephrotoxicity, including pathological kidney condition, can be reversed upon discontinuation

 Ototoxicity, both auditory (hearing loss) and vestibular (vertigo), may be permanent

✴ Neuromuscular blocking, including respiratory paralysis

✴ CNS symptoms including headache, tremor, lethargy, numbness, seizures

　Blurred vision, rash, or urticaria

Contraindications or extreme caution with aminoglycosides applies to patients with:

Tinnitus, vertigo, and high-frequency hearing loss

Reduced renal function

Dehydration

Pregnant or nursing women

Infants or older adults

Interactions of aminoglycosides may occur with:

Other ototoxic drugs (e.g., amphotericin B, cephalosporins, polymixin B, bacitracin, and vancomycin)

General anesthetics or neuromuscular blocking agents (e.g., succinylcholine or curare), which can cause respiratory paralysis

Antiemetics—may mask symptoms of vestibular ototoxicity

Patient Education

Patients being treated with aminoglycosides should be instructed regarding:

Extreme importance of close medical supervision during therapy

Careful observation of intake and urinary output

Prompt reporting of any side effects, especially kidney or hearing problems

CEPHALOSPORINS

Cephalosporins are semisynthetic antibiotic derivatives produced by a fungus. They are related to the penicillins and *some* patients allergic to penicillin are also allergic to cephalosporins. In general, cephalosporins are broad-spectrum, active against many gram-positive and gram-negative bacteria. However, there are many different cephalosporins and they vary widely in their activity against specific bacteria.

Cephalosporins are classified as first, second, third, or fourth generation, according to the organisms susceptible to their activity. First-generation drugs, for example, cephalexin, are usually effective against gram-positive organisms, such as those causing some pneumonias or some urinary tract infections. Second-generation drugs, for example, cefaclor, are usually effective against many gram-positive and gram-negative organisms, such as many strains causing bacterial influenza. Third-generation drugs, for example, ceftriaxone, are usually effective against more gram-negative bacteria than the others and are sometimes used for sexually transmitted diseases (STD) such as chancroid or gonorrhea. Cefepime (Maxipime) a parenteral cephalosporin with excellent activity against both gram-positive and gram-negative bacteria, is classified as a fourth-generation cephalosporin.

A C&S is essential to determine which cephalosporin is appropriate. Different drugs are used to treat different infections of the respiratory tract, skin, urinary tract, bones and joints, septicemias, some sexually transmitted diseases, and endocarditis. They are also used prophylactically, especially in high-risk patients, for many types of surgery.

Side effects of cephalosporins can include:

* Hypersensitivity, including rash, edema, or anaphylaxis (especially in those allergic to penicillin)

  Blood dyscrasias (e.g., increased bleeding time or transient leukopenia)

* Renal toxicity, especially in older patients

  Mild hepatic dysfunction

* Nausea, vomiting, and diarrhea

* Phlebitis with IV administration and pain at site of IM injection

  Respiratory distress

  Seizures

Contraindications or extreme caution with cephalosporins applies to:

Renal impairment

Known allergies, especially to penicillin (3%–6% cross-sensitivity)

Prolonged use possibly leading to superinfections or severe colitis

Pregnant or nursing women

Children

Interactions with cephalosporins can include:

Increased effectiveness with probenecid

Disulfiram-like reactions (flushing, tachycardia, shock) with alcohol ingestion

Aminoglycosides or loop diuretics (increased risk of nephrotoxicity)

Patient Education

Patients being treated with cephalosporins should be instructed regarding:

Possible allergic reactions

Avoidance of alcohol

Reporting any side effects to physician

Including buttermilk or yogurt in diet to restore normal intestinal flora

Taking without regard to meals but with food if stomach upset occurs

Attention to signs of abnormal bleeding (checking stools and urine for blood)

MACROLIDES

Macrolides, such as erythromycin, are used in many infections of the respiratory tract and for skin conditions such as acne or for some sexually transmitted infections when the patient is allergic to penicillin. Erythromycins are considered among the least toxic antibiotics and are therefore preferred for treating susceptible organisms under conditions in which more toxic antibiotics might be dangerous (e.g., in patients with renal disease, pregnant patients, or small infants).

Gram-negative bacilli are generally resistant to the macrolides, and some resistant strains of *streptococcus* A are increasing in number.

Clarithromycin, in combination with amoxicillin and lansoprazole (Prevpac Kit), is being used to treat *Helicobacter pylori* in patients with duodenal ulcer. (See Chapter 16 for further discussion.) Unrelated to its antibacterial effect, erythromycin in low doses stimulates gastric emptying. Therefore, it is used in the treatment of gastroparesis and other GI motility disorders.

Side effects from macrolides of a serious nature are rare, and mild side effects, usually dose related, can include:

* Anorexia, nausea, vomiting, diarrhea, and cramps
  Urticaria and rash
* Superinfections
* Serious side effects can occur with some interactions. See below.

Contraindications or caution with macrolides applies to patients with:

Liver dysfunction

Alcoholism

Hypertension (those taking calcium channel blockers)

Interactions of macrolides may occur with potentiation of the following drugs and possible toxicity:

Carbamazepine (Tegretol)—ataxia, dizziness, drowsiness

Cyclosporine (immunosuppressant with kidney/liver transplants)

Theophylline

Triazolam (Halcion)—potentiation of sedative effect of other benzodiazepines theoretically possible also

Warfarin—may prolong prothrombin time and bleeding

Digoxin

* **Warning.** Erythromycin can cause abnormal, potentially fatal, cardiac arrhythmias when combined with the following drugs, which increase its concentration in the blood:

Verapamil or diltiazem (calcium channel blocker antihypertensives)

Fluconazole (Diflucan) antifungal

Always check the label, or ask a pharmacist, for any other dangerous interactions with erythromycin.

Note: Azithromycin (Zithromax) is generally not associated with many of the drug interactions seen with the other macrolides just described.

Patient Education

Patients being treated with macrolides should be instructed regarding:

Common GI side effects to be expected

Importance of reporting side effects for possible dosage adjustment or prescription of medication for symptomatic relief

Taking medication with full glass of water one hour before or two hours after meals, unless stomach upset (some forms can be taken without regard to meals)

Including yogurt or buttermilk in diet to help regulate intestinal flora and reduce incidence of diarrhea

Not taking with other medications (see Interactions)

PENICILLINS

Penicillins are antibiotics produced from certain species of a fungus. They are used to treat many streptococcal and some staphylococcal and meningococcal infections, including respiratory and intestinal infections. Penicillin is the drug of choice for treatment of syphilis and is also used prophylactically to prevent recurrences of rheumatic fever or endocarditis. Amoxicillin has also been used in combination with other drugs to treat *Helicobacter pylori* infection associated with *duodenal* ulcer disease (see discussion in previous section and in Chapter 16).

Some semisynthetic penicillins have a wider spectrum of activity and are called extended-spectrum penicillins, for example, carbenicillin and piperacillin. These wide-spectrum penicillins are used in the treatment of infections due to organisms such as *Pseudomonas*.

Some organisms, including both gram-positive and gram-negative bacteria, for example that cause gonorrhea, have become *resistant* to many forms of penicillin. Culture and sensitivity tests are essential to determine appropriate forms of medication.

Serious side effects of penicillins can include:

✴ Hypersensitivity reactions ranging from rash to fatal anaphylaxis

✴ Superinfections (especially with oral ampicillin)

✴ Nausea, vomiting, and diarrhea

Blood dyscrasias, which are reversible with discontinuance of drug

✴ Renal and hepatic disorders

CNS effects, for example, confusion, anxiety, seizures (especially with penicillin G)

Contraindications or extreme caution with penicillins applies to patients with:

History of allergy, especially to any drugs (anaphylaxis has been reported with parenteral, oral, or intradermal skin testing)

Impaired renal function

Electrolyte imbalance

Treatment for severe reactions includes discontinuance of the drug, immediate administration of appropriate medications (e.g., epinephrine and corticosteroids), and maintenance of a patent airway. Administration of antihistamines with penicillin will *not* prevent hypersensitivity reaction.

Interactions of penicillins include:

Potentiation of penicillin with probenecid (Benemid) and with anti-inflammatory drugs such as phenylbutazone, indomethacin, and the salicylates given concomitantly (at the same time)

Antagonistic effect (delayed absorption) of oral penicillins when given with antacids or with food

Antagonistic effect of some other anti-infectives on penicillin

Penicillin V or ampicillin may inhibit the action of estrogen-containing oral contraceptives.

Patient Education

Patients being treated with penicillin should be instructed regarding:

Discontinuance of medication and *immediate* reporting of any hypersensitivity reactions (e.g., rash, swelling, or difficulty breathing)

Taking medication on time as prescribed on empty stomach, one hour before or two hours after meals, with full glass of water

Avoidance of antacids and alcohol

Effectiveness of estrogen contraceptives may be affected

Including yogurt or buttermilk in diet to help regulate intestinal flora and reduce incidence of diarrhea

See Table 17-1 for a summary of the aminoglycosides, cephalosporins, macrolides, and penicillins.

Table 17-1 Anti-infective Agents: Aminoglycosides, Cephalosporins, Macrolides, and Penicillins

GENERIC NAME	TRADE NAME	AVERAGE DOSAGE
Aminoglycosides		
amikacin	Amikin	IM, IV 15 mg/kg/day in 1–3 divided doses
gentamycin (w ampicillon)	Garamycin	IM, IV 1 mg/kg q8h
tobramycin	Nebcin	IM, IV 1 mg/kg q8h
Cephalosporins		
First-generation		
cephalexin	Keflex ✶	PO Cap, liquid, tab 250–500 mg q6h
cefazolin	Kefzol, Ancef ✶	IM, IV 250 mg q8h to 2 g q8h
Second-generation		
cefaclor	Ceclor ✶	PO 250–500 mg q8h, cap, liq.
cefuroxime	Ceftin ✶	PO tab, liq. 125–500 mg q12h,
	Kefurox, Zinacef	IM, IV 750–1500 mg q6h
Third-generation		
cefdinir	Omnicef ✶	PO cap, susp 300 mg q12h or 600 mg q24h
ceftriaxone	Rocephin ✶	IV, deep IM 250 mg-2 g daily
Fourth-generation (when they're made, more complex)		
cefepime	Maxipime	IV 500 mg–2 g q12h
		IM 500 mg–1g q12h (UTI only)
Macrolides stop production of protein		
erythromycin ✶	E-mycin, Ery-Tab,	PO tab, cap 250 mg q6h-500 mg q12h
	EES, EryPed	PO tab, susp. 400–800 mg q6–12h
	Erythrocin	IV 15–20 mg/kg/day divided q6h
clarithromycin	✶ Biaxin (pneumonia)	PO tab, liq. 250–500 mg q12h
	Biaxin XL	PO tab 1000 mg daily
azithromycin	Zithromax ✶	PO tab, susp. 500 mg × 1, then 250 mg daily
		IV 500 mg daily
Penicillins		
✶ penicillin G IM version	Bycillin L-A, Wycillin	Deep IM 600,000–2.4 million units
✶ penicillin VK pill	Veetids	PO tab, liq. 250–500 mg q6h
✶ amoxicillin	Amoxil, Trimox	PO caps, liq. 250 mg–1g q8h; 875 mg q12h
✶ ampicillin	Principen	PO caps, liq. 250–500 mg q6h
Extended-spectrum		IM, IV 1–2 g q4–6h
amoxicillin-clavulanate (animal bite, lacerations)	✶ Augmentin w/clavulanic acid	PO tab, liq. 250 mg q8h, 500–875 mg q12h
	Augmentin XR	PO tab 2000 mg q12h
piperacillin-tazobactam	Zosyn	IV 2.25–4.5 g q6–8h
carbenicillin	Geocillin	PO 382–764 mg 4 ×/day

Note: Average doses only are listed. In severe infections, higher doses may be indicated. Many other anti-infectives are available. Only a few are represented here. Pediatric doses are computed according to weight and condition of the child.

✶ unasyn IV- infected diabetic foot

antibiotic prophelaxis for spleenectomy

cocktail - PTU/STD - rocephrin, zithromax, doxycycline

QUINOLONES

Quinolones, such as ciprofloxacin (Cipro) or levofloxacin (Levaquin), are used in adults for the treatment of some infections of the urinary tract, sinuses, lower respiratory tract, GI tract, skin, bones, and joints, and in treating gonorrhea. However, these agents have potential serious side effects, especially with children and older adults. Also, some organisms are showing increased resistance to the quinolones. Therefore, these agents should be reserved for infections that are nonresponsive to other antibiotics, or when a *Pseudomonas* infection is involved, or when the patient is allergic to other antibiotics.

Resistance has developed in strains of *Pseudomonas aeruginosa* (use in UTIs only) and *S. aureus* (use cautiously in skin infections). Therefore, culture and sensitivity tests should be drawn to identify the causative organism *before initiating a quinolone,* and therapy adjusted if necessary.

Side effects of the quinolones can include:

* Nausea, vomiting, diarrhea, abdominal pain, colitis (especially older adult patients)
* CNS effects—headache, dizziness, confusion, irritability, seizures, anxiety
* Crystalluria—may require drinking liberal quantities of fluids
* Superinfection—treat infection appropriately, may need to stop drug
* Hypersensitivity reactions or rash—rare
* Phototoxicity—exposure to sunlight can cause severe sunburn
* Possible cartilage or tendon damage

Contraindications or caution with quinolones applies to:

Older adults, especially with GI disease or arteriosclerosis

Children or adolescents—*potential for cartilage damage*

Strenuous exercise during and several weeks after therapy—(*potential for tendon rupture*)

Pregnancy and lactation

Severe renal impairment

Seizure disorders

Cardiac disease

Interactions of quinolones may occur with:

Theophylline—can potentiate serious or fatal central nervous system (CNS) effects, cardiac arrest, or respiratory failure

Probenicid—increased blood levels of Cipro

Antacids—decreased absorption

Coumadin—increased risk of bleeding

Preparations containing Fe, Mg, Zn, Ca—decrease absorption (do not give within two hours)

Sucralfate (Carafate)—contains aluminum ions, which decrease absorption

Patient Education

Patients taking quinolones should be instructed regarding:

Not taking other medication without physician's approval

Drinking liberal quantities of fluids

Restricting caffeine intake—see CNS effects

Avoiding excessive exposure to the sun

Avoiding strenuous exercise during and several weeks after therapy (potential for cartilage or tendon damage)

Reporting all side effects, especially rash or hypersensitivity signs

Geriatric patients should follow preceding instructions, especially reporting GI effects or CNS effects (see Side Effects)

TETRACYCLINES

Tetracyclines are broad-spectrum antibiotics used in the treatment of infections caused by rickettsia, chlamydia, or some *uncommon* bacteria. Diseases such as Rocky Mountain spotted fever, atypical pneumonia, some sexually transmitted diseases and some severe cases of inflammatory acne are treated with tetracycline. Tetracycline has also been used to treat *H. pylori* infection associated with duodenal ulcer disease in combination with bismuth salicylate and metronidazole (Helidac Therapy Kit). See Chapter 16 for further discussion on this topic. However, some organisms are showing increasing resistance to the tetracyclines, and therefore they should be used only when other antibiotics are ineffective or contraindicated.

Side effects of tetracyclines can include:

* Nausea, vomiting, and diarrhea (frequently dose related)
* Superinfections such as vaginitis and stomatitis
* Photosensitivity, with exaggerated sunburn
* Discolored teeth in fetus or young children
* Retarded bone growth in fetus or young children
  Hepatic or renal toxicity (rare)
  CNS symptoms such as vertigo and cerebral edema
  Thrombophlebitis possible with IV therapy
  Allergic hypersensitivity reactions rare

Contraindications with tetracyclines include:

Pregnancy, lactation, and children under age 8

Patients exposed to direct sunlight

Caution in patients with liver or kidney disease

Patients with esophageal obstruction or dysfunction

Interactions of tetracyclines may occur with the following antagonists (which decrease absorption):

Antacids, calcium supplements, or magnesium laxatives

Iron preparations, zinc

Antidiarrhea agents containing kaolin, pectin, or bismuth

Dairy products (doxycycline and minocycline not significantly affected)

Oral contraceptives—breakthrough bleeding or pregnancy may occur

---

Patient Education

Patients being treated with tetracyclines should be instructed regarding:

Avoiding exposure to sunlight

Avoiding this medication if pregnant or nursing or a child under 8 years of age

Administration preferable on an empty stomach with full glass of water, one hour before or two hours after meals, unless there is gastric distress

Avoiding iron, calcium, magnesium, and antidiarrhea agents or dairy foods within two hours of taking tetracyclines

Not taking at bedtime to prevent irritation from esophageal reflux

Discarding any expired drug—nephrotoxicity can result from taking outdated drug

---

ANTIFUNGALS

Antifungal agents are used to treat specific susceptible fungi. The medications are quite different in action and purpose, and are treated separately.

Amphotericin B

Amphotericin B is administered IV for the treatment of severe systemic, potentially fatal infections caused by susceptible fungi. It is sometimes considered the drug of choice to treat severe fungal infections resulting from immunosuppressive therapy (e.g., antineoplastic agents), or in patients with acquired immunodeficiency syndrome (AIDS), or those with severe illness (e.g., meningitis). *Severe side effects* are expected, and therefore close medical supervision (hospitalization) is usually required so that measures are available to provide symptomatic relief (e.g., antipyretics, antihistamines, and antiemetics).

Side effects of amphotericin B commonly include several of the following:

✳ Headache, chills, fever, hypotension, tachypnea

✳ Malaise, muscle and joint pain, and weakness

* Anorexia, nausea, vomiting, and cramps
* Nephrotoxicity—occurs to some degree in most patients

  Anemia
* Hypokalemia—can lead to congestive heart failure

Because of the many severe side effects and certain dose-limiting toxicities associated with conventional amphotericin B, other formulations have been developed. One example is a lipid-based product (Abelcet) that increases the tolerability of the drug without compromising its antifungal effects. Because patient tolerance varies greatly, a test dose is advisable.

Fluconazole

Fluconazole is usually limited to severe candidial infections unresponsive to conventional antifungal therapy. Because of good patient tolerance, and oral dosage, the drug is appropriate for patients requiring prolonged antifungal therapy. It is used in the treatment of oropharyngeal and esophageal candidiasis and serious systemic candidial infections (e.g., urinary tract infections and pneumonia). Patients with recurrent candidiasis, especially those who are immunodeficient, may require maintenance therapy to prevent relapse. A single oral dose of fluconazole is effective treatment for vaginal candidiasis.

Side effects of fluconazole can include:

* Moderate nausea, vomiting, abdominal pain, diarrhea

  Rash
* Hepatic abnormalities

  Dizziness and headache

Contraindications or extreme caution with fluconazole applies to:

  Children under age 13

  Pregnant or nursing women

  Hepatic or renal disease

Interactions of fluconazole may occur with:

  Coumarin anticoagulants—increased prothrombin time could cause hemorrhage

  Oral antidiabetic agents—hypoglycemia can result

  Rifampin—can lead to clinical failure of fluconazole

Griseofulvin

Griseofulvin is administered PO in the treatment of *specific* fungi causing *tinea* infections (e.g., ringworm or athlete's foot) that do not respond to topical agents. Accurate diagnosis of the infecting organism is essential.

Side effects of griseofulvin can include:

✳ Headache—frequent initially

✳ Thirst, nausea, vomiting, and diarrhea

✳ Hypersensitivity reactions—rash, urticaria

✳ Photosensitivity

Hepatic toxicity

Contraindications with griseofulvin include:

Children under age 2

Pregnancy—or women who may become pregnant while taking the drug

Liver dysfunction

Porphyria

Penicillin hypersensitivity (possible cross-sensitivity)

Interactions of griseofulvin may occur with:

Alcohol, causing flushing and tachycardia

Phenobarbital, which is antagonistic to griseofulvin action (impairs absorption)

Coumarin anticoagulants—decreased prothrombin time

Oral contraceptives—may decrease contraceptive efficacy

Nystatin

Nystatin (Mycostatin) is used orally in the treatment of intestinal candidiasis. It is also used as a fungicide in the topical treatment of skin and mucous membranes; for example, diaper area, mouth, or vagina (see Skin Medications).

Side effects of nystatin are rare but may include nausea, vomiting, and diarrhea with high oral doses occasionally.

Caution should be taken in the use of nystatin with pregnant or nursing women.

Patient Education

Patients on antifungal therapy should be instructed regarding:

Taking the medication for prolonged periods as prescribed, even after symptoms have subsided

Reporting relapses promptly to physician

Reporting side effects immediately to the physician for possible dosage adjustment or symptomatic treatment

Not taking any other medications at the same time without physician approval (see Interactions)

ANTITUBERCULOSIS AGENTS

Antituberculosis agents are administered for two purposes: (1) to treat asymptomatic infection (no evidence of clinical disease), for instance, after exposure to active tuberculosis and/or significantly positive PPD (purified protein derivative) skin test; and (2) for treatment of active clinical tuberculosis and to prevent relapse.

For asymptomatic tuberculosis, the *treatment* consists of daily administration of isoniazid (INH) alone for 6–12 months to prevent development of the disease.

For patients who are intolerant of INH, or who are presumed to be infected with INH-resistant organisms, an alternative treatment consists of *rifampin with pyrazinamide*. Treatment of clinical tuberculosis is challenging for two reasons:

1. Increasing incidence of tuberculosis, particularly among certain high-risk populations (e.g., HIV-infected individuals, socioeconomically disadvantaged racial/ethnic minorities, homeless individuals)

2. Organisms have become resistant to many antituberculosis drugs due to patient noncompliance or failure to complete the 6–24-month conventional treatment.

Therefore, the CDC recommends the following treatment regimen:

1. The American Thoracic Society (ATS) and the CDC currently recommend *short-course regimens* (i.e., at least 6 months) for the treatment of uncomplicated pulmonary tuberculosis in adults. According to the ATS, CDC, and American Academy of Pediatrics (AAP), short-course regimens are also suitable in children. Directly observed therapy (DOT) should be used for all regimens administered two or three times per week whenever possible to ensure compliance.

2. The initial regimen for the treatment of tuberculosis should include INH given once daily for two months (in combination with rifampin, pyrazinamide, and either ethambutol or IM streptomycin), followed by isoniazid and rifampin given daily, twice weekly, or three times per week for an additional four months (and at least three months beyond culture conversion). If the likelihood of INH or rifampin resistance is low (i.e., <4%), an initial regimen of INH, rifampin, and pyrazinamide may be considered. HIV-positive patients should always receive induction therapy with four drugs by DOT. When drug susceptibility results are available, the regimen should be altered as appropriate. In addition, treatment may be extended to nine months or longer in HIV-infected patients, dependent upon clinical signs and symptoms or conversion of sputum cultures from positive to negative.

Safe use of all of these drugs during pregnancy has not been established. The CDC recommends that tuberculosis during pregnancy be treated initially with isoniazid, rifampin, and ethambutol for nine months. Streptomycin is not included because it may cause congenital ototoxicity.

Side effects of *INH and rifampin* are usually more pronounced in the first few weeks of therapy and can be treated symptomatically. Pyridoxine (vitamin B$_6$) is often given (25–50 mg PO daily) with INH to reduce the risk of CNS effects and peripheral neuropathy. Dosage regulations are sometimes required in cases of acute toxicity, but the medication must *not* be discontinued. Side effects can include:

- Nausea, vomiting, and diarrhea
- Dizziness, blurred vision, headache, and fatigue
- Numbness, weakness of extremities
- Hepatic toxicity—especially those over 35 and children (see Cautions)
- Excretions colored red-orange with rifampin
- Hypersensitivity reaction, with flulike symptoms (sometimes with rifampin)

Contraindications or caution with INH and rifampin applies to:

Chronic liver disease or alcoholics, periodic laboratory tests required

Impaired renal function

Children's doses of INH and rifampin should be limited to 10 and 15 mg/kg, respectively, to decrease likelihood of hepatic toxicity.

Interactions of INH and rifampin include:

Antagonism by oral hypoglycemics, corticosteroids, digitalis, anticoagulants, and *estrogen* (serum levels of these drugs are reduced when taking rifampin)

Potentiation by phenytoin (Dilantin); increased action (possible toxicity) when taken with isoniazid

Alcohol, which increases possibility of liver toxicity

Side effects of ethambutol can include:

- Optic neuritis—with visual problems (reversible if discontinued early)
- Dermatitis, pruritus, headache, malaise, fever, confusion, joint pain, GI symptoms, peripheral neuritis rarely

Cautions and contraindications with ethambutol include:

Visual testing should be performed before and during therapy

Impaired renal function—reduced doses indicated

Diabetes, especially diabetic retinopathy

Ocular defects

Children under 13—and only in children whose visual acuity can accurately be determined and monitored

Pregnancy—caution

Patients with gout (ethambutol can cause hyperuricemia)

Side effects of pyrazinamide can include:

★ Hepatic toxicity

Gout—increased uric acid

★ Hypersensitivity

GI disturbances

Cautions and contraindications with pyrazinamide include:

Renal failure or history of gout

Diabetes

Severe hepatic disease or alcoholism

Children—potential toxicity

Pregnant or nursing women

Side effects of streptomycin, common to all aminoglycosides, include:

★ Ototoxicity

★ Nephrotoxicity

Streptomycin is administered by deep IM injection, alternating sites. Although not authorized by the manufacturer, it has been administered IV without adverse side effects (IV in at least 100 ml NS over 20–30 minutes).

Patient Education

Patients taking antituberculosis agents should be instructed regarding:

Taking rifampin on empty stomach for maximum absorption, or with food if nauseated

Taking prescribed medication for *lengthy required period of time* even though asymptomatic

Reporting side effects for possible dosage adjustment or prescription of other palliative medications to relieve discomfort

Importance of frequent medical and laboratory checks

Red-orange color of urine, feces, sputum, sweat, and tears with use of rifampin

Not wearing contact lens with rifampin

Interactions with other drugs, (e.g., *birth control pills may be ineffective*)

Avoidance of alcohol

Importance of visual testing periodically with ethambutol

See Table 17-2 for a summary of quinolones, tetracyclines, antifungal, and antituberculosis agents.

Table 17-2 Anti-Infective Agents: Quinolones, Tetracyclines, Antifungals, Antituberculosis Agents, Miscellaneous Anti-Infectives, and Agents for VRE

GENERIC NAME	TRADE NAME	AVERAGE DOSAGE	COMMENTS
Quinolones			
ciprofloxacin	Cipro	PO 250–750 mg q12h; IV 200–400 mg q12h	Do C&S before Rx, cartilage/tendon damage possible, phototoxicity
	Cipro XR	PO 500–1,000 mg/day (UTIs only)	
levofloxacin	Levaquin	PO, IV 250–500 mg q24h *(serum level equal)*	
Tetracyclines			
tetracycline HCl	Sumycin	PO cap, tab, susp. 250–500 mg q6–12h	Phototoxicity, discolored teeth in infants and children
doxycycline	Vibramycin	PO cap, tab, susp., IV 100–200 mg daily divided doses *(pneumonia ache)*	Phototoxicity, discolored teeth in infants and children *(not under 8 yrs old)*
Antifungals			
amphotericin B	Fungizone Abelcet	IV dose varies with condition and product formulation	Special IV precautions, protect from light
fluconazole	Diflucan	PO or IV 50–400 mg daily	Prolonged or maintenance doses frequently
griseofulvin	Gris-Peg	PO tab, 300–750 mg/day or 2–4 divided doses	Administer with fatty meal to increase absorption
nystatin *(thrush)*	Mycostatin	PO tab, susp. 500,000–1 million units 3–4 ×/day, topical cream, oint., or powder	Continue treatment for 48 h after symptoms to prevent relapse
Antituberculosis Agents			
ethambutol		PO 15–25 mg/kg/day (max 1,600 mg)	Always with other medications
isoniazid	INH	PO 5–15 mg/kg/day (max 300 mg)	Preventive alone, or as treatment with other medications
pyrazinamide	PZA	PO 15–30 mg/kg/day (max 2 g)	Always with other medications
rifampin	Rifadin	PO 10 mg/kg/day (max 600 mg)	Initial phase with other drugs
streptomycin		IM (IV) 15 mg/kg/day (max 1 g)	With other medications initial phase
Miscellaneous Anti-infectives			
clindamycin	Cleocin	PO 150–450 mg q6h, Ped 8–25 mg/kg/day divided doses, IM/IV 600 mg–2.7 g/day divided doses	
metronidazole *(Antifungal)*	Flagyl *(Cipro/ GI linked)*	250–500 mg q8h–q6h IV, PO (max 4 g/24 h)	
	Flagyl ER	PO 750 mg/day (for bacterial vaginosis)	
Agents for VRE			
linezolid	Zyvox	PO, IV 600 mg q12h	

Note: Other anti-infectives are available. Only a few are represented here. Pediatric doses are computed according to weight and condition of child.

MISCELLANEOUS ANTI-INFECTIVES

Clindamycin

Clindamycin has a wider spectrum of activity than lincomycin, from which it is derived. It is used in the treatment of serious respiratory tract infections, septicemia, osteomyelitis, serious infections of the female pelvis caused by susceptible bacteria, and for *Pneumocystis carinii pneumonia* associated with AIDS (see AIDS section in this chapter).

Side effects of clindamycin that frequently occur can include:

* Nausea, vomiting, diarrhea (drug should be discontinued if this develops), colitis
* Rash, pruritus, fever, and occasionally anaphylaxis
* Local effects—minimize by deep IM or frequent IV catheter change

Cautions of clindamycin include:

History of GI, hepatic, or renal disease

Older adults

Children

Pregnancy and lactation—contraindicated

Metronidazole

Metronidazole (Flagyl) is a synthetic antibacterial and antiprotozoal agent that is effective against protozoa such as *Trichomonas vaginalis* and against amebiasis and giardiasis. In addition, it is one of the most effective drugs available against anaerobic bacterial infections (intra-abdominal, skin, gynecological, septicemia, bone/joint, lower respiratory tract). Metronidazole is also useful in treating Crohn's disease, antibiotic-associated diarrhea, rosacea, and *H. pylori* infection (in combination with other drugs). It is available in oral, parenteral, and topical formulations. Because of its mechanism of action, metronidazole is a highly lethal antimicrobial. Resistance to metronidazole is almost nonexistent.

Side effects of Flagyl include:

* Abdominal pain, nausea/vomiting
  Anorexia, metallic taste, xerostomia
* Headache, dizziness, ataxia
* Flushing, rash, urticaria
  Peripheral neuropathy (rare) and seizures
* Dark urine (common but harmless)

Contraindications/precautions with Flagyl include:

Avoid alcohol during and 48 h after treatment (disulfiram-like reaction)

History of blood dyscrasias

Pregnancy and lactation

Use in children (except for treatment of amebiasis)

CNS and hepatic disease

Vancomycin

Vancomycin is structurally unrelated to other available antibiotics. IV vancomycin is used in the treatment of potentially life-threatening infections caused by susceptible organisms that cannot be treated with other less toxic anti-infective agents. It is the drug of choice for methicillin-resistant *Staphylococcus aureus* (MRSA), treating gram-positive infections in penicillin-allergic patients, and some endocarditis. However, the CDC reports an increasing percentage (15% or more) of *vancomycin-resistant enterococci (VRE)*. Use of vancomycin should be restricted to cases in which it is absolutely necessary, and it should not be used prophylactically.

Although vancomycin is poorly absorbed after oral administration, it is occasionally given orally to treat GI infections such as pseudomembranous colitis due to overgrowth of *C. difficile*. It is important to note that patients treated with IV vancomycin for systemic infections should not be switched to the oral form (a common practice with other antibiotics), because it is not effective by the oral route for that purpose.

Side effects of vancomycin can include:

* Ototoxicity or nephrotoxicity with IV use—discontinue with tinnitus, may precede deafness
* *Local effects*—give only IV with care, can cause necrosis or thrombophlebitis
* Rash, anaphylaxis, vascular collapse (hypersensitivity reactions reported in 5%–10% of patients)
  Pseudomembranous colitis due to *Clostridium difficile* infection (rare)

Caution for vancomycin with:

Older adults

Hearing impaired

Renal impairment—Serum levels (peak and trough) are often drawn to determine optimal dosing and give the lowest effective dose possible to lessen the risk of side effects. Kidney function is also monitored every two to three days by serum creatinine and BUN

Contraindicated with pregnancy and lactation

AGENTS FOR VRE

Vancomycin has been used as "the last line of defense" against staphylococcal infections, as well as for certain streptococcal and enterococcal infections. However, in recent years, cases of vancomycin-resistant staphylococci (VRSA) and vancomycin-resistant enterococci (VRE) have become more prevalent across the globe. Also, drug-resistant infections, particularly those by gram-positive pathogens, have spread from hospitals and nursing homes to communities.

Linezolid (Zyvox) is the first new antibiotic approved to target MRSA (and VRE) in 35 years. It is indicated for gram-positive infections and is approved for the treatment of bacterial pneumonia skin and skin structure infections, and VRE infections, including those infections due to susceptible organisms that are complicated by bacteremia. Linezolid is effective in treating diabetic foot infections, which are among the most serious complications of diabetes (leading to amputation in severe cases) and are the leading cause of diabetes-related hospitalizations.

Linezolid, administered by IV infusion or orally, is a nonselective inhibitor of monoamine oxidase (MAO) that has implications for medication safety and drug interactions. Inappropriate use, leading to an increase in resistant organisms, is a concern, and treatment alternatives should be carefully considered before using linezolid in outpatient settings.

Side effects of Zyvox can include:

✴ Nausea, headache, diarrhea (stop medication and contact physician with blood in stool or abdominal pain)

✴ Myelosuppression (including anemia and thrombocytopenia)

Lactic acidosis

✴ Pseudomembranous colitis

Contraindications or caution with Zyvox applies to:

Blood dyscrasias

Cardiac disease, hypertension

GI disease, hyperthyroidism

Pregnancy, lactation, infants

Interactions of Zyvox may occur with:

Beta-blockers (worsen bradycardia)

Radiographic contrast media (increased risk of seizures)

Antidepressants (e.g., SSRIs can cause serotonin syndrome)

Migraine medications (triptans)

Sympathomimetics such as phenylephrine, pseudoephedrine (hypertensive reaction)

Foods or beverages with high tyramine content (see discussion in Chapter 20)

See Table 17.2 for Miscellaneous Anti-infectives and Agents for VRE.

ANTIVIRALS

Acyclovir

The **antiviral** *acyclovir* is used predominantly in the treatment of herpes simplex, herpes zoster (shingles), and varicella zoster (chickenpox) infections. Acyclovir does not cure or prevent further occurrence of blister-like lesions. Topical application appears effective only with initial infections in relieving discomfort and shortening healing time of lesions (see Skin Medications.) Oral treatment is most effective in initial treatment of herpes to relieve pain and to speed healing of lesions and is also used to treat recurrent infections in some patients. In immunocompromised patients and children, parenteral treatment is recommended.

Herpes zoster (shingles) is best treated within 24 to 72 h of onset of rash (blisterlike) or intense pain on the skin of one side of the trunk or head. Delayed treatment with an antiviral medication can lead to complications, especially in older adults, such as intense pain, post-herpetic neuralgia (PHN), lasting for weeks or months. PHN is treated with tricyclic antidepressants (e.g., imipramine) or anticonvulsants (e.g., gabapentin). (See Chapter 20, Adjuvant Analgesics.)

Valacyclovir (Valtrex) is a pro-drug that is converted to acyclovir. The adverse reaction profile is the same as for acyclovir, but improved bioavailability means less frequent dosing for valacyclovir. Famciclovir (Famvir) has a similar spectrum of activity to acyclovir, but has a longer duration of action and can be dosed less frequently.

Side effects of acyclovir are not common, but can include:

Impaired renal function, especially with *rapid IV infusion*

* Lethargy, tremors, confusion, and headache, especially with older adults
* Rash, urticaria, pruritus and photosensitivity
* Nausea, vomiting, abdominal pain, and diarrhea

Contraindications or caution with acyclovir include:

Children, pregnant or nursing women

Renal disease (adjust dosage)

Dehydration

Neurological abnormalities with high doses

Patient Education

Patients being treated with acyclovir should be instructed regarding:

The fact that acyclovir is usually effective only with *initial* infection in relieving pain and shortening healing of lesions, but is *not* a cure and there can be recurrences of lesions

Reporting side effects

Taking medicine only as prescribed. Do not share drug with others

Storing capsules and tablets in tight, light-resistant container at 15–25°C

Avoidance of sexual intercourse when visible genital herpes lesions are present and using protection at other times

Amantadine

Another antiviral, *amantadine,* is used for the prophylaxis and symptomatic treatment of respiratory infections caused by influenza A virus strains, especially with high-risk patients. It has no effect on influenza B or other viruses. Amantadine is also used in the treatment of parkinsonian syndrome (see Chapter 22). Prophylactic use should not be considered a substitute for vaccination.

Side effects of amantadine can include:

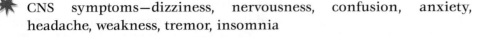

- CNS symptoms—dizziness, nervousness, confusion, anxiety, headache, weakness, tremor, insomnia
- Bluish mottling of skin on legs, eczema
- Anorexia, nausea, constipation, and dry mouth
- Hypotension, edema, urinary retention, dyspnea
- Visual disturbances

Contraindications or caution with amantadine applies to:

- Those with mental disorders
- Seizure disorders
- Cardiovascular disorders, hypotension
- Renal impairment or liver disease
- Older adults—need reduced dosage
- Pregnant or nursing women

Interactions of amantadine with anticholinergics may increase potential for adverse side effects.

Neuraminidase Inhibitors

Oseltamivir (Tamiflu) and zanamivir (Relenza) belong to a class of antivirals called *neuraminidase inhibitors* and are indicated for the treatment of uncomplicated acute illness due to influenza types A and B. Safety and efficacy for the prophylaxis of influenza infection in children are not yet established. Oseltamivir is given orally and zanamivir via inhalation; both will shorten the duration of illness if taken *within 48 h of symptom onset.*

Since zanamivir is given via inhalation, its main *side effect* is airway irritation and *bronchospasm,* especially in patients with asthma and chronic obstructive pulmonary disease (COPD). Oseltamivir causes *nausea, vomiting, and diarrhea* in about one fourth of patients receiving it; these side effects can be lessened by taking the medication with food. Unlike amantadine, neuraminidase inhibitors do not appear to adversely affect the CNS. To date, no clinically significant drug interactions have been identified with either agent.

As with amantadine, vaccination is considered the first line of defense against influenza.

Ribavirin

A drug with the broadest spectrum of antiviral activity, *ribavirin,* is used via nasal and oral inhalation for the treatment of children with severe lower respiratory tract infections. It has also been used orally or parenterally in the treatment of other severe viral infections in adults, for example, Lassa fever, Hantavirus, and hepatitis C (in combination with interferon alfa).

Side effects of ribavirin can include:

* Respiratory complications
* Hypotension, cardiac arrest
    Anemia
    Rash, conjunctivitis

Contraindicated during pregnancy or lactation. Health care workers and visitors who are pregnant or lactating should be warned about the *serious risk of close contact with patients receiving ribavirin inhalation therapy.* Also contraindicated for older adults and those with cardiac disease.

Interactions of ribavirin with NRTIs (agent for HIV), depending on specific agent, can:

    Antagonize antiviral action against HIV
    Cause lactic acidosis
    Cause hepatic failure

TREATMENT OF HUMAN IMMUNODEFICIENCY VIRUS/AIDS INFECTIONS

Treatment of HIV and AIDS infections is a highly specialized field. Those actively practicing in that field must be updated frequently on the many *new* medications and *frequently changing protocols.*

The following information is presented to give health care workers an overview of the complexity of HIV therapy. If you are not actively practicing in this area, you would not be expected to be familiar with all of the many drugs for HIV. (See Table 17-3.). However, all health care workers should be aware that there are numerous side effects and interactions specific to individualized medications. If you are caring for someone with HIV, it is imperative that you familiarize yourself with that particular individual's requirements by researching current information and consulting the pharmacist and/or infectious disease specialists. Additional resources are described following the section, which discusses drugs for HIV.

Acquired immunodeficiency syndrome (AIDS) is due to infection by the human immunodeficiency virus (HIV). Agents approved to treat HIV ("antiretrovirals") are classified by their mechanism of action and include: (1) protease inhibitors (PIs), (2) nucleoside reverse transcriptase inhibitors (NRTIs), (3) non-nucleoside reverse transcriptase inhibitors (NNRTIs), and (4) fusion inhibitors (FIs). The treatment of HIV infection consists of using highly active antiretroviral therapy (HAART) combinations of three or more antiretroviral (ARV) agents and is one of several factors that has led to a decline in the U.S. mortality rate of AIDS. The primary approach to therapy is disruption of the virus at different stages

Table 17-3 Antivirals, Drugs for HIV/AIDS, Sulfonamides, and Urinary Anti-infectives

GENERIC NAME	TRADE NAME	DOSAGE
Antivirals		Take entire Rx even if feeling better.
acyclovir	✱ Zovirax (herpes)	PO 200–800 mg 5×/daily q4h, IV 5 mg/kg q8h
amantadine	Symmetrel	PO 100–200 mg daily
famciclovir	Famvir	PO 500 mg q8h
oseltamivir	✱ Tamiflu	PO 75 mg BID for 5 days
ribavirin	Virazole	Pwdr/sol–inhalation
	Copegus	Oral, dose varies
valacyclovir	✱ Valtrex (herpes)	PO 1,000 mg q8h
zanamivir	Relenza	Inhale 10 mg q12h for 5 days
Drugs for HIV	*Dosage varies with condition.* **Check dosage very carefully.**	
Protease inhibitors (PIs)[a]	(pheno/geno - typed may prescribe 4-5 at one time)	
amprenavir	Agenerase	
fosamprenavir	Levixa	
indinavir	Crixivan	
lopinavir/ritonavir	Kaletra	
nelfinivir	Viracept	
ritonavir	Norvir	
saquinavir	Invirase, Fortovase-SGC	
Nucleoside reverse transcriptase inhibitors (NRTIs)[b]		
abacavir	Ziagen	
didanosine	Videx	
emtricitabine	Emtriva	
lamivudine	Epivir	
lamivudine/zidovudine	Combivir	
stavudine	Zerit	
tenofovir	Viread	
zalcitabine	Hivid	
zidovudine	Retrovir	
Non-nucleoside reverse transcriptase inhibitors (NNRTIs)[c]		
delavirdine	Rescriptor	
efavirenz	Sustiva	
nevirapine	Viramune	
Fusion inhibitors (FIs)		
enfuvirtide	Fuzeon	

[a]May cause GI intolerance with PIs.

[b]May cause renal dysfunction with NRTIs.

[c]May cause hepatic dysfunction with NNRTIs.

Table 17-3 Antivirals, Drugs for HIV/AIDS, Sulfonamides, and Urinary Anti-infectives

GENERIC NAME	TRADE NAME	DOSAGE
Drugs for Opportunistic Diseases of AIDS		
co-trimoxazole	Bactrim, Septra *(Tmp-Smx sulfa drug)*	Adults or peds 15–20 mg/kg/day PO or IV div. doses
clindamycin	Cleocin	1.2–3.6g daily PO or IV div. doses
foscarnet	Foscavir	Slow IV, dose varies
ganciclovir	Cytovene	Slow IV, dose varies
pentamidine	NebuPent	Aerosol inhalation, dose varies
trimetrexate	Neutrexin	IV dose varies
interferon	Roferon A, Intron A	Dose varies
		•Always check **current** literature for dosage and side effects.
		•Other drugs and combinations are being used investigationally in the treatment of HIV- and AIDS-related diseases.
Sulfonamides		
cotrimoxazole	Septra, Bactrim	Tab, suspension, IV 160 mg q12h or 15–20 mg/kg/day in div. doses
Urinary Anti-infective		
nitrofurantoin	Macrodantin, Furadantin	Cap, tab, suspension 50–100 mg 4×/day
trimethoprim	Proloprim, Trimpex	100 mg tab q12–24h

in its reproduction. Eradication of HIV infection *cannot* be achieved with currently available antiretroviral regimens. The *goals of HIV therapy are to achieve maximal and durable suppression of viral load, restore and/or preserve immunological function, improve quality of life, and reduce HIV-related morbidity and mortality.*

The treatment of HIV-infected patients is complex due to the availability of numerous antiretroviral agents and the rapid growth of new information. A patient's clinical condition, readiness for lifelong therapy, CD4 count, and plasma viral load are essential parameters to be used in decisions to initiate or change therapies. Current guidelines for initial treatment of HIV infection recommend the use of two NRTIs with either a protease inhibitor or an NNRTI. A combination of three NRTIs, one of which is abacavir (Ziagen), may be an alternative if other regimens cannot be used.

Antiretroviral Protease Inhibitors (PIs)

The first PI to be approved was saquinavir (Invirase), followed by more than six other antiretroviral protease inhibitors. (See Table 17-3 for names of other PIs.)

Side effects can include:

All PIs are associated with GI intolerance, including nausea, vomiting, and diarrhea

Taste alteration in patients receiving ritonavir, especially the liquid formulation

Fat redistribution, hyperlipidemia, and insulin resistance

Hyperglycemia, new-onset diabetes mellitus, diabetic ketoacidosis, and exacerbation of existing diabetes

Increased spontaneous bleeding episodes in hemophilia patients (joints, soft tissues, intracranial, and GI bleeding)

Indinavir may cause kidney stones (patients should drink at least 1.5 L/day of water to ensure adequate hydration and prevent kidney stones)

Interactions with PIs include:

Oral contraceptives (lose effectiveness) with ritonavir (with or without lopinavir)

Amprenavir, indinavir, and ritonavir should be dosed separately from didanosine, ddI

The following agents are not recommended to be given in combination with any PI: ergot alkaloids, lovastatin, midazolam, simvastatin, or triazolam

Ritonavir should not be given in combination with amiodarone, bepridil, clozapine, flecainide, pimozide, propafenone, or quinidine

Rifampin or St. John's wort should not be given in combination with amprenavir, indinavir, nelfinavir, or saquinavir due to the potential for antiviral failure

Dietary considerations with PIs include:

Ritonavir (with or without lopinavir), atazanavir, nelfinavir, and saquinavir-SGC should be taken with food

Amprenavir and fosamprenavir should be taken consistently with or without food, avoiding high-fat meals

Give indinavir one hour before or two hours after meals

Nucleoside Reverse Transcriptase Inhibitors (NRTIs)

Zidovudine (ZDV, Retrovir) was the first agent to be approved for the treatment of HIV, followed by more than eight other NRTIs. (See Table 17-3 for names of other NRTIs.) Combivir, a combination of zidovudine and lamivudine, allows patients to reduce the number of pills needed daily, which can be upward of 20 a day for certain drug combinations. Most NRTIs are dose adjusted in patients with renal dysfunction.

Side effects of NRTIs can include:

As a class, NRTIs have been associated with lactic acidosis and liver dysfunction (infrequently, but have a high mortality rate)

The major side effect of zidovudine is bone marrow suppression consisting of anemia and/or neutropenia

Didanosine has been associated with pancreatitis

Zalcitabine and stavudine are associated with peripheral neuropathy

Abacavir has been associated with hypersensitivity reactions that can be fatal. Patients who develop signs or symptoms of abacavir hypersensitivity (which may include fever, rash, fatigue, nausea, vomiting, diarrhea, cough, and sore throat) should discontinue abacavir as soon as possible

Tenofovir can cause GI upset and flatulence

Emtricitabine has been associated with hyperpigmentation on the palms and soles

Interactions of NRTIs include:

Alcohol with abacavir

Separate didanosine and zalcitabine 2 hours apart from aluminum and magnesium containing antacids and iron preparations

Didanosine with tenofovir (increased toxicity of both agents)

Dietary considerations with NRTIs include:

Didanosine should be given on an empty stomach

Non-Nucleoside Reverse Transcriptase Inhibitors (NNRTIs)

Nevirapine (Viramune) was the first NNRTI to be approved, followed by delavirdine (Rescriptor) and efavirenz (Sustiva).

Adverse reactions with NNRTIs can include:

Rash is a common toxicity associated with NNRTIs. Approximately 5% of patients receiving NNRTIs may experience severe rashes, and potentially fatal cases of Stevens-Johnson syndrome have been reported.

All NNRTIs may cause increased transaminase levels. Nevirapine has been associated with hepatitis.

Side effects of NNRTIs can include:

Efavirenz causes CNS symptoms, which may include dizziness, somnolence, insomnia, abnormal dreams, confusion, abnormal thinking, impaired concentration, amnesia, agitation, hallucinations, depersonalization, and euphoria

Interactions with NNRTIs include:

NNRTIs and protease inhibitors affect the metabolism of each other; the degree of which depends upon which agents are used in combination

All NNRTIs decrease effectiveness of oral contraceptives

Efavirenz and delavirdine should not be given in combination with midazolam, pimozide, triazolam, or ergot alkaloids. In addition, efavirenz should not be given with H_2 blockers, lovastatin, proton pump inhibitors, or simvastatin

Fusion Inhibitors (FIs)

A new class of antiviral agents, called fusion inhibitors, has been shown to block entry of HIV into cells, which may keep the virus from reproducing. Enfuvirtide (Fuzeon) is the first fusion inhibitor approved for treatment–experienced patients with ongoing HIV replication despite current ARV use. It is administered by subcutaneous injection twice daily.

Almost all patients develop local site reactions to enfuvirtide, usually consisting of mild or moderate pain, erythema, itching, induration, nodules, and cysts. It is important to remember to rotate injection sites.

Although highly active antiretroviral therapy (HAART) is a significant advance in the treatment of HIV, it is still not a cure. Other factors such as high cost, complicated regimens, patient adherence, and interactions with other therapies may limit the utility of these regimens.

HIV INFORMATION AND RESOURCES

Current recommendations for the clinical use of antiretrovirals (ARVs) in the management of HIV-infected adults, adolescents, children, and infants may be found at HIV/AIDS Education and Resource Center at (800) 448-0440 or at http://www.aidsinfo.nih.gov. These guidelines are developed by the U.S. Department of Health and Human Services and the Henry J. Kaiser Family Foundation.

Patient Education

Patients taking antiretrovirals should be instructed regarding:

No cure for HIV, and opportunistic infections may develop

Taking the drug in an upright position with full glass of water

Taking the drug exactly as prescribed

Taking into account dietary considerations

Reporting any change in health status or side effects

Not exceeding the prescribed dosage

Not sharing the drug with others

Not taking any other drugs unless prescribed, for example, acetaminophen contraindicated

Medication does *not* reduce the risk of transmission of HIV to others through sexual contact or blood contamination.

Treatment of the Opportunistic Infections of AIDS

Opportunistic infections are those that occur because the immune system is compromised; for example, Kaposi's sarcoma, *Pneumocystis carinii* pneumonia, and toxoplasmosis.

- *Interferons* are antiviral drugs sometimes used in the palliative treatment of AIDS-related *Kaposi's sarcoma* in selected adults who meet certain criteria; that is, who are otherwise asymptomatic and not severely immunocompromised. Interferon has also been used in the treatment of chronic hepatitis and in some leukemias and other malignancies. *Adverse side effects are common* and varied, depending on dosage and condition treated (see Antineoplastic Drugs).

- *Pneumocystis carinii pneumonia* treatment:

Co-trimoxazole (oral or IV) for prevention in all HIV-infected children and in asymptomatic adults with CD4+ T-cell counts less than 200; for *treatment* of adults and children (see Side Effects, Contraindications, and Interactions under Sulfonamides in this chapter).

Pentamidine aerosolized oral inhalation (antiprotozoal agent) for *prevention* in HIV-infected children and in adults with CD4+ T-cell counts less than 200; for *treatment* of adults and children in patients whose infection does not respond to co-trimoxazole or who cannot tolerate cotrimoxazole because of allergies or adverse side effects.

Side effects of pentamidine can include:

Nephrotoxicity

Cough and bronchospasm

Electrolyte imbalance

Cautions: Health care personnel who administer pentamidine inhalation therapy to HIV-infected patients should be aware of the possibility of exposure to tuberculosis in cough-inducing procedures. Antituberculosis therapy should be initiated before pentamidine treatment in potentially infectious tuberculosis patients. *Use of high-efficiency particulate air filter respirators by health care personnel in such settings is imperative, as well as appropriate isolation procedures.*

Contraindicated (pentamidine) in pregnancy and lactation.

Clindamycin combined with primaquine (alternative treatment). See Side Effects and Cautions of clindamycin under Miscellaneous Anti-infectives in this chapter.

Trimetrexate (Neutrexin)—alternative treatment for patients who have exhibited intolerance to cotrimoxazole. Trimetrexate is a folate antagonist and must be administered with leucovorin to counteract myelosuppression (inhibiting bone marrow function).

Side effects of Neutrexin, with severe toxicity, can include:

Myelosuppression, especially drop in WBC (white blood cell) counts, if not given concurrently with leucovorin

Liver enzyme elevation, fever, rash

GI effects

Contraindications for Neutrexin include:

Pregnant or nursing women

Children under age 18

Interactions of Neutrexin include:

Erythromycin, rifampin, fluconazole, cimetidine, acetaminophen, NNRIs, and PIs increase plasma levels of Neutrexin

- *Toxoplasmosis treatments:*

Cotrimoxazole (Bactrim, Septra) or *pyrimethamine with sulfadoxine* (Fansidar). See Sulfonamides section for side effects of both of these combination drugs.

Clindamycin. See Side Effects and Cautions of clindamycin under Miscellaneous Anti-infectives in this chapter.

- *Cytomegalovirus retinitis treatment:*

Two antiviral agents used to treat this condition are *foscarnet* and *ganciclovir.*

Side effects of foscarnet are common and can be severe, including:

Nephrotoxicity

Nausea, vomiting, and diarrhea

Electrolyte imbalance and cardiac abnormalities

Coughing and dyspnea

Seizures

Blood dyscracias

Side effects of ganciclovir are frequent, but usually reversible, including:

Blood dyscrasias—neutropenia and thrombocytopenia

Headache, confusion, seizure

Renal effects

SULFONAMIDES

Sulfonamides are among the oldest anti-infectives. The increasing resistance of many bacteria has decreased the clinical usefulness of these agents. However, they are used most effectively in combinations with other drugs, for example, with trimethoprim (co-trimoxazole). In combinations such as these, resistance develops more slowly. Co-trimoxazole (Bactrim, Septra) is used for urinary tract infections (UTIs), especially acute, complicated UTIs; enteritis (e.g., travelers' diarrhea); and otitis media, and in the treatment of *Pneumocystis carinii* pneumonia in AIDS patients or prevention of that disease in HIV-infected children (see treatment of HIV/AIDS in this chapter). This combination drug is also used in the treatment of toxoplasmosis in AIDS patients.

Side effects with sulfonamides are numerous and sometimes serious, especially with AIDS patients, and can include:

 Rash, pruritus, dermatitis, and photosensitivity

Nausea, vomiting, and diarrhea

High fever, headache, stomatitis, and conjunctivitis

Blood dyscrasias

✴ Hepatic toxicity with jaundice

✴ Renal damage with crystalluria and hematuria

✴ Hypersensitivity reactions, which can be fatal

Contraindications with sulfonamides include:

Impaired hepatic function

Impaired renal function or urinary obstruction

Blood dyscrasias

Severe allergies or asthma

Pregnancy or lactation

Interactions with sulfonamides include:

Potentiation of anticoagulants and oral antidiabetics

Antagonism of local anesthetics (e.g., procaine may inhibit antibacterial action of sulfa), digitalis, and phenytoin (Dilantin; sulfonamides may inhibit action)

Patient Education

Patients taking sulfonamides should be instructed regarding:

Importance of drinking large amounts of fluid to prevent crystalluria

Discontinuance of sulfa at first sign of rash

Reporting any side effects to physician *immediately*

Avoiding exposure to sunlight

Ingestion of sulfa with food, which delays, but does not reduce, absorption of the drug

URINARY ANTI-INFECTIVES

Urinary anti-infectives are usually bacteriostatic instead of bactericidal in action. Nitrofurantoin (Furadantin and Macrodantin) are the most commonly used for initial or recurrent urinary tract infections caused by susceptible organisms. Treatment must continue for an adequate period of time to be effective and minimize recurrence of infection.

Side effects of Furadantin and Macrodantin can include:

✴ Nausea and vomiting, which are less frequent if taken with milk or food

Numbness and weakness of lower extremities

Headache, dizziness, and weakness of muscles

Respiratory distress with prolonged use

✴ Brown urine

Anemia

Contraindications or caution with Furadantin and Macrodantin applies to:

Renal or hepatic impairment

Anemia

Diabetes

Electrolyte abnormalities

Asthma

Pregnancy and lactation

Children under one month of age

Interactions of Furadantin and Macrodantin (antagonistic) with:

Probenecid and magnesium

Antacids containing magnesium decreasing the effectiveness of these drugs

Quinolones

Patient Education

Patients taking Furadantin or Macrodantin should be instructed regarding:

Importance of taking medication for required number of days and follow-up urine culture

Reporting side effects

Taking medication with milk or food to reduce incidence of nausea and vomiting

Avoiding antacids

Discoloration of the urine, which can stain underpants

See Table 17-3 for a summary of the antivirals, drugs for HIV/AIDS, sulfonamides, and urinary anti-infectives.

Other anti-infective agents in these categories are available. This is a representative sample of drugs most commonly in use. Research is ongoing with these and other new drugs, and the FDA has developed procedures to expedite the review and approval of certain new drugs. When these drugs are being investigated for the treatment of life-threatening or other serious conditions, for example HIV infections, including AIDS, the drugs are classified as investigational new drugs (INDs). Revised government regulations require that INDs receive the highest priority for review in order to make promising new drugs available as soon as possible. Since the status of these drugs changes so rapidly, current information may not be available in the *PDR* or the *American Hospital Formulary Service Drug Information* reference books. However, *it is your responsibility to review all the information obtained from the pharmacist or drug insert before administering any new drugs. The risks are especially great with drugs that have been on the market only a short time, and side effects can be severe, even life-threatening.*

Patient Education

Patients taking antibiotics should be instructed regarding:

Unless directed otherwise, taking all antibiotics with a full glass of water on empty stomach, at least one hour before meals or two hours after meals

Not taking with fruit juice

Not taking with antacids

Not taking with alcohol

If side effects occur, discontinuing medication and consulting the physician or pharmacist

Reporting rash, swelling, or breathing difficulty to the physician *immediately*

Taking antibiotics at prescribed times to maintain blood levels

Taking entire prescription *completely; not* discontinuing when symptoms of infection disappear

Not taking any other medications, prescriptions, or over-the-counter drugs at the same time as antibiotics without checking first with the physician or pharmacist regarding interactions

WORKSHEET FOR CHAPTER 17
ANTI-INFECTIVE DRUGS

List the drugs according to category and complete all columns.
Learn generic or trade names as specified by instructor.

Classifications and Drugs	Purpose	Side Effects	Contraindications or Cautions	Interactions/ Patient Education
Aminoglycosides 1. amikacin 2. gentamycin 3. tobramycin				
Cephalosporins 1. Keflex 2. Ceclor 3. Rocephin 4. maxipime				
Macrolides 1. erythromycin 2. Biaxin 3. Zithromax				
Penicillins 1. penicillin G 2. Amoxil 3. Augmentin				
Quinalones 1. Cipro 2. Levaquin				

Classifications and Drugs	Purpose	Side Effects	Contraindications or Cautions	Interactions/ Patient Education
Tetracyclines 1. tetracycline 2. doxycycline				
Antifungals 1. Fluconazole 2. Griseofulvin 3. Nystatin				
Sulfonamides 1. Septra, Bactrim				
Urinary Anti-infectives 1. macrodantin 2. Trimpex				
Miscellaneous 1. Vancomycin 2. Flagyl				
Agent for VRE 1. Linezolid (Zyvox)				
Anti-TB 1. isoniazid (INH) 2. ethambutol 3. rifampin 4. pyrazinamide (PZA) 5. streptomycin				
Antiviral 1. acyclovir 2. ribavirin 3. amantadine				

A. Case Study for Anti-infective Drugs

Mrs. Madre, a 19-year-old pregnant woman, allergic to penicillin, calls her physician and requests some tetracycline for her acne and some Keflex for a "sore throat." The following information would be useful to her.

1. Tetracycline is contraindicated under all of the following circumstances EXCEPT
   a. Pregnancy
   b. Children under age 8
   c. Working indoors
   d. Nursing a baby

2. Sometimes organisms build up resistance to drugs. The following practices could lead to resistance EXCEPT
   a. Too frequent antibiotic use
   b. Combination antibiotics
   c. Antibiotic for minor URI
   d. Stopping drug after two days

3. If she has fever, productive cough, or trouble swallowing, the physician might order a throat culture to determine all of the following EXCEPT
   a. Causative organisms
   b. Possible allergies
   c. Resistance to drugs
   d. Drug sensitivity

4. Those allergic to penicillin might also be sensitive to cephalosporins. The following are signs of allergic reaction EXCEPT
   a. Rash
   b. Hives
   c. Trouble breathing
   d. Vomiting

5. Cephalosporins can cause superinfections manifested by all of the following EXCEPT
   a. Diarrhea
   b. Vomiting
   c. Sore mouth
   d. Vaginitis

B. Case Study for Anti-infective Drugs

Tom Brown, a 35-year-old prison guard, has a significantly positive skin test for tuberculosis. He has a cough. Active infection is confirmed by sputum test. The following information will be important to him.

1. He will need to take medicines for a minimum of
   a. 1 month
   b. 3 months
   c. 6 months
   d. 2 years

2. Family members will be treated prophylactically with which one of the following medications?
   a. Rifampin
   b. Isoniazid
   c. Ethambutol
   d. Streptomycin

3. While taking the antituberculosis drugs, which one of the following should be avoided?
   a. Milk
   b. Orange juice
   c. Alcohol
   d. Sunlight

4. He will take at least four drugs initially, including all of the following EXCEPT
   a. Isoniazid
   b. Rifampin
   c. Pyrazinamide
   d. Zidovudine

5. Side effects of INH and rifampin are more pronounced at first and can include all of the following EXCEPT
   a. Diarrhea
   b. Dizziness
   c. Hearing problems
   d. Nausea and vomiting

CHAPTER REVIEW QUIZ

Match the medication in the first column with the condition in the second column that it treats. Conditions may be used more than once.

Medication	**Condition**
1. _____ Macrodantin	**a.** Herpes zoster and herpes simplex
2. _____ Mycostatin	**b.** MRSA and VRE
3. _____ Amantadine	**c.** Urinary tract infections
4. _____ Diflucan	**d.** Tuberculosis
5. _____ Zyvox	**e.** Acne
6. _____ Ethambutol	**f.** Fungus
7. _____ Valacyclovir	**g.** Influenza A
8. _____ Erythromycin	

Choose the correct answer.

9. The goals of HIV therapy include all of the following EXCEPT:
   a. Restore immune function
   b. Improve quality of life
   c. Eradicate the virus
   d. Reduce morbidity

10. All of the following are possible side effects of sulfonamides EXCEPT:
    a. Kidney stones
    b. Hypersensitivity
    c. Photosensitivity
    d. Confusion

11. Which statement is not true of aminoglycosides, for example gentamycin?
    a. Usually given PO
    b. Contraindicated for older adults
    c. Can cause vertigo
    d. Can cause deafness

12. **Which statement is not true of clarithromycin, a macrolide?**
    a. Can cause superinfections
    b. Used to treat *H. pylori*
    c. Many resistant bacilli
    d. Few interactions

13. The following statements are true of penicillin interactions EXCEPT?
    a. Potentiated with Benemid
    b. Penicillin inhibits contraceptives
    c. Potentiated with food
    d. Potentiated with NSAIDs

14. The quinolones, for example Cipro, can have all of the following side effects EXCEPT:
   a. Tendon rupture
   b. Sunburn
   c. Constipation
   d. Confusion

15. The following statements are true of tetracyclines EXCEPT:
   a. Discolor children's teeth
   b. Accelerate bone growth
   c. Used to treat acne
   d. Used to treat *H. pylori*

16. Interactions of INH and rifampin with specific other drugs can have the following specific results EXCEPT:
   a. Ineffective birth control
   b. Lower effect with hypoglycemics
   c. Optic neuritis
   d. Hepatic toxicity

17. The following statements are true of metronidazole (Flagyl) therapy EXCEPT:
   a. For *Trichomonas vaginalis*
   b. In combination for *H. pylori*.
   c. Avoid alcohol
   d. Causes constipation

18. The following statements apply to vancomycin therapy EXCEPT:
   a. Kidney side effect
   b. Used prophylactically
   c. Deafness possible
   d. VRE possible

19. The following statements apply to treating herpes zoster (shingles) with acyclovir EXCEPT:
   a. Start within 72 h
   b. Relieves discomfort
   c. Shortens healing
   d. Prevents recurrence

20. Which statement is true of amantadine (Symmetrel)?
   a. Replaces flu vaccine
   b. Appropriate for older adults
   c. Treats influenza A
   d. Treats influenza B

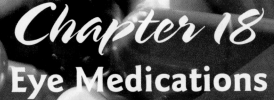

Chapter 18
Eye Medications

Objectives

Upon completion of this chapter, the learner should be able to

1. Define the Key Terms

2. Demonstrate the administration technique for instillation of ophthalmic medication to reduce systemic absorption

3. List the five categories of ophthalmic medication

4. Identify side effects, contraindications, and interactions for each category of ophthalmic medication

5. Explain appropriate patient education necessary for each category of eye medication

Key Terms

Antiglaucoma agents

Anti-infective

Anti-inflammatory

Beta-adrenergic blocker

Carbonic anhydrase inhibitors

Cycloplegic

Intraocular pressure

Miotics

Mydriatics

Medications for the eye can be classified into five categories: anti-infectives, anti-inflammatory agents, antiglaucoma agents, mydriatics, and local anesthetics.

ANTI-INFECTIVES

Many **anti-infective** ophthalmic topical ointments and solutions are available for treatment of superficial infections of the eye caused by susceptible organisms. It is important to determine the causative organism so that the appropriate medication is used. Ophthalmic antibiotic preparations include erythromycin, gentamycin, quinolones, sulfonamides, neomycin, polymixin B, and others. Resistance and cross-resistance have been demonstrated with many antibiotics. When treating infections, if there is no improvement in two to three days, suspect microbial resistance, inappropriate choice of drug, or incorrect diagnosis.

In general, topical therapy should not exceed 10 days. Prolonged use may result in overgrowth of nonsusceptible organisms including fungi. Always check the latest literature regarding resistant organisms and check the patient's history regarding allergies. See Chapter 17 for further details on anti-infective agents, resistance, and allergies.

Patient Education

Patients being treated with anti-infective ophthalmic preparations should be instructed regarding:

Using only as directed; check dosage for frequency

Careful instillation into the lower conjunctival sac to avoid contamination of the tip of the dropper or ointment tube (see Figure 18-1)

Possible hypersensitivity reactions in patients with allergies of any kind

Discontinuance of the medication and reporting immediately to a physician any signs of sensitivity (e.g., burning and itching)

Careful handwashing to prevent spread of infection to other eye or other persons

Not using eye makeup or not wearing contact lenses while treating eye infections

When using more than one ophthalmic product at the same time, administer the more viscous preparation (i.e., ointment, suspension) *last*.

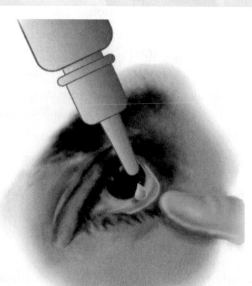

Figure 18-1 Instilling eye medication. Gently press the lower lid down and have the patient look upward. Opthalmic solution is dropped inside the lower eyelid.

Side effects of anti-infectives can include hypersensitivity reactions such as conjunctivitis, local burning, stinging, blurred vision, rash, and urticaria in allergic persons.

Contraindications for anti-infectives apply to:

Anyone allergic to the drug

Viral and fungal diseases of the ocular structure

Interactions may occur with prolonged use of corticosteroids, which can result in secondary ocular infections caused by suppression of immune response.

Antiviral ophthalmic preparations, used topically in the treatment of herpes simplex, keratitis, or conjunctivitis include trifluridine (Viroptic) ophthalmic solution. Dose is 1 drop to the lower conjunctival sac of the infected eye up to nine times daily at two-hour intervals while awake.

ANTI-INFLAMMATORY AGENTS
Corticosteroids

Anti-inflammatory ophthalmic agents are used to relieve inflammation of the eye or conjunctiva in allergic reactions, burns, postoperatively, or irritation from foreign substances. Various topical forms of the corticosteroids are also useful in the *acute* stages of eye injury to prevent scarring but are not used for extended periods because of the danger of masking the symptoms of infection or slowing the healing process. Application of ophthalmic corticosteroids topically does not generally cause systemic effects. However, systemic absorption can be minimized by gentle pressure on the inner canthus of the eye following instillation of corticosteroid ophthalmic drops or ointment (see Figure 18-2).

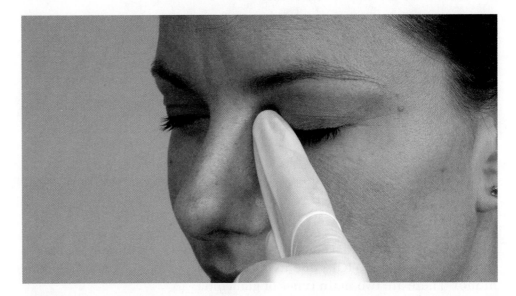

Figure 18-2 Gentle pressure on the inner canthus following administration of ophthalmic medications. Systemic absorption is thus minimized with medications such as corticosteroids, miotics, and mydriatics.

Side effects of corticosteroids can include:

 Increased intraocular pressure (depends on dose, frequency, and length of treatment)

 Reduced resistance to bacteria, virus, or fungus

 Delayed healing of corneal wounds, thinning of cornea, corneal ulceration

 Stinging, burning, or ocular pain

Contraindications or extreme caution with corticosteroids applies to:

Acute bacterial, viral, or fungal infections

Primary open-angle glaucoma

Pregnancy

Prolonged use

Nonsteroidal Anti-inflammatory Drugs (NSAIDs)

NSAIDs such as flurbiprofen (Ocufen) and ketorolac (Acular) ophthalmic drops are used to treat postoperative inflammation following cataract surgery. NSAIDs are not generally first-line agents for other eye conditions with inflammation, but are an alternative to corticosteroids if a contraindication exists.

Caution applies to those who may be allergic to aspirin and other NSAIDs.

Patient Education

Patients being treated with anti-inflammatory ophthalmic drugs should be instructed regarding:

Following directions carefully regarding time and amount

Lowered resistance to infection—do not use long term

Administration (i.e., pressure on tear duct at inner corner to reduce systemic absorption (see Figure 18-2)

Not using leftover drug for new eye inflammation—discard drug when no longer needed

See Table 18-1 for a summary of anti-inflammatory ophthalmic drugs.

ANTIGLAUCOMA AGENTS

Glaucoma is an abnormal condition of the eye in which there is increased intraocular pressure (IOP) due to obstruction of the outflow of aqueous humor. There are two main types of glaucoma:

1. *Acute (angle-closure) glaucoma.* Characterized by a sudden onset of pain, blurred vision, and a dilated pupil. If untreated,

Table 18-1 Anti-inflammatory Ophthalmic Drugs

GENERIC NAME	TRADE NAME	DOSAGE
Corticosteroids		
fluorometholone	FML	Oint, susp; varies with condition
prednisolone	Econopred, Pred Forte	Oint, sol, susp; varies with condition
	Many combinations with antibiotics	Oint, sol, susp; varies with condition
dexamethasone	Many combinations with antibiotics	Oint, sol, susp; varies with condition
Nonsteroidal Anti-inflammatory Drugs		
flurbiprofen	Ocufen	Sol; varies with condition
ketorolac	Acular	Sol; varies with condition

Note percent and dose ordered **carefully!** Follow directions. Do not use for longer than prescribed.

This is a representative sample; many other products available.

blindness can result in a few days. Treatment consists of miotics (e.g., pilocarpine), osmotic agents (e.g., mannitol) (see Diuretics, Chapter 15), carbonic anhydrase inhibitors (e.g., Diamox), and surgery to open a pathway for release of aqueous humor.

2. *Chronic (open-angle) glaucoma.* Much more common, often bilateral, and develops slowly over a period of years with few symptoms except a gradual loss of peripheral vision and possibly blurred vision. Halos around lights and central blindness are late manifestations. *Treatment* consists of miotics, carbonic anhydrase inhibitors, and a local beta-adrenergic blocker, such as timolol (Timoptic) eye drops; sometimes epinephrine eye drops are given *with the miotics.*

Note: Epinephrine ophthalmic drops are *contraindicated in angle-closure glaucoma.*

Antiglaucoma drugs, given to lower **intraocular pressure,** can be divided into six main categories based on their mode of action:

1. *Carbonic anhydrase inhibitors,* for example, Diamox. Act by decreasing the formation of aqueous humor and have a diuretic effect.

2. *Miotics,* for example, pilocarpine. Act by increasing the aqueous humor outflow.

3. *Beta-adrenergic blockers,* for example, timolol. Act by decreasing rate of aqueous humor production.

4. *Sympathomimetics,* for example dipivefrin, a pro-drug of *epinephrine,* usually combined with other antiglaucoma drugs. Increase outflow and decrease production of aqueous humor.

5. *Alpha agonists,* for example brimonidine (Alphagan-P). Decrease production of aqueous humor.

6. *Prostaglandin analogs,* for example latanoprost. Act by increasing aqueous outflow.

Drugs in different categories are sometimes given concomitantly. Combination products are sometimes available as well, for example, timolol combined with dorzolamide (Cosopt).

Carbonic Anhydrase Inhibitors (CAIs)

Acetazolamide (Diamox)

Carbonic anhydrase inhibitors such as acetazolamide (Diamox) reduce the hydrogen and bicarbonate ions and have a diuretic effect. Acetazolamide (Diamox) is administered orally in the treatment of open-angle glaucoma or short-term preoperatively to reduce intraocular pressure in angle-closure glaucoma, and is given with miotics or epinephrine products.

Side effects of CAIs, infrequent and usually dose related, can include:

 Nausea, vomiting, diarrhea, and constipation

Thirst, taste alteration

Drowsiness, fatigue, confusion, and seizures

Numbness, muscular weakness, and tingling with high doses

Blood dyscrasias

Hepatic and renal disorders

Photosensitivity (avoid excessive sunlight exposure)

Contraindications or caution with CAIs applies to:

Chronic obstructive pulmonary disease (COPD)

Diabetes

Electrolyte, hematological, hepatic, pulmonary, and renal disorders

Sulfonamide hypersensitivity

Pregnancy and lactation

Interactions with CAIs are frequent because of increasing or decreasing excretion of other drugs and can include:

Decreased effects of lithium, phenobarbital, and oral antidiabetics

Increased effects of procainamide, quinidine, amphetamines, and other diuretics

Hypokalemia with thiazides and corticosteroids

Potentiates risk of salicylate toxicity

Dorzolamide (Trusopt)

Dorzolamide is a CAI that is applied topically to treat open-angle glaucoma.

Side effects of dorzolamide can include:

Burning or stinging

Bitter taste

Caution applies to:

Those with sulfonamide hypersensitivity

Patient Education

Patients being treated with carbonic anhydrase inhibitors should be instructed regarding:

Reporting side effects and response to the physician for appropriate dosage regulation

Importance of follow-up with the physician

Checking with the physician regarding dosage before taking any other medication

Miotics

Miotics are medications that cause the pupil to contract. Miotics reduce intraocular pressure by increasing the aqueous humor outflow. They act by contracting the ciliary muscle. Miotics (e.g., pilocarpine) are used in the treatment of open-angle glaucoma or in short-term treatment of angle-closure glaucoma before surgery. Pilocarpine is also used after ophthalmic examinations in glaucoma patients to *constrict the pupil* and counteract the *mydriatic* (pupil-dilating) effect. Miotics are usually administered with acetazolamide, dipivefrin, and/or timolol. Because of its increased duration of effect and less frequent administration, pilocarpine hydrochloride gel may provide some advantages over ophthalmic solutions, especially long term with noncompliant patients.

Pilocarpine has cholinergic action and side effects. (See Chapter 13, Cholinergics.)

Side effects of pilocarpine, usually dose related, can include:

* Blurred vision and myopia
* Twitching, stinging, and burning
* Ocular pain and headache
* Photophobia and poor vision in dim light
  Aggravation of inflammatory processes of the anterior chamber of the eye

Systemic effects with frequent or prolonged use or high doses of pilocarpine, especially in children, can include:

* Nausea, vomiting, and diarrhea
* Increased lacrimation, salivation, and sweating
* Hypotension, bradycardia
* Bronchospasm

Contraindications or caution with pilocarpine applies to:

Angle-closure glaucoma

History of retinal detachment or retinal degeneration

Acute inflammatory processes

Soft contact lenses in place

Corneal abrasion

Interactions of pilocarpine may occur with:

Topical epinephrine, timolol, and acetazolamide, which potentiate effectiveness (desired)

Topical NSAIDs, which reduce effectiveness

Topical atropine and phenylephrine, which reduce effectiveness

Patient Education

Patients being treated with miotics should be instructed regarding:

Following directions carefully regarding time and amount

Administration by closing tear duct after instillation (see Figure 18-2)

Reporting side effects to the physician for possible dosage adjustment

Administration at bedtime to reduce side effects

Not driving at night

Beta-Adrenergic Blockers

Timolol (Timoptic)

Timolol is a **beta-adrenergic blocker.** It is used topically to lower intraocular pressure in open-angle glaucoma. Other beta-blockers are also used topically to reduce IOP by decreasing the rate of aqueous humor production.

Side effects of beta-blockers are infrequent but may include:

Ocular irritation, conjunctivitis, or diplopia

Aggravation of *preexisting* cardiovascular or pulmonary disorders, which may cause bradycardia, hypotension, and vertigo, or bronchospasm

Contraindications or extreme caution with beta-blockers applies to:

Bradycardia and heart block

Patients receiving oral beta-blocker drugs

Asthma and chronic obstructive pulmonary disease (COPD)

Children, pregnancy, and lactation

Diabetes and hyperthyroidism

Closed-angle glaucoma

Interactions of beta-blockers may occur with:

Other antiglaucoma drugs to help lower IOP

Oral beta-blockers to increase chances of hypotension, bradycardia, and heart block

Betaxolol (Betoptic)

Betaxolol is a cardioselective beta-blocker that can be used with caution in patients with bronchospastic pulmonary disease.

Patient Education

Patients being treated with beta-adrenergic blockers should be instructed regarding:

Administration by closing tear duct after instillation to reduce systemic effects (see Figure 18-2)

Caution in patients with cardiac or pulmonary disorders or who are taking oral beta-blockers

Importance of regular eye examinations

Continuous use of medications for glaucoma; *do not discontinue abruptly*

When administering more than one ophthalmic medication, allowing time interval (at least five minutes) between medications

---

Sympathomimetics

Drugs that mimic the action of the sympathetic nervous system are called sympathomimetics or adrenergics. (See Chapter 13 Autonomic Nervous System Drugs.) Adrenergic action includes dilation of the pupils (mydriatic).

Epinephrine has a mydriatic effect in patients with open-angle glaucoma but is ineffective as a mydriatic in normal eyes, except during surgery. Epinephrine is sometimes combined with miotics in the treatment of open-angle glaucoma (not for angle-closure glaucoma). Epinephrine augments the action of miotics. Instill the miotic first.

Because of the frequent adverse side effects of epinephrine, a *pro-drug* of epinephrine, dipivefrin (Propine), is used more frequently to reduce elevated IOP in the treatment of chronic open-angle glaucoma. A pro-drug is a group of chemicals that exhibit their pharmacological activity after biotransformation. Therefore, less of the drug is required and side effects occur less frequently and are milder with dipivefrin than with epinephrine. It is usually combined with one or more other antiglaucoma drugs.

Side effects, frequent with topical application of epinephrine, and milder with dipivefrin, include:

* Burning, stinging, pain, and headache
* Blurred vision and photophobia

Allergic reactions (e.g., dermatitis and edema)

 Systemic effects, including palpitation, tachycardia, and tremor

Contraindications or extreme caution with epinephrine drugs applies to:

Narrow-angle glaucoma

Cardiac disorders and hypertension

Diabetes

Thyroid disorders

Cerebral arteriosclerosis

Alpha Agonist

Brimonidine (Alphagan-P) is a selective alpha-agonist that decreases formation of aqueous humor with minimal effects on cardiovascular or pulmonary hemodynamics. It is an alternative for those for whom topical beta-blocker therapy is contraindicated.

Side effects of alpha agonists can include dizziness and headache.

Patient Education

Patients being treated with sympathomimetics should be instructed regarding reporting side effects to the physician immediately.

Prostaglandin Analogs

Lantanoprost (Xalatan), travoprost (Travatan), and others, are prostaglandin analogs that cause the greatest reduction in IOP by increasing the outflow of aqueous humor. They may be used concomitantly with other topical ophthalmic drugs to lower IOP (administer the drugs at least five minutes apart).

Side effects of prostaglandin analogs include:

 Blurred vision, burning, and stinging

Slow, gradual change in the color of the iris (resultant color change may be permanent)

Change in length, thickness, and pigmentation of eyelashes

 Systemic effects, including upper respiratory tract infection, muscle and joint pain

Contraindications or extreme caution with prostaglandin analogs applies to:

Contact lens wearers

Hepatic and renal disease

Pregnancy, lactation, use in children

Drug interaction of prostaglandin analogs with eye drops containing the preservative thimerosal (precipitation occurs). If such drugs are used, administer with an interval of at least five minutes between applications. There are no other clinical significant drug interactions.

More frequent administration of prostaglandin analogs than the dosage indicated in Table 18-2 may actually decrease their IOP lowering effect. Refrigerate unopened bottle of Xalatan; once opened the container may be stored at room temperature for six weeks. Travatan does not require refrigeration.

Patient Education

Inform patients about the possibility of iris color change (increase of the brown pigment).

Contact physician immediately if ocular reactions develop.

Prostaglandin analogs contain a preservative that may be absorbed by contact lenses. Remove lenses prior to administration of the drug and wait 15 min before reinserting.

See Table 18-2 for a summary of antiglaucoma agents.

Table 18-2 Antiglaucoma Agents

GENERIC NAME	TRADE NAME	DOSAGE
Carbonic Anhydrase Inhibitors		
acetazolamide	Diamox	Cap, tab, IV, 250–500 mg 4×/day (max 1 g/day)
dorzolamide	Trusopt	Ophthalmic sol. 1 gtt TID
Miotics[a]		
pilocarpine HCl	Isopto Carpine, Pilocar	Ophthalmic sol. 0.25–8%[b], dose varies
pilocarpine gel	Pilopine HS	Ophthalmic gel 4% at bedtime
Beta-Adrenergic Blockers		
timolol	Timoptic, Timoptic-XE	Ophthalmic sol. gel 0.25–0.5% 1 gtt BID
timolol w/dorzolamide	Cosopt	Ophthalmic sol, 1 gtt BID
betaxolol	Betoptic, Betoptic-S	Ophthalmic sol. 0.5%, susp 0.25% 1–2 gtt BID
Sympathomimetic		
dipivefrin	Propine	Ophthalmic sol. 0.1% 1 gtt q12h
Alpha Agonist		
brimonidine	Alphagan-P	Ophthalmic sol. 0.15%; 1 gtt TID (8 h apart)
Prostaglandin Analogs		
latanoprost	Xalatan	Ophthalmic sol. 0.005%, 1 gtt at bedtime
travoprost	Travatan	Ophthalmic sol. 0.004%, 1 gtt at bedtime

[a]Constrict the pupil.

[b]**Wide variation in strengths available. Check carefully for correct percentage.**

Other antiglaucoma agents and combination drugs are available. This is a representative list.

MYDRIATICS

Mydriatics (e.g., atropine) are used topically to *dilate the pupil* for ophthalmic examinations. Atropine also acts as a **cycloplegic** (paralyzes the muscles of accommodation). It is the drug of choice in eye examinations for children. However, other mydriatics, for example cyclopentolate, are more often used for adults because of faster action and faster recovery time.

Side effects of mydriatics, more likely in older adult patients, may include:

* Increased IOP
* Local irritation, burning sensation transient
* Blurred vision common
* Flushing, dryness of skin, and fever
* Confusion (caution in older adults)

Contraindications for mydriatics apply to:

> Angle-closure glaucoma
>
> Infants

Phenylephrine (Neo-Synephrine) is a sympathomimetic that produces mydriasis without cycloplegia. Side effects and contraindications are similar to those of epinephrine.

Patient Education

Patients being treated with mydriatics should be instructed regarding:

Administration by closing tear duct after instillation (see Figure 18-2)

Aseptic technique to prevent contamination of medicine

Blurred vision and sensitivity to light to be expected (wear dark glasses or stay out of bright light)

See Table 18-3 for a summary of the mydriatics.

Table 18-3 Mydriatics and Local Anesthetics for the Eye

GENERIC NAME	TRADE NAME	DOSAGE	COMMENTS
Mydriatics[a]			
atropine	Atropine	Oint, sol 0.5–2%[b]	Administered 40–60 min before exam
cyclopentolate	Cyclogyl	Ophthalmic sol, 0.5–2%[b]	Check carefully for percent
phenylephrine	Neo-Synephrine	Ophthalmic sol, 0.12%, 2.5%, 10%[b]	
Local Anesthetics			
tetracaine	Pontocaine	Sol, 0.5%	Apply eye patch
proparacaine	Ophthetic	Sol, 0.5%	Apply eye patch

[a]Dilate the pupil.

[b]**Wide variations in strengths available. Check carefully for correct percentage!**

LOCAL ANESTHETICS

Local ophthalmic anesthetics, such as tetracaine *(Pontocaine)*, are applied topically to the eye for minor surgical procedures, removal of foreign bodies, or painful injury.

Side effects of local anesthetics are rare, except with prolonged use but may include *hypersensitivity* (transient stinging), reactions such as *anaphylaxis in those allergic to the "-caine" local anesthetics* (ester type).

Contraindicated for prolonged use because of the danger of corneal erosions.

Patient Education

Patients given local ophthalmic anesthetics should be instructed regarding:

Necessity of wearing an eye patch after use of Pontocaine because of loss of blink reflex

Avoidance of touching or rubbing the eye until the anesthesia has worn off

Patient Education

Patients taking ophthalmic medications should be instructed regarding:

Making certain the correct medication and correct percent solution are used as prescribed

Proper aseptic technique to prevent contamination of the other eye, the dropper, or the ointment tube

Instillation of the *correct number of drops* or amount of ointment into the conjunctival sac (see Figure 18-1)

Closing the eye gently so as not to squeeze the medication out

Applying gentle pressure to inner canthus after instillation to minimize systemic effects (see Figure 18-2)

Use of an eyecup as an aid to administration is discouraged due to risk of contamination. Monitor expiration dates closely—do not use outdated medication.

WORKSHEET FOR CHAPTER 18
EYE MEDICATIONS

List the drugs according to category and complete all columns.
Learn generic or trade names as specified by instructor.

Classifications and Drugs	Purpose	Side Effects	Contraindications or Cautions	Patient Education
Anti-inflammatory Corticosteroids 1. 2. NSAIDs				
Carbonic Inhibitors (CAIs) 1. Diamox 2. Trusopt				
Miotics 1. 2.				
Beta-Adrenergic Blocker 1. Timoptic 2. Betoptic				

Classifications and Drugs	Purpose	Side Effects	Contraindications or Cautions	Patient Education
Sympathomimetic 1.				
Prostaglandin Analogs 1. 2.				
Mydriatics 1. 2.				
Local Anesthetic 1. Pontocaine 2. Ophthetic				

A. Case Study for Eye Medications

Ida Lake, age 35, has been using corticosteroid eye drops for one week for "bloodshot eyes." She now has a purulent drainage from the left eye. She needs the following information.

1. Corticosteroid ophthalmic drops are used to treat all of the following EXCEPT
   a. Inflammation
   b. Allergies
   c. Infection
   d. Burns

2. Eye infections can be treated with all of the following EXCEPT
   a. Viroptic
   b. Prednisolone
   c. Gentamycin
   d. Polymixin B

3. The choice of antibiotic product would include consideration of the following EXCEPT
   a. Allergies
   b. Resistance
   c. Sensitivity of organism
   d. Age of the patient

4. Side effects of corticosteroid products with extended use could include the following EXCEPT
   a. Increased IOP
   b. Stinging
   c. Premature healing
   d. Fungal infections

5. Administration of antibiotic drops would include the following instruction EXCEPT
   a. Wash hands first
   b. Instill in inner canthus
   c. Avoid contaminating tip
   d. Discontinue with itching

B. Case Study for Eye Medications

Sol Gold, age 70, has been diagnosed with open-angle glaucoma. He will need the following information.

1. Treatment could include all of the following EXCEPT
   a. Isopto Carpine
   b. Timoptic
   c. Atropine
   d. Propine

2. The purpose of antiglaucoma drugs can include all of the following EXCEPT
   a. Reduce IOP
   b. Dilate pupil
   c. Reduce aqueous formation
   d. Increase aqueous outflow

3. The following statements are true of Diamox EXCEPT
   a. Diuretic effect
   b. Given PO
   c. Reduces IOP
   d. Given alone

4. Side effects of pilocarpine could include all of the following EXCEPT
   a. Photophobia
   b. Headache
   c. Urinary retention
   d. Blurred vision

5. Side effects of Timoptic can include all of the following EXCEPT
   a. Palpitations
   b. Bronchospasm
   c. Hypotension
   d. Vertigo

CHAPTER REVIEW QUIZ

Match the medication in the first column with the condition in the second column that it is used to treat. Conditions may be used more than once.

Medication		Condition
1. _____	Cosopt	**a.** To dilate pupils
2. _____	Acular	**b.** Glaucoma
3. _____	Pontocaine	**c.** Allergic reaction of eyes
4. _____	Atropine	**d.** Postoperative inflammation
5. _____	Prednisolone	**e.** Eye injury pain
6. _____	Pilocarpine	
7. _____	Timoptic	
8. _____	Diamox	
9. _____	Propine	
10. _____	Neo-Synephrine	

Choose the correct answer.

11. When using more than one ophthalmic product at the same time, the following rules apply EXCEPT:
a. Give five minutes apart
b. Give drops before ointment
c. Give one with highest % last
d. Close the tear duct after instillation

12. Patients being treated with anti-infective eye preparations should be given the following instructions EXCEPT:
a. Do not use makeup
b. Discontinue if burning occurs
c. Do not wear contact lenses
d. Use eyecup for administration

13. Corticosteroid ophthalmic products could cause all of the following EXCEPT:
a. Ocular pain   c. Thinning of cornea
b. Inflammation   d. Corneal ulceration

14. The following statements are true of carbonic anhydrase inhibitors, for example Diamox, EXCEPT:
a. Used to treat glaucoma   c. Have diuretic effect
b. For diabetic retinopathy   d. Combined with miotics

15. The following statements are true of prostaglandin agonists, for example Xalatan, EXCEPT:
a. Contain thimerosal preservative
b. Increase aqueous humor outflow
c. Can change eye color
d. Can affect eyelashes

Chapter 19
Analgesics, Sedatives, and Hypnotics

Objectives

Upon completion of this chapter, the learner should be able to

1. Define the Key Terms

2. Compare and contrast the purpose and action of nonopioid, opioid, and adjuvant analgesics, sedatives, and hypnotics

3. List the side effects of the major analgesics, sedatives, and hypnotics

4. Describe the necessary information for patient education regarding interactions and cautions

5. Explain the contraindications to administration of the CNS depressants in this chapter

Key Terms

Adjuvant	Opioid antagonists
Analgesics	Opioids
Antipyretic	Paradoxical
Coanalgesic	Placebo effect
Dependence	Sedatives
Endogenous	Subjective
Endorphins	Tinnitus
Hypnotics	Tolerance
Objective	

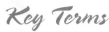 Analgesics, sedatives, and hypnotics depress central nervous system (CNS) action to varying degrees. Some drugs can be classified in more than one category, depending on the dosage.

Analgesics are given for the purpose of relieving pain.

Sedatives are given to calm, soothe, or produce sedation.

Hypnotics are given to produce sleep.

ANALGESICS

Pain is subjective (i.e., it can be experienced or perceived only by the individual subject). Health care workers can view the patient's pain only in an objective way (i.e., observing the patient's reaction to pain in terms of vital signs, position, and emotional response). Pain has both psychological and physiological components. Some persons have a higher pain threshold than others because of conditioning, ethnic background, sensitivity, or physiological factors (e.g., endorphin release).

Endorphins are endogenous analgesics (produced within the brain) as a reaction to severe pain or intense exercise (e.g., "runner's high"). Endorphins block the transmission of pain. Endorphin release may be responsible for a placebo effect: relief from pain as the result of suggestion without the administration of an analgesic.

Opioid Analgesics

Analgesics can be classified as opioid, nonopioid, and adjuvant. Opioids are classified as full or pure agonists, partial agonists, or mixed agonist-antagonists depending on the specific receptors they bind to and their activity at the receptor. Full agonists are commonly used because their action is similar to that of opium in altering the perception of pain, and they do not have a ceiling to analgesic effects, that is, medication level at which there is no enhanced analgesia. These opioids (e.g., morphine, hydromorphone, meperidine, oxycodone, and fentanyl) will not reverse analgesia like the other classes (e.g., pentazocine, butorphanol, and nalbuphine). Opioids are listed under the controlled substance schedule and include both the natural opium alkaloids, for example, morphine and codeine, and the synthetics, for example, meperidine (Demerol) and propoxyphene (Darvon). Opioids tend to cause tolerance (i.e., a larger dose of opioid is needed to achieve the same level of analgesia) and physiological dependence (i.e., physical adaptation of the body to the opioid and withdrawal symptoms after abrupt drug discontinuation) with chronic use.

Addiction or psychological dependence is not a problem for patients who require opioids for pain management. The majority of people stop taking opioids when their pain stops. Because of tolerance, the potential for developing dependence, and the potential for developing undesirable side effects, opioids are not used for extended periods except to relieve chronic pain, for example, cancer pain, terminal illness, and in selected patients with nonmalignant pain who do not benefit from other pain relief methods. Adequate pain control is important for the terminally ill. Dependence is irrelevant for dying patients and should not be a consideration. More effective pain control can be achieved by combining opioids with nonopioid and adjuvant drugs. Analgesics should be given to the terminally ill patients *around-the-clock,* with additional "as needed" doses, for breakthrough pain, and dosages adjusted to achieve pain relief with an acceptable level of side effects. Around-the-clock dosing prevents pain from developing.

Chronic pain therapy, for example, for back pain, sometimes includes the addition of a tricyclic antidepressant or anticonvulsant to the analgesic regimen. These drugs that enhance analgesic effects are called *adjuvant* analgesics and are explained later in this chapter. This addition can reduce the dosage of opioids.

Side effects of opioids can include:

✳ Sedation

✳ Confusion, euphoria, restlessness, and agitation

✳ Headache and dizziness

✳ Hypotension and bradycardia

Urinary retention

✳ Nausea/vomiting (usually resolves within a few days), and constipation (frequently requires treatment)

✳ Respiratory depression (appropriate dose titration reduces risk)

✳ Physical and/or emotional dependence

Blurred vision

Seizures with large doses
Flushing, rash, and pruritus (opiate agonists cause histamine release)

Contraindications or extreme caution with opioids applies to:

Head injury (i.e., conditions associated with increased intracranial pressure)

Cardiac disease, hypotension

CNS depression

Hepatic, renal, and thyroid disease

Chronic obstructive pulmonary disease (COPD), asthma

Pregnancy, lactation, and pediatrics

Older adults and debilitated

Addiction prone, suicidal, and alcoholic

Hypersensitivity

Higher doses in opioid-naïve patients

Interactions include potentiation of effect of opioids with all CNS depressants, including:

Psychotropics

Alcohol

Sedatives and hypnotics

Muscle relaxants

Antihistamines

Antiemetics

Antiarrhythmics or antihypertensives

Preoperatively, an opioid, for example, meperidine (Demerol) 50–100 mg, is frequently combined in a syringe with the anticholinergics (see Chapter 13), to reduce the number of injections given concurrently. Check compatibilities. Preoperative medications are usually administered intramuscularly 30–60 min before the start of anesthesia, according to directions of the anesthesiologist.

Meperidine is frequently combined with Phenergan postoperatively to potentiate analgesic effect. Morphine is better for older adults.

Opioid agonists are available in various strengths, as concentrated oral solutions and in combination products. Carefully note product/strength to be administered.

See Table 19-1 for a summary of the opioid analgesics.

Opioid antagonists are used in the treatment of opioid overdoses and in the delivery room and newborn nursery for opiate-induced respiratory depression. Two opiate antagonists are naloxone and naltrexone.

GENERIC NAME	TRADE NAME	COMMENTS
naloxone	Narcan	For all conditions listed above
naltrexone	ReVia	To treat opiate and alcohol dependence

Caution: Naltrexone is used only *after* withdrawal from opiates, such as heroin and morphine, to help avoid relapses. It acts by robbing the drugs of their pleasurable effects. If given to someone currently dependent on opiates, it can send the addict *instantly into severe, life-threatening withdrawal.*

Nonopioid Analgesics

Nonopioid analgesics, many of which are available without prescription as over-the-counter (OTC) medications, are very popular in this nation of "pill poppers." Therefore, it is extremely important that the health care worker be informed and responsible for patient education in this very important area of public health. The lay public needs to become aware of the dangers of self-medication, overdosage, side effects, and interactions, as well as the grave danger of poisoning to children and older adults by inappropriate use of these readily available drugs.

The nonopioids are given for the purposes of relieving mild to moderate pain, fever, and anti-inflammatory conditions, for example, arthritis. This group of analgesics is also used as a **coanalgesic** in severe acute or chronic pain requiring opioids. The salicylates (aspirin, salsalate, choline magnesium trisalicylate) are most commonly used for their *analgesic* and **antipyretic** properties, as well as for their anti-inflammatory action. Other anti-inflammatory drugs, for example, ibuprofen, are also used for their analgesic properties. The nonsteroidal anti-inflammatory drugs (NSAIDs) are discussed in Chapter 21. Acetaminophen has analgesic and antipyretic properties but very little effect on inflammation. Aspirin and acetaminophen are frequently combined with opioids (see Table 19-1) or with other drugs for more effective analgesic action. See Table 19-2 for a representative sample of nonopioid analgesics and antipyretics. There are many other combination analgesic products available OTC. Patients should be instructed to check all ingredients in these

Table 19-1 Opioid Analgesics*

GENERIC NAME	TRADE NAME	DOSAGE	USES
butorphanol	Stadol Stadol NS	1–4 mg IM, or 0.5–2 mg IV, or 1 mg (one spray) nasal spray q 3–4h PRN	Moderate to severe acute pain (e.g., migraine)
codeine	Codeine[a]	15–60 mg PO/IM q4h PRN; SubQ q4h PRN; PO 10–20 mg q4–6h PRN	Mild to moderate acute, chronic, and cancer pain Antitussive
fentanyl citrate	Sublimaze Duragesic	PO 200–400 mcg q4–6h PRN; or 25–100 mcg slow IV/IM Transdermal q72h	Moderate to severe acute, chronic, or cancer pain Not for acute pain
hydrocodone	Lorcet[b]	PO 5–10 mg q4–6h PRN	Moderate acute, chronic, cancer pain, or antitussive
with acetaminophen	Lortab Vicodin	Max 4 g acetaminophen per day	
hydromorphone	Dilaudid	PO 1–4 mg q3–4h PRN IM, IV, SubQ 1–2 mg q3–4h PRN R 3 mg q6–8h PRN	Moderate to severe acute, chronic, or cancer pain
meperidine	Demerol	50–150 mg PO/IM/SubQ, q3–4h PRN	Moderate to severe acute pain, not for chronic pain, not for older adults
methadone	Dolophine	2.5–10 mg IM/SubQ/PO initially q3–4h PRN; maint. 5–20 mg PO q6–8h PRN	Severe acute, chronic, and cancer pain; also for narcotic withdrawal
morphine sulfate	Morphine MS Contin SR Avinza SR cap MS/R (immediate release)	PO 10–30 mg or R 10–20mg q4h PRN PO, R 15–100 mg q8–12h PO 30–120 mg q24h IV 2.5–15 mg over 4–5 min IM/SubQ 2.5–20 mg q4h PRN	Moderate to severe acute, chronic, or cancer pain Don't crush! OD can be fatal May open cap for NG admin.
oxycodone	Oxycontin Roxicodone	PO 10–80 mg SR q8–12h PO 5–10 mg q6h PRN PO 1–2 tab or 5–10 ml	Serious abuse potential, overdose can be fatal; Do not crush. Moderate to severe acute, chronic, or cancer pain
with aspirin	Percodan[c]	q4–6h PRN;	
with acetaminophen	Tylox, Percocet	Max 4 g acetaminophen/day	
pentazocine	Talwin-NX	PO 50–100 mg q3–4h PRN	Moderate to severe pain; not for older adults
propoxyphene HCL	Darvon	PO 65–100 mg q4h PRN	Mild to moderate acute, chronic, or cancer pain
with acetaminophen	Darvocet[d]	Max 4 g acetaminophen/day	Not for older adults

Combination Opioid Products (Check for allergies, especially aspirin combinations.)

[a]Tylenol with Codeine tabs contain 300 mg acetaminophen plus codeine;
#2 tab 15 mg codeine, #3 tab 30 mg, #4 tab 60 mg (max acetaminophen dose 4 g/day).
Tylenol with codeine elixir: 120 mg acetaminophen and 12 mg codeine per 5 ml.
[b]Lorcet-HD caps; Lortab, or Vicodin tabs: 500 mg acetaminophen and 5 mg hydrocodone.
Lorcet Plus tabs: 650 mg acetaminophen and 7.5 mg hydrocodone.

Vicodan ES tabs: 750 mg acetaminophen and 7.5 mg hydrocodone.
Vicodin HP tabs: 660 mg acetaminophen and 10 mg hydrocodone.
Lortab elixir: 167 mg acetaminophen and 2.5 mg hydrocodone per 5 ml.
[c]Percodan or Endodan tabs: 325 mg aspirin and 5 mg oxycodone.
Percocet, Roxicet, or Endocet: 325 mg acetaminophen and 5 mg oxycodone.
Tylox or Roxilox: 500 mg acetaminophen and 5 mg oxycodone.
[d]Darvocet-N 50: 325 mg acetaminophen and 50 mg propoxyphene.
Darvocet-N 100: 650 mg acetaminophen and 100 mg propoxyphene.
Darvocet-A 500: 500 mg acetaminophen and 100 mg propoxyphene.

Table 19-2 Nonopioid Analgesics and Antipyretics

GENERIC NAME	TRADE NAME	DOSAGE	COMMENTS
acetylsalicylic acid[a]	Aspirin, ASA, Ecotrin, Ascriptin, Bufferin	5–10 gr PO or rectal supp q4h PRN; large doses for arthritis	Give with milk or food
acetaminophen	Tylenol, Panadol, Tempra	325–650 mg PO or rectal supp q4h PRN (max 4 g/day)	No anti-inflammatory action
combinations[b] ASA and caffeine	Anacin	2 tabs PO q6h PRN, max 8/day	
ASA and meprobamate	Equagesic	1–2 tabs PO 3–4×/day	Used to treat pain accompanied by anxiety and/or tension
ASA, acetaminophen, and caffeine	Excedrin	2 tabs/caps PO q6h PRN, max 8/day	Also for pain of migraine headaches
butalbital, caffeine, and acetaminophen	Esgic, Fioricet	1–2 tabs/caps PO q4h PRN, max 6/day	See Equagesic
tramadol	Ultram	50–100 mg PO q4–6h PRN, max 400 mg daily	Strong analgesic, not controlled
with acetaminophen	Ultracet	2 tabs q4–6h, max 8 tabs/24 h	

[a]Other nonsteroidal anti-inflammatory drugs with analgesic action are listed in Table 21-2.
[b]Representative sample.

combination products because of potentially serious adverse side effects, for example, aspirin allergy or acetaminophen contraindications.

Salicylates and Other NSAIDS

Salicylate analgesic and anti-inflammatory actions are associated primarily with preventing the formation of prostaglandins. The salicylates, for example, aspirin (ASA) and other NSAIDs, are also discussed in Chapter 21.

Side effects of salicylates and other NSAIDs, especially with prolonged use and/or high dosages, can include:

 Prolonged bleeding time

Bleeding and frequent bruising

Gastric distress, ulceration, and bleeding (which may be silent)

Tinnitus (ringing or roaring in the ears) and hearing loss with overdose

Hepatic dysfunction

Renal insufficiency, decreased urine output with sodium and water retention, renal failure

Drowsiness, dizziness, headache, sweating, euphoria, depression

Rash

✳ Coma, respiratory failure, or anaphylaxis, which can result from hypersensitivity or overdosage, especially with children (watch for aspirin allergy)

✳ Gastrointestinal (GI) symptoms, which can be minimized by administration with food, milk, or by using an aspirin buffered with antacids or in enteric-coated form

Poisoning—keep out of reach of children (especially flavored children's aspirin)

Contraindications for salicylates and other NSAIDs include:

GI ulcer and bleeding

Bleeding disorders in patients taking anticoagulants

Asthma

Children younger than 15 with influenza-like illness (because of the danger of Reye's syndrome)

Pregnancy

Lactation

Vitamin K deficiency

Allergy to ASA

Caution in use of salicylates and other NSAIDs with the following:

Anemia

Hepatic disease

Renal disease

Hodgkin's disease

Pre/postoperatively (discontinue five to seven days before elective surgery)

Interactions of salicylates may also occur with NSAIDs and the following:

Alcohol (may increase potential for ulceration and bleeding)

Anticoagulants (potentiation)

Corticosteroids (gastric ulcer)

Antacids in high doses (decreased effect)

NSAIDs (decreased effect, increased GI side effects)

Do not give salicylates and NSAIDs together.

Insulin or oral antidiabetic agents (increased effects); may interfere with certain urinary glucose tests

Methotrexate (increased effects)

Probenecid (decreased effects)

Antihypertensives: angiotensin-converting enzyme (ACE) inhibitors, beta-blockers and diuretics (decreased effects)

Carbonic anhydrase inhibitors (toxic effects)—for example, Diamox

Acetaminophen

Acetaminophen (Tylenol) is used extensively in the treatment of mild to moderate pain and fever. It has very little effect on inflammation. However, acetaminophen has fewer adverse side effects than the salicylates (e.g., does not cause gastric irritation or precipitate bleeding). Therefore, it is sometimes used only for its analgesic properties in treating the chronic pain of arthritis so that the salicylate dosage may be reduced to safer levels with fewer side effects in these patients.

Side effects of acetaminophen are rare, but large doses can cause:

* Severe liver toxicity
* Renal insufficiency (decreased urine output)
   Rash or urticaria
   Blood dyscrascias

Caution must be used with frequent acetaminophen use and alcohol ingestion because of potential liver damage. Caution also with pregnancy and breast-feeding.

Contraindicated for repeated administration with anemia, cardiac or asthmatic conditions, renal or hepatic disease.

> *Note:* Acetaminophen (Tylenol) is frequently combined with opioid analgesics when stronger pain relief is required. Some examples of such combinations include Tylenol #3, Lorcet, Lortab, Vicodin, Tylox, Percocet, Roxicet, and Darvocet. For examples of other opioid combinations, and for information regarding the proportion of the ingredients in each product, see Table 19-1 and Combination Opioid Products, below the table. Remember, all opioids are controlled substances.

Tramadol

Tramadol (Ultram) is a centrally acting synthetic analgesic compound similar in effect to the opioids, but is chemically unrelated. It is nonopioid and is not a controlled substance. It produces analgesia by inhibiting the reuptake of norepinephrine and serotonin.

Side effects of Ultram can include:

* Dizziness, somnolence, malaise, headache
   Nausea, constipation
   Sweating and pruritus
* Orthostatic hypotension
   Anxiety, confusion
* Rash, allergic reactions

Contraindications with Ultram include:

>   Increased intracranial pressure or head injury
>
>   Renal and hepatic disease
>
>   Seizure disorders
>
>   Pregnant or nursing women
>
>   Children under 16
>
>   Abrupt discontinuation
>
>   Opiate agonist hypersensitivity (especially to codeine)

Caution with Ultram in older adults and with anyone driving or operating machinery. May impair mental or physical abilities.

Interactions of Ultram with:

>   Monoamine inhibitors (MAOIs) or neuroleptics—may increase seizure risk
>
>   Carbamazepine (Tegretol) antagonizes Ultram action
>
>   Selective serotonin reuptake inhibitors (SSRIs) (especially Paxil, Zoloft)—may cause serotonin syndrome and increase seizure risk

See Table 19-2 for a summary of the nonopioid analgesics and antipyretics.

Adjuvant Analgesics

These drugs were originally intended for treatment of conditions other than pain. **Adjuvant** analgesics may enhance analgesic effect with opioids and nonopioids, produce analgesia alone, or reduce the side effects of analgesics. Two classes commonly used for analgesia include anticonvulsants and tricyclic antidepressants. Lidocaine is available topically in a patch (Lidoderm) for those patients in whom oral analgesics may not be a viable option for pain control. See Table 19-3 for a summary of adjuvant analgesics.

Tricyclic Antidepressants

Tricyclic antidepressants are used in the treatment of nerve pain associated with herpes, arthritis, diabetes, and cancer, migraine or tension headaches, insomnia, and depression. Often, the patient will describe the pain as "burning." Tricyclic antidepressant actions are associated with increasing available norepinephrine and serotonin, which blocks pain transmission. Drugs used commonly for pain include Elavil, Pamelor, and Tofranil. Allow two to three weeks to see therapeutic effects.

Side effects of tricyclic antidepressants can include:

*   Dry mouth, urinary retention, delirium, constipation
*   Sedation (take at bedtime)
*   Orthostatic hypotension
*   Tachyarrhythmias
    Heart block in cardiac patients

Table 19-3 Adjuvant Analgesics and Local Anesthetic

GENERIC NAME	TRADE NAME	DOSAGE	COMMENTS
Tricyclic Antidepressants			
amitripytyline	Elavil	PO 10–100 mg at bedtime	Caution combining with opioids
nortriptyline	Pamelor	PO 10–150 mg at bedtime	
imipramine	Tofranil	PO 10–150 mg at bedtime	
Anticonvulsants			
carbamazepine	Tegretol	PO 200 mg BID 4×/day	Especially for trigeminal neuralgia Monitor serum levels periodically
gabapentin	Neurontin	PO 600–3600 mg/day div. doses 3–4×/day	For nerve pain, especially postherpetic neuralgia
lamotrigine	Lamictal	PO 25–200 mg BID	Use when unresponsive to others
Local Anesthetic			
Lidocaine	Lidoderm	1–3 Patches 5% daily	For postherpetic neuralgia (on 12 h/off 12 h

[a]*Note:* All adjuvants should be started at the lower end of the dosage range and titrated upward in small increments weekly according to clinical response.

The degree of side effects varies with each antidepressant. Side effects may be additive with opioids (e.g., increased constipation, hypotension, sedation, etc.).

Caution with tricyclics if used with prostatic hypertrophy, urinary retention, increased intraocular pressure, and glaucoma.

Contraindications for tricyclics with hypersensitivity and recovery phase of myocardial infarction.

Anticonvulsants

Anticonvulsants (i.e., Neurontin and Tegretol), like tricyclic antidepressants, are commonly used for the management of nerve pain associated with neuralgia, herpes zoster (shingles), and cancer. Anticonvulsant therapy is implemented when the patient describes the pain as "sharp," "shooting," "shocklike pain," or "lightning-like." Neurontin is generally considered a first-line *anticonvulsant* for neuropathic pain therapy, followed by Tegretol and Lamictal.

Side effects of anticonvulsants can include the following:

* Sedation, dizziness, and confusion
* Nausea, vomiting, constipation, and anorexia
* Hypotension and unsteadiness (Tegretol)
  Hepatitis

Rash, Stevens-Johnson syndrome (Lamictal—start low, slow titration upward)

✴ Bone marrow suppression

Nystagmus, diplopia (double vision), and blurred vision

Gingivitis (Neurontin)

Caution with anticonvulsants if used with allergies, hepatitis, cardiac disease, and renal disease.

> CAUTION: **Do not confuse** *Lamictal* **(anticonvulsant) with** *Lamisil* **(antifungal).**

Contraindications with anticonvulsants include:

Hypersensitivity

Psychiatric conditions

Pregnancy

SA (sinoatrial) and AV (atrioventricular) block (Tegretol)

Hemolytic disorders (Tegretol)

Abrupt discontinuation

Interactions of anticonvulsants occur with:

Alcohol (decreased effects)

Antacids (decreased effects) (Neurontin)

Antineoplastics (decreased effects) (Tegretol)

CNS depressants (decreased effects) (Tegretol)

Folic acid (decreased effects) (Lamictal)

Dilantin with any drug in solution or syringe

Antiretrovirals (increased or decreased effects) with Lamictal and Tegretol

LOCAL ANESTHETIC

The lidocaine patch (Lidoderm) is approved for the management of postherpetic neuralgia, although it can provide significant analgesia in other forms of neuropathic pain, including diabetic neuropathy and musculoskeletal pain such as osteoarthritis and low back pain. Topical lidocaine provides pain relief through a peripheral effect and generally has little if any central action. The penetration of topical lidocaine into intact skin is sufficient to produce an analgesic effect, but less than the amount necessary to produce anesthesia.

The lidocaine patch must be applied to intact skin. Patches may be cut into smaller sizes with scissors before removal of the release liner. To reduce the potential for serious adverse effects, patches are worn only once for up to 12 h within a 24-h period, then removed.

Side effects of the lidocaine patch, local in nature, are generally mild and transient, and include:

* Erythema, edema and hives
* Allergic reactions

Precautions and contraindications for the lidocaine patch include:

Sensitivity to local anesthetics

Hepatic disease

Nonintact skin

Pregnancy, breast-feeding, and pediatric use

Handling and disposal to prevent access by children or pets

Drug interactions of the lidocaine patch with:

Antiarrhythmic drugs such as tocainaide and mexiletene

Local anesthetics

Antimigraine Agents

Migraine is the most common neurovascular headache and may include nausea, vomiting, and sensitivity to light or noise. Migraines (and most other forms of headache) respond best when treated early. Simple analgesics (see Table 19-2), NSAIDs (see Chapter 21) and opioid analgesics can be effective, especially if they are taken at the initial sign of migraine.

Serotonin Receptor Agonists (SRAs)

For those patients unresponsive to the aforementioned treatments, serotonin agonists were developed based on the observation that serotonin levels decrease, while vasodilation and inflammation of blood vessels in the brain increase, as the migraine symptoms worsen during an attack. SRAs also effective in treating the nausea and vomiting associated with migraines because serotonin receptors are also found in the GI tract.

The first "triptan" approved was sumatriptan (Imitrex), followed by (among others) rizatriptan (Maxalt) and eletriptan (Relpax). SRAs are indicated for the acute treatment of migraines in adults and have no therapeutic value for the prophylactic management of migraine headaches.

Side effects of SRAs include:

* Malaise, fatigue, dizziness, drowsiness
* Nausea, vomiting, diarrhea
* Asthenia, tingling, paresthesias, flushing
* Pain or pressure in the chest, neck, or jaw
* Arrythmias, angina, palpitations, myocardial infarction, cardiac arrest

Contraindications and precautions with SRAs include:

Patients with cerebrovascular or cardiovascular disease

Hepatic or renal disease

Use in older adults (who are more likely to have decreased hepatic function and more pronounced blood pressure increases and are at risk for coronary artery disease)

Pregnancy, lactation, use in children

Drug interactions of SRAs with:

Ergot alkaloids (i.e., methylergonovine)—additive vasopastic effects

MAOIs elevate plasma levels of most triptans (do not use within two weeks of discontinuing use of the MAOI)

Most antidepressants potentiate the effects of serotonin (including SSRIs and tricyclics) resulting in serotonin syndrome (mental status changes, diaphoresis, tremor, hyperreflexia, and fever)

Macrolide antibiotics, antiretroviral protease inhibitors, and "azole" antifungals with eletriptan (increased plasma levels)—do not use within at least 72 h of each other.

See Table 19-4 for information on antimigraine agents.

Table 19-4 Antimigraine Agents

GENERIC NAME	TRADE NAME	DOSAGE FORMS	INITIAL DOSE ADULT	REPEAT TIME (HOURS)	DAILY MAXIMUM DOSE (MG)
eletriptan	Relpax	Tablet	20–40 mg	2	80
rizatriptan	Maxalt	Tablet	5–10 mg	2	30
	Maxalt-MLT	OD tablet	5–10 mg	2	30
sumatriptan	Imitrex	SubQ	6 mg	1	12
		Nasal	20 mg	2	40
		Tablet	25–100 mg	2	200

OD, orally disintegrating tablet.

Note: Representative sample; other products are available.

SEDATIVES AND HYPNOTICS

Sedatives and **hypnotics** are controlled substances used to promote sedation in smaller doses and promote sleep in larger doses. The sedative-hypnotics are classified as barbiturates and nonbarbiturates. Some psychotropic drugs (see Chapter 22) and some antihistamines (see Chapter 26) are also used as sedative-hypnotics.

Antihistamines, for example, diphenhydramine (Benadryl, Nytol, Sominex) have an extended half-life, remaining in the system longer. Because of slower metabolism and impaired circulation, the older or debilitated patient is particularly susceptible to *side effects,* such as dizziness, hypotension, confusion, and decreased coordination. These effects can continue for a longer time, resulting in "morning-after" problems. Therefore, antihistamines are not as effective as other available sedative-hypnotics.

None of these medications should be used for extended periods of time except under close medical supervision, as in the treatment of epilepsy, because of the potential for psychological and physical dependence. In addition, these medications depress the REM (rapid eye movement, or dream) phase of sleep, and withdrawal after prolonged use can result in a severe rebound effect with nightmares and hallucinations. The nonbarbiturates depress REM sleep to a lesser degree than the barbiturates. Abrupt withdrawal of hypnotics, even after short-term therapy, for example, one week, may result in rebound insomnia. Therefore, gradual reduction of dosage is indicated.

✳ Before starting pharmacological treatment, patients should be encouraged to use more natural methods of combating insomnia. These include exercise during the day, avoiding daytime naps, avoiding heavy meals and activating medications near bedtime, warm milk, back rubs, soft music, and other calming influences. Additionally, avoidance of caffeine and alcohol should be stressed. Alcohol may help to initiate sleep but results in early awakening.

Barbiturates

Barbiturates have been implicated in many suicides and fatalities due to accidental overdoses, especially when combined with other CNS depressants or alcohol. They are particularly dangerous because they are metabolized and excreted slowly; that is, they have an extended half-life, remaining in the system longer.

Because of the many serious, potentially dangerous, *side effects*, especially *CNS depression,* barbiturates are used infrequently now as sedative-hypnotics. Phenobarbital is still used in the treatment of seizure disorders (see Chapter 22). However, there are many other safer and more effective hypnotics available. Therefore, the use of barbiturates for sedation is restricted to specific, limited circumstances in which the patient can be closely monitored.

Nonbarbiturates

Nonbarbiturates have supplanted barbiturates as sedative-hypnotics and have less potential for abuse. However, withdrawal effects are observed after long-term use and *respiratory depression* (when taken with alcohol) can be potentially fatal. As mentioned earlier, the cause of insomnia should be established and underlying factors treated before a hypnotic is prescribed. Only short-term use (7–10 days) is recommended.

Older nonbarbiturate hypnotics include chloral hydrate. Newer drugs include the benzodiazepine temazepam (Restoril) and nonbenzodiazepine hypnotics like zolpidem (Ambien) and zaleplon (Sonata).

Side effects of chloral hydrate include:

✳ Nausea, vomiting, diarrhea

    Rash

✳ Dizziness

Ataxia

Dependence, withdrawal symptoms

Side effects of benzodiazepines can include:

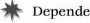 Daytime sedation, confusion, and headache—hangover effect

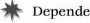 Increased risk of falls (especially in older adults or with long-acting hypnotics)

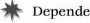 Dependence/withdrawal symptoms

 Amnesia, hallucinations, and bizarre behavior may occur more often with triazolam (Halcion) than with other benzodiazepines

Contraindications for all the sedative-hypnotics include:

Hypersensitivity

Severe liver impairment

Coadministration of ketoconazole or itraconazole with triazolam

Severe renal impairment

Porphyria

Abrupt discontinuation

Caution with all sedative hypnotics for the following:

Older adults

Debilitated

Addiction prone

Renal impairment

Liver impairment

Depressed and mentally unstable

Suicidal individuals

Pregnancy and lactation

Children

COPD and sleep apnea

Interactions of all the sedative hypnotics with the following drugs can be dangerous and potentially fatal:

Psychotropic drugs

Alcohol

Muscle relaxants

Antiemetics

Antihistamines

Analgesics

See Table 19-5 for a summary of the sedatives and hypnotics.

Table 19-5 Sedatives and Hypnotics (Use Hypnotics Short Term Only)

GENERIC NAME	TRADE NAME	DOSAGE	COMMENTS
Nonbarbituarates			
chloral hydrate		PO 500 mg–1 g or R ½ h before bedtime	Short-term treatment of insomnia only (loses effectiveness within 2 weeks) Preop sedation especially for children
estazolam	Prosom	PO 0.5–2 mg at bedtime	Rapid onset, intermediate duration
flurazepam	Dalmane	15–30 mg PO at bedtime	Rapid onset, long half-life
temazepam	Restoril	7.5–30 mg PO at bedtime	Intermediate onset, duration
triazolam	Halcion	0.125–0.25 mg PO at bedtime	Can cause amnesia, hallucinations, bizarre behavior, rapid onset, short duration
zolpidem	Ambien	5–10 mg PO	Rapid induction 30 min Short half-life (less than 3 h)
zaleplon	Sonata	PO 5–10 mg at bedtime	Rapid onset, very short half-life

Patient Education

Patients taking analgesics, sedatives, or hypnotics should be instructed regarding:

Potential for physical and psychological dependence and tolerance with opioids, sedatives, and hypnotics

Taking only limited doses for short periods of time, *except* to relieve pain in terminal illness (in terminal cases, analgesics should be given on a regular basis around the clock to prevent or control pain)

Caution with interactions; *not* taking any medications (except under close medical supervision) that potentiate CNS depression (e.g., psychotropics, *alcohol,* muscle relaxants, antihistamines, antiemetics, cardiac medications, and antihypertensives)

Serious potential side effects with prolonged use or overdose of opioids, sedatives, and hypnotics (e.g., oversedation, dizziness, headache, confusion, agitation, nausea, constipation, urinary retention, and *potentially fatal* respiratory depression, bradycardia, or hypotension)

Tolerance with prolonged use, with increasingly larger doses required to achieve the same effect

Potential for overdose of sedatives or hypnotics and paradoxical reactions with older adults (e.g., confusion, agitation, hallucinations, and hyperexcitability)

Withdrawal after prolonged use of sedatives and hypnotics possibly leading to rebound effects with nightmares, hallucinations, or insomnia

Mental alertness and physical coordination impairment causing accidents or falls

Caution regarding OTC analgesic combinations and checking ingredients on the label; being aware of possible side effects with those containing aspirin (e.g., gastric distress or bleeding)

Not discontinuing abruptly

WORKSHEET FOR CHAPTER 19
ANALGESICS, SEDATIVES, AND HYPNOTICS

List the drugs according to category and complete all columns.
Learn generic or trade names as specified by instructor.

Classifications and Drugs	Purpose	Side Effects	Contraindications or Cautions	Patient Education
Opioids 1. codeine				
2. hydrocodone (Vicodin)				
3. meperidine (Demerol)				
4. morphine (MS Contin) (MSIR)				
5. oxycodone (Percodan) (Oxycontin) (Tylox)				
6. methadone (Dolophine)				
7. Darvon, Darvocet				
8. Fentanyl				
9. Dilaudid				
Opioid Antagonist 1. Narcan				

Classifications and Drugs	Purpose	Side Effects	Contraindications or Cautions	Patient Education
Nonopioid Analgesics 1. aspirin (combinations) 2. acetaminophen (Tylenol) (combinations) 3. tramadol (Ultram)				

Adjuvant Analgesics
1. tricyclics
   Elavil, Tofranil
 	
2. anticonvulsants
   Tegretol
   gabapentin (Neurontin)				

Sedative-Hypnotic Nonbarbiturates 1. chloral hydrate 2. estazolam (Prosom) 3. temazepam (Restoril) 4. zolpidem (Ambien) 5. zaleplon (Sonata)				

A. Case Study for Analgesics

Sarah Payne, a 45-year-old terminal cancer patient, is discharged from the hospital to her home with hospice care. Her husband is concerned that she be pain-free, but worries that she will become "addicted" to her pain medicines. He needs the following information.

1. Opioids, for example, morphine, are given regularly with all of the following conditions EXCEPT
   a. Cancer pain
   b. Arthritis pain
   c. Short-term acute pain
   d. Terminally ill

2. Morphine is frequently combined with other drugs to enhance pain relief. Which one would NOT potentiate effect?
   a. Ibuprofen
   b. Tofranil
   c. Narcan
   d. Neurontin

3. Analgesics are *most* effective for terminally ill patients when given
   a. As necessary
   b. During waking hours
   c. Before meals
   d. Around-the-clock

4. Side effects of opioids can include all of the following EXCEPT
   a. Dizziness
   b. Diarrhea
   c. Nausea
   d. Confusion

5. Opioids are frequently given with nonopioids for better analgesic action. Which one is NOT considered a coanalgesic?
   a. Acetaminophen
   b. Aspirin
   c. Elavil
   d. Ambien

B. Case Study for Hypnotics

Freda Stone, a 70-year-old patient with arthritis pain, has been taking Restoril for sleep for years. She wants to change to Halcion now. She needs the following information.

1. Which statement is generally true of most hypnotics?
   a. Rapid elimination usual
   b. Safe for older adults
   c. Effective long term
   d. Side effects common

2. Halcion can have all of the following side effects EXCEPT
   a. Amnesia
   b. Hallucinations
   c. Palpitations
   d. Bizarre behavior

3. Which of the following would be LEAST susceptible to ill effects?
   a. Children
   b. Debilitated
   c. Obese
   d. Older adults

4. Common side effects of many hypnotics can include all of the following EXCEPT
   a. Dizziness
   b. Diuresis
   c. Confusion
   d. Hangover

5. Hypnotic interactions can be potentially dangerous with all of the following EXCEPT
   a. Alcohol
   b. Antidepressants
   c. Analgesics
   d. Antacids

CHAPTER REVIEW QUIZ

Match the medication in the first column with the classification in the second column. Classifications may be used more than once.

Medication	Classification
1. ____ Amitripytline	**a.** Antitussive
2. ____ Vicodin	**b.** Opioid antagonist
3. ____ Ultram	**c.** Opioid analgesic with aspirin
4. ____ Methadone	**d.** Tricyclic antidepressant (adjuvant)
5. ____ Percodan	**e.** Opioid analgesic with acetaminophen
6. ____ Duragesic	**f.** Nonopioid analgesic (not controlled)
7. ____ Demerol	**g.** Anticonvulsant (adjuvant analgesic)
8. ____ Codeine	**h.** Synthetic analgesic for acute pain
9. ____ Narcan	**i.** Opioid analgesic and narcotic withdrawal
10. ____ Tegretol	**j.** Transdermal analgesic for chronic pain
	k. Opium alkaloid for severe, acute, or cancer pain

Choose the correct answer.

11. Diphenhydramine (Benadryl, Nytol) can cause all of the following side effects EXCEPT:
    a. Dizziness
    b. Hypertension
    c. Confusion
    d. Decreased coordination
12. The following statements are true of barbiturates, for example, phenobarbital, EXCEPT:
    a. Interact with alcohol
    b. Extended half-life
    c. CNS depressant
    d. Insomnia remedy
13. The following statements are true of opioids containing acetaminophen, for example, Tylox, EXCEPT:
    a. Antipyretic
    b. Anti-inflammatory
    c. Analgesic
    d. Many interactions
14. Tricyclic antidepressants, used as adjuvant analgesics, can have the following side effects EXCEPT:
    a. Frequency
    b. Tachycardia
    c. Constipation
    d. Dry mouth
15. Anticonvulsants, for example, Neurontin, are used for nerve pain associated with the following conditions, EXCEPT:
    a. Neuralgia
    b. Cancer
    c. Shingles
    d. Polymyalgia

Chapter 20
Psychotropic Medications, Alcohol, and Drug Abuse

Objectives

Upon completion of this chapter, the learner should be able to

1. Define the Key Terms

2. Categorize the most commonly used psychotropic medications according to the following four classifications: CNS stimulants, antidepressants, anxiolytics, and antipsychotic medications

3. List the purpose, action, side effects, interactions, and contraindications for psychotropic medications in common use

4. Describe the physiological effects of prolonged alcohol use

5. Explain treatment of acute and chronic alcoholism

6. Compare and contrast drug addiction and habituation

7. Describe the effects of three commonly used illegal drugs

8. List the responsibilities of the health care worker in combating drug abuse

Key Terms

Addiction

Antidepressant

Antipsychotic

Anxiolytics

Ataxia

Atypical antipsychotics

Bipolar disorders

Chemical dependency

Extrapyramidal

Heterocyclic

Neurotransmitters

Psychotropic

SSRIs

Tardive dyskinesia

Tricyclics

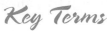**Psychotropic** refers to any substance that acts on the mind. Psychotropic medications are drugs that can exert a therapeutic effect on a person's mental processes, emotions, or behavior. Drugs used for other purposes

can have psychotropic effects. Examples of other medications that affect mental functioning are anesthetics, analgesics, sedatives, hypnotics, and antiemetics, which are discussed in other chapters.

Psychotropic medications can be classified according to the purpose for administration. The four classes are CNS stimulants, antidepressants, anxiolytics, and antipsychotic medications.

Psychotropic medications are frequently prescribed concurrently with psychotherapy or professional counseling.

CNS STIMULANTS

CNS (central nervous system) stimulant medications are given for the purpose of promoting CNS functioning. One drug in this category, caffeine citrate, has been used in the treatment of neonatal apnea.

Prolonged, high intake of caffeine in any form may produce tolerance, habituation, and psychological dependence. Physical signs of withdrawal such as headaches, irritation, nervousness, anxiety, and dizziness may occur upon abrupt discontinuation of the stimulant.

Since caffeine crosses the placenta and is also distributed into the milk of nursing women, most clinicians recommend that those who are pregnant or nursing avoid or limit their consumption of foods, beverages, and drugs containing caffeine; for example, over-the-counter (OTC) analgesics or decongestants.

Other CNS stimulant drugs include controlled substances, such as the amphetamines (e.g., Adderall) and methylphenidate (Ritalin), which are used to treat attention-deficit hyperactivity disorder (ADHD) or attention-deficit disorder without hyperactivity (ADD) in children over age 6, and for narcolepsy. Ritalin is also occasionally used in the treatment of senile apathy and major depression refractory to other therapies. The use of amphetamines to reduce appetite in the treatment of obesity is *not* recommended because tolerance develops rapidly and physical or psychic dependence may develop within a few weeks. *These drugs have a high potential for abuse and should be used only under medical supervision for diagnosed medical disorders.* However, when these drugs are used appropriately, as ordered by the physician, abuse potential and dependence appear to be minimal.

Side effects of the controlled CNS stimulants can include:

* Nervousness, insomnia, irritability, seizures, or psychosis from overdose
* Tachycardia, palpitations, hypertension, and cardiac arrhythmias
  Dizziness, headache, and blurred vision (dilated pupils with photophobia)
* Gastrointestinal (GI) disturbances, including anorexia, nausea, vomiting, abdominal pain, and dry mouth
* Habituation and dependence possible with prolonged use

Contraindications or caution with CNS stimulants applies to:

Treatment for obesity (never more than three to six weeks)—without diet and exercise modifications, weight gain resumes after discontinuation of medication

Patients with anxiety or agitation

History of drug dependence, alcoholism, or eating disorders

Hyperthyroidism

Cardiovascular disorders

Closed-angle glaucoma (not modafinil)

Pregnant or nursing women

Abrupt withdrawal, depression results

Use with monoamine oxidase inhibitors (MAOI) may cause hypertensive crisis

Caution with sustained release preparations differing designations (CD, ER, LA, SR) and their respective dosing requirements (see Table 20-1).

Pediatric precautions: Prolonged administration of CNS stimulants to children with ADD has been reported to cause at least a temporary suppression of normal weight and/or height patterns in some patients, and therefore close monitoring is required. Growth rebound has been observed after discontinuation, and attainment of normal adult weight and height do not appear to be compromised. CNS stimulants, including amphetamines, have been reported to exacerbate motor and vocal tics

Table 20-1 Central Nervous System Stimulants and SNRI for ADHD

GENERIC NAME	TRADE NAME	DOSAGE	COMMENTS
caffeine citrate	Cafcit	PO 20–30 mg/kg X1, then 5–8 mg/kg/daily	For neonatal apnea Caution: Do *not* use caffeine and sodium benzoate
amphetamines	Adderall Adderall XR	PO 5–30 mg daily–BID PO 5–30 mg daily	For narcolepsy, ADHD, ADD, (>3 yr old)
methylphenidate	Ritalin Ritalin SR Metadate ER Medadate CD Ritalin LA Concerta	PO 5–20 mg BID-TID 10–20 mg BID-TID (Note 8-h duration of action) PO 20–60 mg q A.M. PO 18–54 mg q A.M. ER tab PO 18–54 mg q A.M.	For narcolepsy, ADHD, ADD, (>6 yr), senile apathy, major depression For once-daily treatment of ADHD or ADD ER tab for once-daily treatment of ADD, ADHD
modafinil	Provigil	PO 100–400 mg daily	For narcolepsy, sleep apnea, and shift-work sleep disorder (>16 yr)
SNRI atomoxetine	Strattera	PO 20–50 mg BID	For ADHD (black box warning: suicidal tendencies)

and Tourette's disorder, and clinical evaluation for these disorders in children and their families should precede use of the drugs. Children should also be observed carefully for development of tics while receiving these drugs.

There is some evidence that medication use only during school days may be tried in children with controlled ADHD, but only if no significant behavior or social difficulties are noted. Once controlled, dosage reduction or interruption may be possible during weekends, holidays, or vacations.

(See also *SNRIs* in Table 20-2 for a *nonstimulant noncontrolled* drug for ADHD.)

Abuse of amphetamines: Signs and symptoms of chronic amphetamine abuse and acute toxicity are discussed later in this chapter in the section entitled Drug Abuse. Treatment of acute toxicity is also described in that section.

Modafinil (Provigil) is a newer psychostimulant medication approved for narcolepsy, sleep apnea, and shift-work sleep disorder in adults and adolescents (>16 years old). The potential for abuse and dependence appears to be lower than that for the amphetamines and methylphenidate. Modafinil does not appear to be effective in treating ADHD in adults and has not been demonstrated to promote weight loss.

Side effects of modafinil (Provigil) are infrequent. Only about 1% of people complain of mild headache and nausea.

Cautions for the use of modafinil include: Possible causes of fatigue and sleepiness should be determined before stimulant medicines are prescribed to increase wakefulness. Without adequate investigation, some common disorders, such as diabetes and sleep apnea, might go undiagnosed.

Reducing the necessary amount of restorative sleep for prolonged periods of time can result in mental and physical problems, especially neurological and cardiovascular effects.

Patient Education

Patients receiving controlled CNS stimulants should be warned about the potential side effects.

They should be cautioned about the potential for abuse and should take them only according to physician's orders.

Medication should be taken early in the day to reduce insomnia.

Abrupt withdrawal may result in depression, irritability, fatigue, agitation, and disturbed sleep.

Parents of children receiving amphetamines and methylphenidate should watch for signs of tics, gastric disturbance, insomnia, weight loss, or nervousness, and report to the physician.

Older adults should be warned particularly about dangerous cardiovascular side effects.

Do not chew or crush sustained release products.

Those taking modafinil should be cautioned about the necessity for regular sleep in sufficient amounts to restore mental and physiological functioning to an optimal level.

SELECTIVE NOREPINEPHRINE REUPTAKE INHIBITOR (SNRI)

Atomoetine (Strattera) is a selective norepinephrine reuptake inhibitor (SNRI) and the first *nonstimulant, noncontrolled* drug approved for attention-deficit hyperactivity disorder (ADHD). Atomoxetine, structurally related to fluoxetine, does not have a potential for abuse and has been shown to be safe and effective in adolescents and children more than six years old and adults with ADHD.

Side effects of SNRIs include:

* Dry mouth, reduced appetite, fatigue
* Nausea, vomiting, constipation, dyspepsia
  Urinary hesitation/retention
* Possible suicidal tendencies (black box warning)

Contraindications and Cautions for SNRIs include:

Narrow-angle glaucoma

Cerebrovascular, heart, or hepatic disease

Possible growth disturbance during treatment

Interactions of SNRIs with:

Beta-agonists, MAOIs, vasopressor agents

Fluoxetine, paroxetine, quinidine

See Table 20-1 for a summary of the CNS stimulants and nonstimulant medication for ADHD.

ANTIDEPRESSANTS

Depression is frequently described as a chemical imbalance. In many depressed patients, certain chemicals in the brain may be in short supply. Chemicals in the brain, like dopamine, serotonin, and norepinephrine are known as **neurotransmitters.** Substances that travel across the synapse (contact point of two neurons) transmit messages between nerve cells. If these neurotransmitters are reabsorbed by one nerve ending before they have had a chance to make contact with the next nerve cell, they cannot perform their function. In depression, there may be a shortage of the neurotransmitters dopamine, serotonin, or norepinephrine.

Antidepressant medications, sometimes called mood elevators, are used primarily to treat patients with various types of depression. The four categories in general use are the tricyclic antidepressants, the MAOIs, the selective serotonin reuptake inhibitors (**SSRIs**), and the heterocyclic antidepressants.

Tricyclics

The mechanism of antidepressant action of the **tricyclics** involves potentiation of norepinephrine and serotonin activity by blocking their reuptake presynaptically. Their pharmacology also includes strong *anticholinergic* activity that is responsible for many of the side effects seen.

The tricyclics have delayed action, elevating the mood and increasing alertness after two to four weeks. They are frequently given at bedtime because of a mild sedative effect. They are used more frequently than the MAOIs because of milder and fewer side effects, except with older adults. Tricyclics may be more effective than SSRIs in some severe depression and are used as an adjunct in neurogenic pain control (see Chapter 19, Analgesics, Sedatives, and Hypnotics).

Side effects of the tricyclics, such as imipramine (Tofranil), are anticholinergic in action and can include:

* Dryness of the mouth

  Increased appetite and weight gain
* Drowsiness and dizziness

  Blurred vision
* Constipation and urinary retention, especially with benign prostatic hypertrophy (BPH)
* Postural hypotension, cardiac arrhythmias, and palpitation
* Confusion, especially in older adults

Contraindications or extreme caution with tricyclics applies to:

Cardiac, renal, GI, and liver disorders

Older adults

Glaucoma

Obesity

Seizure disorder

Pregnancy and lactation

Concomitant use with MAOIs

SSRIs—increase tricyclic blood levels

Interactions of tricyclics can include:

Clonidine—causing hypertensive crisis

CNS drugs and alcohol

Monoamine Oxidase Inhibitors (MAOIs)

MAOIs were discovered as part of research with isoniazid (INH), an anti-tubercular drug. The mechanism of antidepressant action of MAOIs involve increasing the concentrations of serotonin, norepinephrine, and dopamine in the neuronal synapse by inhibiting the MAO enzyme.

The MAOIs, for example phenelzine (Nardil), are rarely used today because of potential serious side effects and food and drug interactions. They cannot be given until two weeks after tricyclics and other interacting drugs have been discontinued. These agents are typically reserved for refractory or atypical depressions or those associated with panic disorder or phobias.

Side effects of MAO inhibitors are adrenergic in action and can include:

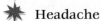 Nervousness, agitation, and insomnia

Headache

Stiff neck

Hypertension or hypertensive crisis (can be fatal)

Tachycardia, palpitation, and chest pain

Nausea, vomiting, and diarrhea

Blurred vision

Contraindications for MAOIs apply to:

Patients with cerebrovascular, heart, liver, and renal disease

Children under 16 yr

Pregnancy and lactation

Abrupt discontinuation

Interactions of the MAOIs with some drugs and foods can cause *hypertensive crisis,* manifested by severe headache, palpitation, sweating, chest pain, possible intracranial hemorrhage, and even death. Interactions may also occur with:

Adrenergic drugs, diuretics, insulin, and levodopa

Any antidepressant, resulting in seizures, fever, hypertension, and confusion

CNS depressants, resulting in circulatory collapse

Foods containing tryamine, tryptamine, or tryptophan, such as yogurt, sour cream, all cheeses, liver (especially chicken), pickled herring, figs, raisins, bananas, pineapple, avocados, broad beans (Chinese pea pods), meat tenderizers, *alcoholic beverages* (especially red wine and beer), and all fermented or aged foods (e.g., corned beef, salami, and pepperoni)

Selegilene (Eldepryl) is a selective MAOI (type-B) used as adjunctive treatment for Parkinson's disease (see Chapter 22, Anticonvulsants and Antiparkinsonian Drugs, for interactions and contraindications).

Selective Serotonin Reuptake Inhibitors (SSRIs)

SSRIs are considered to be the first-line medications for treatment of depression. They are preferred because of fewer side effects, greater safety in cases of overdose, and increased patient compliance.

The antidepressants in this category selectively block the reabsorption of the neurotransmitter serotonin, thus helping to restore the brain's chemical balance. Drugs in this class include fluoxetine (Prozac) and sertraline (Zoloft). Therapy may be required for several months or longer. Symptomatic relief may require one to four weeks and there is prolonged elimination of the drug. SSRIs do not have a significant effect of cognition in older adults.

Side effects of the SSRIs may include:

    Sexual dysfunction

    Nausea, anorexia

    Diarrhea, sweating

    Insomnia, anxiety, nervousness, tremor, drowsiness, fatigue, dizziness, headache

    Other side effects have been reported in less than 1% to 3% of patients receiving them.

Caution with SSRIs applies to patients with the following conditions:

    Liver or renal impairment

    Suicide prone

    Diabetes

    Bipolar disorders—may precipitate manic attacks

    Underweight, eating disorders

    Pregnancy, lactation

Recent studies in children with depression, especially at the beginning of treatment with SSRIs, appear to suggest an increased risk of suicidal thought and actions. There were no suicides in any of these studies. It is not clear whether the SSRIs contribute to the emergence of suicidal thinking and behavior, but patients should be observed closely for behaviors associated with these drugs (e.g., anxiety, agitation, panic attacks, insomnia, irritability, hostility, impulsivity, severe restlessness, hypomania, and mania). Physicians have been asked to be especially vigilant with patients who have bipolar disorder.

Interactions of SSRIs possible with:

    Other CNS drugs—lower doses of tricyclics may be needed; monitor for toxicity

    MAOIs—never take concurrently

    Antiarrhythmics, anticoagulants, beta-blockers, and calcium channel blockers

Another SSRI, different in structure but similar in action, enhancing serotonin and norepinephrine, is venlafaxine (Effexor).

Side effects and cautions for Effexor are similar to those of other SSRIs.

However, an increase in blood pressure, which could be dose related, is possible. Therefore, it is recommended that patients receiving venlafaxine have regular monitoring of blood pressure. Constipation and dry mouth are also possible.

Heterocyclic Antidepressants

The second-generation **heterocyclic** antidepressants are comparable in efficacy to the first-generation tricyclic antidepressants, but have differing effects on dopamine, norepinephrine, and serotonin, and distinctly different adverse effect profiles. Buproprion (Wellbutrin) is considered an *activating antidepressant* (like the SSRIs) and can be useful in cases of severe depression characterized by extreme fatigue, lethargy, and psychomotor retardation. It is also useful in helping to reduce relapse rates in persons who are quitting smoking (see Zyban in Chapter 26) and those patients who experience sexual dysfunction with other antidepressants.

Mirtazapine (Remeron) is a *calming antidepressant* that can be useful in treating agitated depression, mixed anxiety and depression, and fibromyalgia. A common side effect of mitrazapine is weight gain, which can be helpful in patients with a poor appetite. Trazodone (Desyrel) is highly sedating and is used in low doses as a hypnotic. It can be useful in higher doses in older adult patients for agitation secondary to dementia and to treat activation side effects caused by the SSRIs.

Side effects of heterocyclic antidepressants can include:

* Drowsiness—common (except buproprion)
* Insomnia, restlessness, agitation, anxiety (with buproprion)
* Dry mouth, nausea, dizziness, confusion
  Priapism or impotence—discontinue the drug (trazodone)
* Weight gain (mirtazapine, trazodone)

Interactions of heterocyclics with other CNS depressants, including alcohol, may potentiate sedation. Taking medication with food may decrease incidence of lightheadedness.

Caution with heterocyclics applies to:

Suicide prone

Seizure disorder

Cardiac or liver disorders

Interactions of heterocyclics possible with:

Other CNS drugs

Antidiabetic agents

MAOIs—never take concurrently

ANTIMANIC AGENTS
Lithium

Lithium salts are antimanic agents, not recommended for depression alone. **Bipolar disorders** (manic-depressive) are treated *long term* with lithium salts. A maintenance dose is established by monitoring blood levels. Serum levels are checked initially and every few months thereafter to maintain a level of 0.8–1.5 mEq/ml. Patients must be monitored and alerted for signs of toxicity.

Side effects of lithium can include:

* GI distress (usual initially and resolves)—take medicine with meals
* Cardiac arrhythmias and hypotension

Thirst and polyuria (dehydration may cause acute toxicity)

* Tremors—can be treated with propranolol

Thyroid problems

Signs of lithium toxicity can include:

* Drowsiness, confusion, blurred vision, and photophobia
* Tremors, muscle weakness, seizures, coma, and cardiovascular collapse

Caution with lithium must be used with:

Seizure disorders, Parkinsonism

Cardiovascular and kidney disorders

Older adults and debilitated patients

Thyroid disease

Interactions of lithium with CNS drugs, diuretics, nonsteroidal anti-inflammatory drugs (NSAIDs), angiotensin-converting enzyme (ACE) inhibitors, and sodium salts.

The anticonvulsants valproate (Depakote, Depakene) and carbamazepine (Tegretol) are also used for mood stabilization in bipolar illness (see Chapter 22, Anticonvulsants, for details on these drugs).

Symbyax, a combination of the atypical antipsychotic olanzapine and the SSRI fluoxetine, is the first FDA-approved combination product for the depressive phase of bipolar disorder. In addition, the atypical antipsychotics olanzapine, quetiapine, and risperidone are now approved to treat the manic phase of bipolar disorder. Refer to the discussion of these agents in this chapter for further details.

See Table 20-2 for a summary of antidepressants and antimanic agents.

Table 20-2 Antidepressants and Antimanic Agents

GENERIC NAME	TRADE NAME	DOSAGE	COMMENTS
Tricyclics			
amitriptyline	Elavil	PO 50–300 mg daily	All of these drugs interact with CNS drugs. Give at bedtime.
desipramine	Norpramin	PO 50–300 mg daily	Less sedation, anticholinergic S.E., and orthostatic hypotension
doxepin	Sinequan, Adapin	PO 50–300 mg daily	Also used topically for eczema
imipramine	Tofranil	PO 50–300 mg daily	Also effective for enuresis
nortriptyline	Aventyl, Pamelor	PO 25–150 mg daily	Older adults and adolescent patients need lower dose
MAOIs			
isocarboxazid	Marplan	PO 10–60 mg daily in div. doses	All of these drugs interact with many foods and other drugs, resulting in serious reactions
phenelzine	Nardil	PO 45–90 mg daily in div. doses	
tranylcypromine	Parnate	PO 20–60 mg daily in div. doses	
SSRIs			
citalopram	Celexa	PO 20–60 mg daily	Take A.M. or P.M. with or without food
escitalopram	Lexapro	PO 10–20 mg daily	May be better tolerated than Celexa
fluoxetine	Prozac	PO 10–80 mg daily	Delayed response, long half-life; take A.M.
paroxetine	Paxil	PO 10–60 mg daily	Older adults ½ dose; take in A.M.
	Paxil CR	PO 12.5–62.5 mg daily	Do not give with antacids
sertraline	Zoloft	PO 25–200 mg daily	Take in A.M.
venlafaxine	Effexor	PO 75–375 mg div. doses	Take PC to lessen nausea
	Effexor-XR	PO 37.5–225 mg daily	Do not chew or crush, swallow whole
Heterocyclics			
buproprion	Wellbutrin	PO 100–150 mg BID–TID	Take early in the day; space doses at
	Wellbutrin SR	PO 150–200 mg daily–BID	least 6 h apart to minimize seizure risk
	Wellbutrin XL	PO 150–400 mg	8 A.M.
mirtazapine	Remeron	PO 15–45 mg daily	Take at bedtime, sedation common
trazodone	Desyrel	PO 25–100 mg at bedtime for insomnia	Take PC to decrease dizziness and nausea; if drowsiness occurs, may
		PO 150–600 mg in div. doses for depression	give large portion of dose at bedtime
Antimanic Agents			
lithium	Lithobid, Eskalith	900–1,800 mg div. doses	0.8–1.5 mEq/ml (desired serum level)
carbamazepine	Tegretol	PO 600–1,600 mg in div. doses	4–12 mcg/ml (desired serum level)
valproate	Depakote, Depakene	PO 15–60 mg/kg/day (div. doses)	50–100 mcg/ml (desired serum level)
	Depakote ER	PO 250–1,000 mg/day	For migraine prophylaxis
olanzapine/fluoxetine	Symbyax	PO q P.M. (various strengths)	For bipolar depression

Note: All tricyclics have a delayed response and mild tranquilizing effect. SSRIs also have delayed response.

ANXIOLYTICS

Antianxiety medications (e.g., benzodiazepines) are sometimes referred to as **anxiolytics** or minor tranquilizers. They are useful for the *short-term* treatment of (1) anxiety disorders, (2) neurosis while making the patient amenable to psychotherapy, (3) some psychosomatic disorders and insomnia, and (4) nausea and vomiting. Benzodiazepines, such as Valium, are also used as muscle relaxants, anticonvulsants, or preoperatively. Anxiolytics, when given in small doses, can reduce anxiety and promote relaxation without causing sedation. Larger doses are sometimes prescribed at bedtime for their sedative effect. Minor tranquilizers should *not* be taken for prolonged periods of time because *tolerance, and physical and psychological dependence* may develop. *Sudden withdrawal after prolonged use may result in seizures, agitation, psychosis, insomnia, and gastric distress.*

Compounds with a long half-life, such as diazepam (Valium), should be avoided in older adults. Oxazepam (Serax), lorazepam (Ativan), and alprazolam (Xanax) have medium to short half-lives and inactive metabolites, and are less prone to accumulation in older adult patients or those with liver disease.

Side effects of the benzodiazepines may include:

- Depression, hallucinations, confusion, agitation, bizarre behavior, amnesia
- Drowsiness, lethargy, and headache
- **Ataxia,** tremor, and **extrapyramidal** reactions
- Rash and itching
- Sensitivity to sunlight

Contraindications or extreme caution with benzodiazepines applies to:

Mental depression

Suicidal tendencies

Depressed vital signs

Pregnancy, lactation, and children

Liver and kidney dysfunction

Older adults and debilitated patients (paradoxical reactions), prolonged elimination time

Persons operating machinery

Interactions of benzodiazepines with potentiation of effect may occur with:

CNS depressants (e.g., analgesics, anesthetics, sedative hypnotics, other muscle relaxants, antihistamines, and alcohol)

Digitalis and phenytoin

Grapefruit juice can potentiate the effects of diazepam (Valium) and should not be taken concurrently.

Midazolam (Versed) is a potent benzodiazepine. It is used preoperatively to relieve anxiety and provide sedation, light anesthesia, and amnesia of operative events. Because of its more rapid onset of sedative effects and more pronounced anxiolytic effects during the first hour following administration, it is considered the drug of choice for short surgical procedures. Midazolam is usually administered IM and the duration of amnesia is about one hour. It has also been used IV or orally for preoperative sedation and to relieve anxiety with good results.

Midazolam is also used IV for *conscious sedation* and relief for anxiety, either alone or in combination with an opioid, for example meperidine, for short-term procedures such as endoscopy, cardiac catheterization, or coronary angiography. Midazolam is also used IV for induction of general anesthesia, along with an opioid. This potent sedative requires individualized dosage with adjustment for age, weight, clinical condition, and procedure.

Side effects of midazolam (Versed) can include:

Depressed respiration with large doses, especially in older adults and those with COPD (chronic obstructive pulmonary disease)

Paradoxical reactions (agitation or involuntary movements) occur occasionally

Nausea and vomiting occasionally

Cautions with Versed:

Watch for apnea, hypoxia, and/or cardiac arrest

Respiratory status should be monitored continuously during parenteral use

Facilities and equipment for respiratory and cardiovascular support should be readily available

Vital signs should be monitored carefully for changes in blood pressure or decrease in heart rate

Patients with electrolyte imbalance, renal impairment, and congestive heart failure, and children are at increased risk of complications

Contraindicated in pregnancy and comatose patients and those with narrow-angle glaucoma

Interactions of Versed apply to:

CNS depressants, including alcohol, potentiate possibility of respiratory depression

Cimetidine (Tagamet) and ranitidine (Zantac) can potentiate respiratory depression

Erythromycin, ketoconazole, itraconazole, diltiazem, and verapamil can potentiate respiratory depression

Other anxiolytics, not related to the benzodiazepines, include buspirone (BuSpar). Unlike the benzodiazepines, it has no anticonvulsant or muscle relaxant activity, does not substantially impair psychomotor function, and has little sedative effect. Limited evidence suggests that buspirone may be more effective for cognitive and interpersonal problems, including anger and hostility associated with anxiety, whereas the benzodiazepines may be more effective for somatic symptoms of anxiety.

Buspirone has a slower onset of action than most anxiolytics (two to four weeks for optimum effect). Therefore, it is ineffective on a PRN basis. It has little potential for tolerance or dependence and has been used without unusual adverse effects or decreased efficiency for as long as a year.

Side effects of buspirone (fewer and less severe) may include:

Dizziness, drowsiness, and headache

GI effects (e.g, nausea)

Caution with buspirone applies to renal and hepatic impairment.

Another short-term anxiolytic, chemically different from the benzodiazepines, is hydroxyzine (Vistaril, Atarax).

Side effects of hydroxyzine may include:

Drowsiness, ataxia, dizziness

Urinary retention, mydriasis

Caution with hydroxyzine applies to:

GI, hepatic, and respiratory disorders

Closed angle glaucoma

See Table 20-3 for a summary of antianxiety medications.

Table 20-3 Antianxiety Medications (Anxiolytics)

GENERIC NAME	TRADE NAME	DOSAGE	COMMENTS
Benzodiazepines (short-term only)			
alprazolam	Xanax	PO 0.125–0.5 mg BID–TID	Abrupt withdrawal may cause severe side effects
	Xanax XR	PO 0.5–6 mg q A.M.	For panic disorder
chlordiazepoxide	Librium	PO 5–25 mg TID or 4×/day	Larger doses IV/IM with severe anxiety or ethanol withdrawal
chlorazepate	Tranxene	PO 15–60 mg daily div. doses 7.5–15 mg daily div. doses	For older adult patients no more than 15 mg daily
diazepam	Valium	PO 2–10 mg TID, IV	Do not mix in syringe with other medications, also used as muscle relaxant or IV in status epilepticus
lorazepam	Ativan	PO or IM 2–3 mg daily div. doses	For older adults who are agitated
oxazepam	Serax	PO 10–15 mg TID or 4×/day	For older adults who are agitated
Other Anxiolytics			
buspirone	Buspar	PO 15–60 mg daily div doses	Slow onset of action, may be used long term
hydroxyzine (antihistamine)	Atarax, Vistaril	PO 25–100 mg 4×/day or 25–100 mg deep IM	Antiemetic, antipruritic, or preoperative

ANTIPSYCHOTIC MEDICATIONS/MAJOR TRANQUILIZERS

Antipsychotic medications, or major tranquilizers, such as haloperidol (Haldol), are sometimes called *neuroleptics*. They are useful in three major areas:

> Relieving symptoms of psychoses or severe neuroses, including delusion, hallucinations, agitation, and combativeness

> Relieving nausea and vomiting; for example, prochlorperazine (Compazine) (see Chapter 16)

> Potentiation of analgesics; for example, promethazine (Phenergan)

Many of the typical antipsychotics are classified chemically as phenothiazines; for example, chlorpromazine (Thorazine). Dosage can be regulated to modify disturbed behavior and relieve severe anxiety in many cases without profound impairment of consciousness. These agents work by blocking dopamine receptors, resulting in unbalanced cholinergic activity, which causes frequent extrapyramidal side effects (EPS) and tardive dyskinesia (TD).

Another class of antipsychotics, the **atypical antipsychotics,** for example risperidone, are chemically different from the phenothiazines, blocking both serotonin and dopamine receptors. This mechanism results in less potential for adverse effects, especially EPS and TD.

Although helpful in treating behavioral and psychological symptoms of dementia, *atypicals* are not approved for the treatment of patients with dementia-related psychosis. Cerebrovascular adverse events (strokes, transient ischemic attacks, and cerebrovascular accidents), including fatalities, were reported in older adults with dementia (Alzheimer's, vascular and mixed) being treated with the atypical antipsychotics.

Side effects of all antipsychotics may include:

> Postural hypotension, tachycardia, bradycardia, and vertigo

> Insomnia, agitation, depression, headaches, seizures

> Dry mouth, blurred vision, and fever

> Jaundice, rash, photosensitivity or hypersensitivity reactions

> Confusion, drowsiness, restlessness, and weakness

> Constipation, urinary retention, and anorexia

> Agranulocytosis with clozapine

> Increased risk of hyperglycemia and diabetes with the atypicals

> Weight gain with clozapine and olanzapine

> Extrapyramidal reactions (EPS), severe CNS adverse effects, include:

> > • Parkinsonian symptoms, for example, tremors, drooling, dysphagia— more common in older adults

- **Tardive dyskinesia** (TD) (involuntary, and often irreversible, movements such as tics)—more common in older adults, especially females
- Dystonic reactions (spasms of the head, neck, or tongue)—more frequent in children
- Akathisia (motor restlessness)—more common in children

Note: Parkinsonian symptoms and tardive dyskinesia may become permanent and irreversible. Therefore, patients receiving antipsychotic agents should be assessed frequently for these conditions. Dosage should not be terminated abruptly in those receiving high doses for prolonged periods of time.

Treatment of parkinsonian symptoms includes concomitant administration of an anticholinergic antiparkinsonian agent; for example, Artane or Cogentin (see Chapter 22). *Prophylactic administration of these drugs will not prevent extrapyramidal symptoms. These drugs will not alleviate symptoms of TD and can make them worse.* Dystonic reactions usually appear early in therapy and usually subside rapidly when the antipsychotic drug is discontinued. Artane, Cogentin, or Benadryl are used to treat dystonic reactions. Patients receiving antipsychotic medication should be assessed for TD at the start of treatment and *at least* every six months with the Abnormal Involuntary Movement Scale (AIMS) (see Figure 20-1 and Figure 20-2) or Dyskinesia Identification System: Condensed User Scale (DISCUS) available from SANDOZ Pharmaceuticals Corporation.

Contraindications for antipsychotics include:

Seizure disorders

Parkinsonian syndrome

Cerebral vascular disease

Severe depression

Pregnancy

Blood dyscrasias

Caution with antipsychotics applies to older adults, children, hepatic, cardiovascular, renal disease, prostatic hypertrophy, and diabetes.

Interactions of the antipsychotics may include:

Potentiation with CNS depressants, anticholinergics, antihypertensives

Antagonism with anticonvulsants (seizure activity may increase)

See Table 20-4 for a summary of the antipsychotic medications. See Figure 20-3 for a summary of psychotropic drugs.

INSTRUCTIONS: Complete Examination Procedure (reverse side) before making ratings.

Code: 0 = None, 1 = Minimal, may be extreme normal, 2 = Mild, 3 = Moderate, 4 = Severe

FACIAL AND ORAL MOVEMENTS:	**1. Muscles of Facial Expression** e.g., movements of forehead, eyebrows, periorbital area, cheeks; include frowning, blinking, smiling, grimacing	(CIRCLE ONE) 0 1 2 3 4
	2. Lips and Perioral Areas e.g., puckering, pouting, smacking	0 1 2 3 4
	3. Jaw e.g., biting, clenching, mouth opening, lateral movement	0 1 2 3 4
	4. Tongue Rate only increase in movement both in and out of mouth, NOT inability to sustain movement	0 1 2 3 4
EXTREMITY MOVEMENTS:	**5. Upper (arms, wrists, hands, fingers)** Include choreic movements (i.e., rapid, objectively purposeless, irregular, spontaneous), athetoid movements (i.e., slow, irregular, complex, serpentine). Do NOT include tremor (i.e., repetitive, regular, rhythmic)	0 1 2 3 4
	6. Lower (legs, knees, ankles, toes) e.g., lateral knee movement, foot tapping, heel dropping, foot squirming, inversion and eversion of foot	0 1 2 3 4
TRUNK MOVEMENTS:	**7. Neck, shoulder, hips** e.g., rocking, twisting, squirming, pelvic gyrations	0 1 2 3 4
GLOBAL JUDGEMENTS:	**8. Severity of abnormal movements**	0 1 2 3 4
	9. Incapacitation due to abnormal movements	0 1 2 3 4
	10. Patient's awareness of abnormal movements Rate only patient's report	No awareness 0 Aware, no distress 1 Aware, mild distress 2 Aware, moderate distress 3 Aware, severe distress 4 No = 0 Yes = 1
DENTAL STATUS:	**11. Current problems with teeth and/or dentures**	No = 0 Yes = 1
	12. Does patient usually wear dentures?	

It is always preferable to perform the entire AIMS Examination. This establishes consistent testing conditions and allows test results to be compared. Nonambulatory residents may be observed informally for abnormal involuntary movements while in bed or in a wheelchair. Uncooperative residents should be observed during normal activities.

You must check one of these boxes: ☐ Full examination conducted and scored
☐ Scores from informal observations—Resident was:
☐ Not ambulatory—observed in   ☐ bed   ☐ wheelchair
☐ Not cooperative

RATER	DATE:	PATIENT	Resident #

Figure 20-1 Abnormal Involuntary Movement Scale (AIMS). This test, or a comparable one, is performed every three to six months with all patients receiving antipsychotic medication to identify any signs of tardive dyskinesia.

AIMS EXAMINATION PROCEDURE

Either before or after completing the examination procedure observe the patient unobtrusively, at rest (e.g., in waiting room).

The chair to be used in this examination should be a hard, firm one without arms.

1. Ask patient whether there is anything in his/her mouth (i.e., gum, candy, etc.) and if there is, to remove it.

2. Ask patient about the current condition of his/her teeth. Ask patient if he/she wears dentures. Do teeth or dentures bother patient now?

3. Ask patient whether he/she notices any movements in mouth, face, hands, or feet. If yes, ask to describe and to what extent they currently bother patient or interfere with his/her activities.

4. Have patient sit in chair with hands on knees, legs slightly apart, and feet flat on floor. (Look at entire body for movements while in this position.)

5. Ask patient to sit with hands hanging unsupported. If male, between legs, if female and wearing a dress, hanging over knees. (Observe hands and other body areas.)

6. Ask patient to open mouth. (Observe tongue at rest within mouth.) Do this twice.

7. Ask patient to protrude the tongue. (Observe abnormalities of tongue movement.)

♦ 8. Ask patient to tap thumb, with each finger, as rapidly as possible for 10–15 seconds; separately with right hand, then with left hand. (Observe facial and leg movements.)

9. Flex and extend patient's left and right arms (one at a time). (Note any rigidity and rate on DOTES.)

10. Ask patient to stand up. (Observe in profile. Observe all body areas again, hips included.)

♦ 11. Ask patient to extend both arms outstretched in front with palms down. (Observe trunk, legs, and mouth.)

♦ 12. Have patient walk a few paces, turn, and walk back to the chair. (Observe hands and gait.) Do this twice.

♦ Activated movement, some practitioners score these movements differently.

INTERPRETATION OF THE AIMS SCORE

- Individuals with no single score exceeding 1 are at very low risk of having a movement disorder.

- A score of 2 in only one of the seven body areas is borderline and the patient should be monitored closely.

- A patient with score of 2 in two or more of the seven body areas should be referred for a complete neurological examination.

- A score of 3 or 4 in only one body area warrants referring the patient for a complete neurological examination.

Figure 20-2 Abnormal Involuntary Movement Scale (AIMS). Examination procedure.

Table 20-4 Antipsychotic Medications/Major Tranquilizers

GENERIC NAME	TRADE NAME	DOSAGE[a]	COMMENTS
Typical (These drugs frequently cause EPS with long-term use. Monitor closely.)			
chlorpromazine	Thorazine	PO 200–800 mg daily, also R, deep IM, or IV	Primarily for agitation; also for nausea and vomiting and severe behavior problems
haloperidol[b]	Haldol	PO or IM 1–20 mg daily	For agitation, especially with schizophrenia and delusions in older adults
	Haldol decanoate IM	50–300 mg q 4 wk	
prochlorperazine	Compazine	PO, supp, IM, IV 5–10 mg PR 25 mg 3–4 ×/d BID	For agitation; primarily for nausea and vomiting in adults
thioridazine	Mellaril	PO 10–200 mg 4 ×/d	For psychoneurosis, agitation, or combativeness
trifluoperazine	Stelazine	PO 2–40 mg BID	Tranquilizer for psychotic disorders
thiothixene[b]	Navane	PO 2–10 mg BID	For chronic schizophrenic or behavioral management of withdrawn patients
fluphenzine HCl	Prolixin	PO 2.5–20 mg daily div. doses	For older adults, reduce dose to ½ or ¼
perphenazine	Trilafon	PO 8–64 mg daily div. doses	For psychosis, nausea, and vomiting in adults
Atypical			
aripiprazole	Abilify	PO 5–30 mg daily	For schizophrenia
clozapine	Clozaril	PO 12.5–900 mg (div. doses)	Monitor WBC, agranulocytosis risk
olanzapine	Zyprexa	PO 5–20 mg daily IM 10 mg (max. dose 30 mg/day)	Reduce dose by ½ for older adults For acute agitation
quetiapine	Seroquel	PO 50–750 mg daily (div. doses)	Monitor for orthostatic hypotension
risperidone	Risperdal	PO 1–4 mg BID	Reduce dose by ½ for older adults
	Risperdal Consta	IM 25–50 mg q2wk	For schizophrenia
ziprasidone	Geodon	PO 20–80 mg BID IM 10–20 mg q2–4h (max. dose 40 mg/day)	Greater risk of cardiac disorders For acute psychosis/agitation

[a]Varies with condition (divided doses).

[b]These drugs are not phenothiazines. All of the other typical drugs listed are phenothiazines.

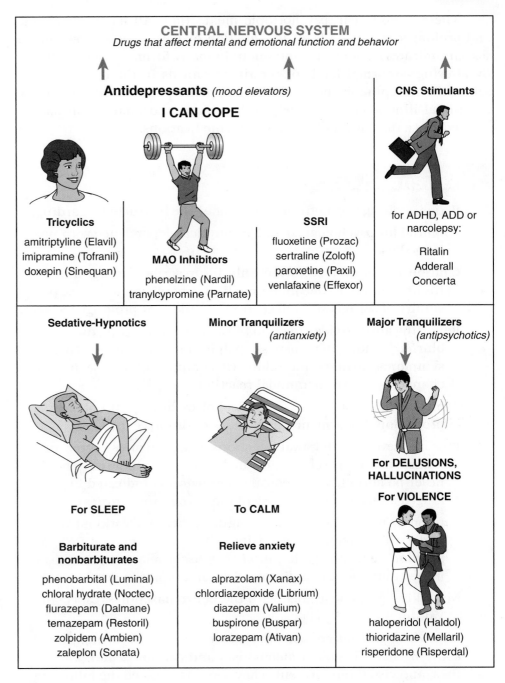

Figure 20-3 Summary of psychotropic drugs.

There is no "ideal" psychotropic medication. All have side effects, and prolonged use often leads to addiction or habituation. However, research indicates a chemical component in many forms of mental illness. By altering abnormal levels of certain chemicals in the brain, such as serotonin, norepinephrine, or dopamine, many patients with mental or emotional illness have been helped. Psychiatric hospitalization has decreased since the advent of psychotropic medications.

Patient Education

Patients taking psychotropic drugs should be instructed regarding:

Potential for psychological and/or physical dependence with prolonged use

Caution in taking medication only in prescribed dosage and for limited period of time under medical supervision to reduce possibility of serious side effects from overdose or prolonged use

Reporting adverse side effects to physician at once (e.g., dizziness, blurred vision, nervousness, palpitations and other cardiac symptoms, urinary retention, GI symptoms, adverse mental changes, and extrapyramidal reactions)

Avoiding chemical abuse (e.g., alcohol or drugs) and obtaining professional treatment when these conditions exist

Possible severe withdrawal reactions (e.g., seizures) after prolonged use of psychotropic medications (withdrawal should never be abrupt, and medical supervision is indicated for prolonged administration of any of the psychotropic drugs)

Caution with interactions; *not* taking any other medications (except under close medical supervision) that can potentiate CNS depression (e.g., analgesics, *alcohol,* muscle relaxants, antihistamines, antiemetics, cardiac medications, or antihypertensives)

Not taking grapefruit juice with the benzodiazepines, especially Valium

Older adult patients are more at risk for the side effects mentioned above because of slowed metabolism and cardiovascular, kidney, liver, and visual impairment. They should be issued the following cautions:

Rise slowly because of potential for hypotension.

Avoid operating machinery or driving while taking these drugs. Report to the physician immediately any side effects, especially dizziness, confusion, sleep disturbances, or weakness.

Avoid taking any OTC drugs or alcohol.

Tell the prescribing physician about all other medicines you are taking, including eyedrops.

ALCOHOL

Alcohol (ethyl alcohol, ethanol) can be classified as a psychotropic drug and a CNS depressant. It is the number one drug problem in the United States, accounting for 100,000 deaths per year and is directly responsible for more than half of traffic accidents (30% of all U.S. traffic fatalities).

Alcohol is a fast-acting depressant, pharmacologically similar to ether. The body reacts to alcohol with excitement, sedation, and finally anesthesia. Large amounts of alcohol can result in alcoholic stupor, cerebral edema, and depressed respiration.

Alcohol is rapidly absorbed from the GI tract into the bloodstream. Alcohol depresses primitive areas of the cortex first and then decreases control over judgment, memory, and other intellectual and emotional functioning. Within a few hours, motor areas are affected, producing unsteady gait, slurred speech, and incoordination. Prolonged use can cause permanent CNS damage and result in peripheral neuritis, convulsive disorders, Wernicke's syndrome, and Korsakoff's psychosis with mental deterioration, memory loss, and ataxia.

Prolonged alcohol use affects almost all organs of the body. Chronic drinking causes liver damage and pancreatitis. Alcohol irritates the mucosa of the digestive system, leading to possible esophageal varices, gastritis, ulceration, and hemorrhage. Alcohol can also lead to malabsorption of nutrients and malnutrition.

Cardiovascular effects include peripheral vasodilation (producing the flushing and sweating seen with intoxication) and vasoconstriction of the coronary arteries. Alcohol increases the heart rate and, with chronic use, can cause cardiac myopathy, either directly or through metabolic and electrolyte imbalances. Potassium deficiency can cause cardiac arrhythmias.

Recent studies have shown an inverse association between consumption of wine and coronary heart disease. In another study, it was determined that consumption of one or two drinks per day (five to six days each week) resulted in a substantially reduced risk of MI compared with nondrinkers. All this must be tempered with the deleterious effects of alcohol and the potential for abuse.

Alcohol Poisoning

Symptoms of acute alcoholic poisoning include cold, clammy skin; stupor; slow, noisy respirations; and alcoholic breath.

Mortality associated with acute alcohol poisoning alone is uncommon, but can be an important factor when mixed with recreational drugs.

Treatment includes close observation for:

Respiratory problems. Establish and maintain airway.

Vomiting. Gastric lavage if indicated.

Convulsions. Phenytoin sometimes given prophylactically to decrease seizure activity.

Cerebral edema. Diuretics sometimes required (e.g., mannitol).

Electrolyte imbalance. IV fluids with thiamine, folic, and vitamins added.

Delirium tremens. Chlordiazepoxide (Librium) sometimes given.

Fetal alcohol syndrome (FAS) is a teratogenic effect of ethanol. As few as two drinks early in pregnancy has been associated with FAS, although more commonly seen in infants whose mothers consumed four or five drinks per day.

Chronic Alcoholism

Symptoms of chronic alcoholism include:

Frequent falls and accidents

Blackouts and memory loss

Dulling of mental faculties

Neuritis and muscular weakness

Irritability

Tremors

Conjunctivitis

Gastroenteritis

Neglect of personal appearance and responsibilities

Treatment of chronic alcoholism can include an intensive in-house rehabilitation program in a special facility for a period of 28 days. Treatment frequently includes:

Vitamin B (thiamine) IM or PO, multiple vitamins, and folic acid

Low-carbohydrate and high-protein diet to combat hypoglycemia

Elimination of caffeine (in coffee, tea, chocolate, and soft drinks)

Reeducation of the patient, with intensive individual, group, and family counseling, including Alcoholics Anonymous techniques

Sometimes disulfiram (Antabuse) is used, with patient cooperation, as part of *behavior modification.* Patients receive daily doses of disulfiram and are taught to expect a very unpleasant reaction if even a small amount of alcohol is ingested. There is some evidence that drinking frequency is reduced, but minimal evidence that it facilitates abstinence. This treatment is used less frequently because of severe reaction potential and poor compliance.

Disulfiram-alcohol reactions can include:

Flushing and throbbing headache

Nausea and vomiting

Sweating and dyspnea

Palpitation, tachycardia, and hypotension

Vertigo and blurred vision

Anxiety and confusion

Patient Education

Patients taking disulfiram should be instructed regarding:

Avoidance of cough syrups, sauces, vinegars, elixirs, and other preparations containing alcohol

Caution with external applications of liniments, lotions, after-shave, or perfume

Signs of disulfiram-alcohol reaction

Reporting to emergency facility if effects do not subside or with severe reaction

Carrying identification card noting therapy

Avoiding other medications that may interact with disulfiram (e.g., anticoagulants and phenytoin)

Another treatment for alcoholism includes the use of daily maintenance doses of naltrexone (ReVia), as part of counseling programs, to *keep* alcoholics sober after detoxification. Naltrexone acts by blocking the pleasurable sensations associated with alcohol, and therefore lessens the desire or craving to drink. Naltrexone reduces the frequency and risk of heavy drinking, but does not necessarily enhance abstinence.

Naltrexone is also used in treatment programs for opiate addicts (e.g., heroin and morphine). *After* withdrawal from the drugs, it helps to prevent relapses. It acts by robbing the drugs of their pleasurable effects.

Caution: If naltrexone is given to someone currently dependent on opiates, it can send the addict *instantly into severe, life-threatening* withdrawal.

Side effects of naltrexone are usually minor and include:

Nausea and joint pains

Liver damage can occur with doses larger than recommended dose of 50 mg daily

Contraindications for use of naltrexone include:

Patients with acute/chronic hepatitis and liver failure

More recent research has identified a drug that has proven more effective than other drugs for reducing or eliminating problematic alcohol consumption. Topiramate (Topamax) is an anticonvulsant typically used to treat partial seizures. Topamax can be taken while still drinking alcohol and acts by eliminating excess dopamine released by drinking alcohol. (See Chapter 22, Anticonvulsants for dosage.)

DRUG ABUSE

Drug abuse can be defined as the use of a drug for other than therapeutic purposes. Drug **addiction** is a common problem, (9.4% of the U.S.

population) and consists of the combination of all four of the following side effects: tolerance, psychological dependence, physical dependence, and withdrawal reaction with physiological effects. *Habituation* consists of psychological dependence only. **Chemical dependency** is the term in common usage today to describe a condition in which alcohol or drugs have taken control of an individual's life and affect normal functioning.

Health care workers have ready access to many prescription drugs and, therefore, sometimes become involved in illegal misuse of psychotropic drugs. Prescription drugs most often abused by medical personnel are hydrocodone, oxycodone, and the benzodiazepines. Counteractive measures include accurate record keeping of all controlled substances and recognition of the side effects and symptoms associated with drug abuse. (See Chapter 19 for discussion of narcotic analgesics and discussion earlier in this chapter of the anxiolytics.) Report suspected abuse to the person in authority.

This section describes four types of drugs that can be produced illegally: marijuana, cocaine, the hallucinogens (LSD and PCP), and the amphetamines.

Amphetamines

While amphetamines can be produced and prescribed legally, they are also produced in illegal labs. Two examples are methamphetamine ("crystal," "crank," "meth," "speed") and methylenedioxymethamphetamine (MDMA, "Ecstasy"). At normal dosage levels, administration of an amphetamine may produce tolerance within a few weeks. However, in hypersensitive individuals, psychotic syndrome may occur within 36–48 h of a single large dose of amphetamine. Some emotionally unstable individuals come to depend on the pleasant mental stimulation the drugs offer.

Symptoms of chronic abuse of amphetamines include:

 Emotional lability, irritability

Anorexia

 Mental impairment, confusion, amnesia, neurotoxicity

Occupational deterioration, social withdrawal

Continuous chewing or teeth grinding resulting in trauma or ulcers of the tongue and lip

Photophobia—frequently wearing sunglasses indoors

Paranoid syndrome with hallucinations with prolonged use of high doses

Tooth decay ("meth mouth")

Symptoms of acute toxicity from amphetamines can include:

 Strokes, cardiovascular symptoms including flushing or pallor, palpitation, tachypnea, tremor, extreme fluctuations of pulse and blood pressure, cardiac arrhythmias, chest pain, circulatory collapse

Dilated pupils, diaphoresis, and hyperpyrexia

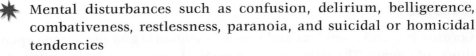

✴ Mental disturbances such as confusion, delirium, belligerence, combativeness, restlessness, paranoia, and suicidal or homicidal tendencies

✴ Fatigue and depression usually follow CNS stimulation

Treatment: There is no specific antidote for amphetamine overdosage. Treatment of overdose is symptomatic and includes administration of sedative drugs and a cathartic, and isolation of the patient to avoid possible external stimuli. General physiological supportive measures include treatment for shock or cardiac irregularities as appropriate. Emesis or gastric lavage and administration of activated charcoal may help if applied soon enough. Hypothermic measures or drugs to reduce intracranial pressure may be employed if appropriate.

Abrupt withdrawal of amphetamines may unmask mental problems. Therefore, patients require careful supervision during withdrawal and long-term follow-up may be required since some manifestations (e.g., depression) may persist for prolonged periods.

Marijuana

Tetrahydrocannabinol (THC) is the active ingredient in marijuana. Although classified technically as a CNS depressant, it also possesses properties of a euphoriant, sedative, and hallucinogen. Marijuana is currently under investigation as a possible treatment for glaucoma. Marinol (dronabinol—a synthetic form of THC) is approved for prevention of chemotherapy-induced nausea and vomiting, and is also used as an appetite stimulant in cachexia associated with AIDS or cancer.

The *Cannabis* plant grows over the entire world, especially in tropical areas. Potency varies considerably from place to place and time to time.

THC, the active ingredient released when marijuana is smoked, is fat-soluble and is stored in many fat cells, especially in the brain and reproductive organs. THC metabolizes slowly. A week after a person smokes one marijuana cigarette, 30%–50% of the THC remains in the body, and four to six weeks are required to eliminate all of the THC.

Side effects of marijuana include:

✴ Short-term memory loss, impaired learning, and slowed intellectual performance

✴ Perceptual inaccuracies, impaired reflex reaction (dangerous with driving)

✴ Apathy, lethargy, and decreased motivation

Increased heart rate

Lung irritation and chronic cough

Reduced testosterone level and sperm count

Reduced estrogen level, crossing of placental barrier, and transmission through mother's milk; miscarriage and stillbirth possible

✴ Delayed development of coping mechanisms in children and adolescents

Cocaine

Cocaine is a CNS stimulant and produces euphoria and increased expenditure of energy. The only approved medical use is as a local anesthetic, usually for nasal procedures, *applied topically only*.

Cocaine is highly addictive, causing dependence after even short-time use. It is abused by intranasal application (sniffing or snorting), intravenous injection, or by inhalation (smoking "crack"). Nasal application can damage mucous membranes and/or the nasal septum. The effects of intravenous use are extremely rapid and dangerous and can be fatal. Smoking causes the most rapid addiction, sometimes after only one use. Cocaine crosses the placental barrier and has resulted in babies who are irritable, jittery, anorexic, and seizure prone. Cocaine use has caused numerous crimes and deaths. Severe depression can be associated with withdrawal, which is a lengthy and difficult process.

Side effects of cocaine, which are serious, include:

 Euphoria, agitation, and excitation

Hypertension, tachycardia, cardiac arrhythmias, or cardiac failure

Anorexia, nausea, and vomiting

Tremor and seizures

Hallucinations, possible psychosis, and possible violent behavior

Possible death from circulatory collapse

Perforated nasal septum from prolonged nasal use

Hallucinogens

Lysergic acid (LSD) and phencyclidine (PCP), an animal tranquilizer, are hallucinogens. They produce bizarre mental reactions and distortion of physical senses. Hallucinations and delusions are common with confused perceptions of time and space (e.g., the user can walk out of windows because of the impression that he or she can fly). PCP is also an amnesic.

Side effects of hallucinogens include:

 Increased pulse and heart rate and rise in blood pressure and temperature

Possible "flashbacks" months later

Panic or paranoia (lack of control)

 Possible psychotic episodes

Possible physical injury to self or others

An illegal drug of a different type, flunitrazepam (Rohypnol), is a potent benzodiazepine that is approved for use in Central and South America for ethanol withdrawal. Not approved in the United States, it is being used here as a recreational drug (sometimes snorted to offset cocaine withdrawal) and is known on the street as "roofies." It has also acquired the title "date-rape drug" due to its ability to induce amnesia, preventing the victim from recalling specific events while under the influence of the drug.

The Role of the Medical Personnel

The role of the medical personnel in combating drug abuse includes:

Thorough knowledge of psychotropic drugs, action, and side effects

Willingness to participate in education of the patient, the patient's family, and others in the community

Giving competent care to those under the influence of drugs in a nonjudgmental way

Recognizing drug abuse and making appropriate referrals *without exception*

Complete and accurate record keeping of controlled stocks of drugs that could be considered potential drugs of abuse

It is the responsibility of all medical personnel not only to recognize drug abuse, but also to report any observed drug abuse to the *proper person in authority*. To look the other way not only enables the individual to continue to harm himself or herself but also endangers those in his or her care.

There are many services available to help medical personnel deal with drug abuse problems. Check with your state licensing agency or certification board for information about programs in your area, such as the Impaired Nurse program. Local mental health clinics or psychiatric facilities can also provide assistance and information. Other agencies that can provide information include:

Department of Health and Human Services
Public Health Service
Alcohol, Drug Abuse, and Mental Health Administration
Washington, DC 20402

National Clearinghouse for Drug Abuse Information
P.O. Box 1706
Rockville, MD 20850

WORKSHEET 1 FOR CHAPTER 20
PSYCHOTROPICS

Note the drugs listed according to category and complete all columns. Learn generic or trade names as specified by instructor. Fill in the first column with names of other drugs common in your area.

Classifications and Drugs	Purpose	Side Effects	Contraindications or Cautions	Patient Education
CNS Stimulants 1. Adderall 2. Ritalin				
Tricyclics 1. Elavil 2. Tofranil 3. Sinequan				
MAOIs 1. Marplan 2. Nardil				
SSRIs 1. sertraline (Zoloft) 2. fluoxetine (Prozac) 3. paroxetine (Paxil) 4. venlafaxine (Effexor)				
Heterocyclics 1. Wellbutrin 2. Remeron 3. Desyrel				

Classifications and Drugs	Purpose	Side Effects	Contraindications or Cautions	Patient Education
Antimanic 1. Lithium				
Antianxiety Medications 1. Ativan 2. Valium 3. Xanax				
Antipsychotic Medications 1. Thorazine 2. Haldol 3. Mellaril 4. Risperdal 5. Zyprexa				

WORKSHEET 2 FOR CHAPTER 20
DRUG ABUSE

Complete the columns.

Drugs	Side Effects and Signs of Abuse
Amphetamines	
Marijuana	
Cocaine	
Hallucinogens	

A. Case Study for Psychotropic Medications

Miss Blue, a 25-year-old secretary, presents in the physician's office with a history of depression for one month. She complains of crying frequently, loss of appetite, and insomnia. The physician prescribes Tofranil. The patient should be given the following information:

1. She should expect to feel better
- a. In a few days
- b. In a few weeks
- c. One hour after taking medicine
- d. One day after taking medicine

2. The medicine should be taken
- a. Before meals
- b. With meals
- c. In the morning
- d. At bedtime

3. She can expect all of the following side effects EXCEPT
- a. Increased appetite
- b. Improved sleep
- c. Weight loss
- d. Dry mouth

4. She should be told to report any of the following side effects EXCEPT
- a. Dizziness
- b. Palpitations
- c. Blurred vision
- d. Increased thirst

B. Case Study for Psychotropic Medication

Mr. Elzware, a 90-year-old nursing home resident with Alzheimer's, Parkinson's, and enlarged prostate, has been pacing the hall talking loudly in a confused way. He is wringing his hands. The nurse calls the physician's office and requests Haldol "to calm him down." Both the nurse in the nursing home and the medical assistant in the physician's office should be aware of the following facts about Haldol:

1. Haldol is only an appropriate medication for which condition listed below?
- a. Nervousness
- b. Confusion
- c. Uncooperativeness
- d. Combativeness

2. Haldol is appropriate in which of the following conditions?
- a. Seizure disorder
- b. Parkinson's disease
- c. Prostatic hypertrophy
- d. Paranoid psychosis
- e. Depression

3. Agitation can be caused by all of the following EXCEPT
- a. Pain
- b. Constipation
- c. Senility
- d. Urinary retention

4. Geriatric patients receiving antipsychotic medication are at increased risk of having extrapyramidal reactions including all of the following EXCEPT
- a. Dystonia
- b. Diaphoresis
- c. Tardive dyskinesia
- d. Parkinsonian syndrome

5. The following statements are true of tardive dykinesia EXCEPT
- a. Can be permanent
- b. Cured with medicine
- c. Assessed with AIMS test
- d. Manifested by tics

6. Side effects of antipsychotics, like Haldol, can include all of the following EXCEPT
- a. Depression
- b. Weakness
- c. Blurred vision
- d. Increased appetite

CHAPTER REVIEW QUIZ

Match the medication in the first column with the classification in the second column. Classifications may be used more than once.

Medication

Classification

1. _____ Xanax   **A.** Antipsychotic

2. _____ Lithium   **B.** Anxiolytic

3. _____ Risperdal   **C.** Antidepressant

4. _____ Elavil   **D.** CNS stimulant

5. _____ Prozac   **E.** Antimanic

6. _____ Adderall

7. _____ Buspar

8. _____ Zyprexa

9. _____ Ativan

10. _____ Wellbutrin

Choose the correct answer.

11. Ritalin and Adderall, prescribed for ADHD, can cause all of the following EXCEPT:
    a. Motor tics   c. Headache
    b. Growth spurt   d. Anorexia

12. Modafinil (Provigil) is approved for the following conditions EXCEPT:
    a. Sleep disorders   c. Obesity
    b. Narcolepsy   d. Sleep apnea

13. SSRIs, for example Zoloft and Effexor, can have the following side effects EXCEPT:
    a. Sexual dysfunction c. Diarrhea
    b. Weight gain   d. Dizziness

14. Remeron would be used to treat patients with the following conditions EXCEPT:
    a. Depression   c. Anxiety
    b. Bipolar disorder   d. Agitation

15. Signs of lithium toxicity could include all of the following EXCEPT:
    a. Hypertension   c. Tremors
    b. Blurred vision   d. Confusion

16. Benzodiazepines, for example Xanax, used long term, can cause the following side effects EXCEPT:
    a. Photosensitivity   c. Depression
    b. Tachycardia   d. Confusion

17. Which of the following statements is NOT true of tardive dyskinesia caused by antipsychotics?

a. Can be permanent

b. AIMS test detects

c. More in females

d. Artane treats

18. Chronic alcoholism can result in all of the following EXCEPT:

a. Memory loss

b. Esophageal varices

c. Bradycardia

d. Neuritis

19. Chronic amphetamine abuse can cause all of the following EXCEPT:

a. Cardiac irregularities

b. Increased appetite

c. Photophobia

d. Psychosis

20. Side effects of frequent marijuana use can include all of the following EXCEPT:

a. Reduced testosterone

b. Slowed reflexes

c. Memory loss

d. Irritability

Chapter 21
Musculoskeletal and Anti-inflammatory Drugs

Objectives

Upon completion of this chapter, the learner should be able to

1. Define the Key Terms

2. Identify commonly used skeletal muscle relaxants

3. Describe the side effects to be expected with muscle relaxants

4. List the drugs that can interact with the muscle relaxants and cause serious potentiation of effect

5. Differentiate among the anti-inflammatory drugs, antirheumatic drugs, and drugs used to treat acute episodes of gout

6. Explain the serious side effects of NSAIDs

7. List drug interactions with NSAIDs

8. Explain appropriate patient education for those taking skeletal muscle relaxants and NSAIDs

9. Describe the new medications for osteoporosis therapy

10. Compare and contrast COX-2 inhibitors and other NSAIDs

Key Terms

Anti-inflammatory

COX-2 inhibitors

Gout

Hormone replacement therapy

NSAIDs

Osteoporosis therapy

Skeletal muscle relaxants

Disorders of the musculoskeletal system are rather common. Drugs used to treat such conditions may be classified in two broad categories: skeletal muscle relaxants and nonsteroidal anti-inflammatory drugs (NSAIDs). Corticosteroid therapy for inflammatory conditions is discussed in Chapter 23.

SKELETAL MUSCLE RELAXANTS

Some disorders of the musculoskeletal system can be attributed to structural defects (e.g., ruptured disks) that may require surgical intervention rather than medication. However, many disorders associated with pain, spasm, abnormal contraction, or impaired mobility do respond to medications classified as **skeletal muscle relaxants.** Acute, painful musculoskeletal conditions, such as backache or neck strain, are treated with a combination of muscle relaxants, rest, physical therapy (e.g., hot or cold packs), and mild analgesics (e.g. nonsteroidal anti-inflammatory drugs [NSAIDs]). Muscle relaxants are given only on a short-term basis, and, after the acute pain subsides, exercises are usually prescribed by the physician to strengthen the weak muscles.

Most muscle relaxant drugs affect the spinal cord and brain, with no direct effect on skeletal muscle. The resulting action reduces muscle spasm, causes alterations in the perception of pain, and produces a sedative effect, promoting rest and relaxation of the affected part. Drugs used to treat acute, painful musculoskeletal conditions include diazepam (Valium) and methocarbamol (Robaxin).

A different type of muscle relaxant, dantrolene, causes a direct effect on skeletal muscles and is used in the management of spasticity resulting from upper motor neuron disorders such as multiple sclerosis or cerebral palsy. This medication is ineffective for amyotrophic lateral sclerosis and is not indicated for the treatment of muscle spasms resulting from rheumatic disorders or musculoskeletal trauma.

Another type of muscle relaxant includes *neuromuscular blocking agents (NMBAs)* such as succinylcholine or tubocurarine, used during surgical, endoscopic, or orthopedic procedures. These drugs are potentially very dangerous and can result in respiratory arrest. Neuromuscular blocking agents are administered only by anesthesiologists or specially trained personnel skilled in intubation and cardiopulmonary resuscitation.

NMBAs must be used with caution because of possible serious central nervous system (CNS) problems, such as respiratory arrest and allergic reactions. Antidotes such as neostigmine (Prostigmin) or edrophonium (Tensilon) may be indicated. Prostigmin may also be used in the treatment of myasthenia gravis and Tensilon in the diagnosis of myasthenia gravis. See Chapter 13 for discussion of cholinergic drugs.

Side effects of skeletal muscle relaxants can include:

* Drowsiness, dizziness, or dry mouth
* Weakness, tremor, ataxia
  Headache
* Confusion and nervousness
  Slurred speech
  Blurred vision
* Hypotension
  Gastrointestinal (GI) symptoms, including nausea, vomiting, diarrhea, or constipation
  Urinary problems, including enuresis, frequency, or retention
* Hypersensitivity reactions including liver toxicity with dantrolene and tizanidine
* Respiratory depression

Contraindications with skeletal muscle relaxants and:

Muscular dystrophy

Myasthenia gravis

Pregnancy or lactation

Children under 12 years old

Caution with skeletal muscle relaxants and:

History of drug abuse

Impaired kidney function

Liver disorders

Blood dyscrasias

Chronic obstructive pulmonary disease (COPD)

Cardiac disorders

Older adults

Abrupt discontinuation

Closed-angle glaucoma

Interactions with potentiation of effect with skeletal muscle relaxants and:

Alcohol

Analgesics

Psychotropic medications

Antihistamines

Patient Education

Patients taking skeletal muscle relaxants should be instructed regarding:

Potential side effects (e.g., drowsiness, dizziness, weakness, tremor, blurred vision, hypotension, respiratory distress, or GI disorders); care with driving

Avoidance of other CNS depressants at the same time (e.g., tranquilizers, antihistamines, or alcohol), which can cause serious CNS depression, and care with analgesics, only as prescribed by a physician

Importance of following the physician's orders regarding rest and physical therapy (e.g., heat and firm mattress or bed board with back problems) and exercises as prescribed (after the acute pain subsides) to strengthen the weak muscles

The acronym RICE (rest, ice, compression [elastic bandage], elevation) represents appropriate care for musculoskeletal injuries to extremities

Taking the medication only as long as absolutely necessary and observing caution regarding prolonged use, which could lead to physical or psychological dependence and withdrawal symptoms (e.g., seizures from Valium withdrawal after prolonged use)

See Table 21-1 for a summary of the skeletal muscle relaxants.

Table 21-1 Skeletal Muscle Relaxants

GENERIC NAME	TRADE NAME	DOSAGE	COMMENTS
carisoprodol	Soma	PO 350 mg 3–4 ×/day	Caution with asthma; watch for abuse potential
cyclobenzaprine	Flexeril	PO 15–30 mg/day in div. doses	For acute painful musculoskeletal conditions
diazepam	Valium	2–10 mg PO 3–4 ×/day IM/IV 5–10 mg q3–4h	Abrupt withdrawal after prolonged use may cause seizures
methocarbamol	Robaxin	4–8 g PO daily div. doses also IM, IV	For acute painful musculoskeletal conditions
dantrolene	Dantrium	PO 25–100 mg 2–4 ×/day	For multiple sclerosis and cerebral palsy, not for trauma or rheumatic disorders
baclofen	Lioresal	PO 10–20 mg 3–4 ×/day intrathecal 300–800 mcg	May be of some value with spinal cord injury or spinal cord diseases
tizanidine	Zanaflex	PO 2–8 mg 1–3 ×/day (6–8 h intervals)	For increased muscle tone associated w/spasticity, e.g., multiple sclerosis or spinal cord trauma

Note: Representative sample; other products are available.

ANTI-INFLAMMATORY DRUGS

Anti-inflammatory drugs are used to treat disorders in which the musculoskeletal system is not functioning properly due to inflammation. Such conditions as arthritis, bursitis, spondylitis, gout, and muscle strains and sprains can cause swelling, redness, heat, pain, and limited mobility. Analgesics and corticosteroids are used at times for acute stages of these disorders and are discussed in Chapters 19 and 23. The corticosteroids are not used for extended periods of time because of serious side effects. However, nonsteroidal anti-inflammatory drugs (NSAIDs) are frequently given for lengthy time periods in maintenance doses as low as possible for effectiveness.

Nonsteroidal Anti-inflammatory Drugs

NSAIDs inhibit synthesis of prostaglandins, substances responsible for producing much of the inflammation and pain of rheumatic conditions, sprains, and menstrual cramps. No cure has been found for rheumatic disorders, but many medications are used to alleviate the pain and crippling effects. Because of lower metabolic rates and other complications, older adults are particularly susceptible to side effects from NSAIDs (e.g., "silent bleeding") and should be cautioned to report any untoward signs or symptoms to their doctor without delay.

The salicylates (e.g., aspirin) are the oldest drug in this category with analgesic, anti-inflammatory, and antipyretic effects. (See Chapter 19.) Many nonsalicylate NSAIDs are on the market, and some are tolerated better than aspirin by some patients, especially as *short-term* analgesics. However, with large doses and/or long term, they all share many of the same side effects and interactions to a greater or lesser degree. Patients on prolonged therapy with any of the NSAIDs should be monitored carefully. Older adults or debilitated patients do not tolerate ulceration or bleeding (which can be "silent") as well as other individuals, and most reports of fatal GI events are in these populations. If chronic anti-inflammatory therapy must be continued despite ulceration, the patient should be switched to a *partially selective* NSAID (e.g., etodolac, meloxicam, or nambutone) or a *selective* COX-2 inhibitor (see later discussion). When the NSAID must be continued, drugs can be added to inhibit gastric acid. Combination products are available, for example Arthrotec, which combines diclofenac (Voltaren) with Cytotec to protect the gastric mucosa, or Prevacid NapraPAC, which combines naproxen with lansoprazole (Prevacid). (See Chapter 16, Treatment of Ulcers.)

The FDA has issued a warning regarding over-the-counter (OTC) nonselective NSAIDs: They should be used in strict accordance with label directions. If an OTC NSAID is needed for longer than ten days, a physician should be consulted.

COX-2 Inhibitor

Celecoxib (Celebrex) is a nonsteroidal anti-inflammatory drug (NSAID) that exhibits anti-inflammatory, analgesic, and antipyretic activities by *selectively* inhibiting cyclooxygenase-2 (COX-2) prostaglandin synthesis. However, it does *not* inhibit COX-1 and, therefore, does *not* inhibit platelet aggregation (clotting). Consequently, it does not pose the bleeding risks of the other *nonselective* NSAIDs described previously. Due to the specific action inhibiting COX-2 prostaglandin synthesis, Celebrex has the potential to cause fewer gastric problems and pose less risk of GI bleeding.

The selective **COX-2 inhibitor** rofecoxib (Vioxx) was voluntarily withdrawn from the market in 2004 after it was revealed that subjects receiving Vioxx had roughly twice the rate of myocardial infarction and stroke when compared with those receiving placebo. There is concern that this adverse effect may also apply to Celebrex, and warnings are in place.

Subsequently, Bextra, another COX-2 inhibitor, which sometimes caused severe, even fatal, skin reactions, was also taken from the market.

Earlier studies have suggested that there is a "good" and a "bad" prostaglandin as far as the heart is concerned. Suppressing both types in the way nonselective NSAIDs do actually helps the heart. The selective COX-2s shut down only the "good" prostaglandin, raising the risk of high blood pressure, atherosclerosis, and clotting. Until studies defining the cardiovascular safety of the remaining COX-2 agent (Celebrex) are complete, the *benefits and risks* of this agent in terms of pain relief and cardiovascular and GI safety must be weighed carefully for each individual.

The FDA has posted extensive NSAID medication information at http://www.fda.gov/cder/drug/analgesics/default.htm. The health care worker has the responsibility to stay informed of the latest developments in this area.

Side effects of *non-selective* NSAIDs frequently include:

 GI ulceration and bleeding—may not be preceded by warning signs or symptoms

 Epigastric pain, nausea, heartburn, and gastroesophageal reflux disease (GERD)

     Constipation

     Tinnitus and hearing loss

     Headache or dizziness

     Visual disturbances

     Hematuria and albuminuria

 Rash, hypersensitivity reactions, bronchospasm (especially with aspirin)

 Blood dyscrasias, especially prolonged bleeding time

     Liver toxicity

Contraindications or extreme caution with NSAIDs applies to:

     Asthma—may manifest aspirin sensitivity as bronchospasm

     Cardiovascular disorders (e.g., hypertension, congestive heart failure [CHF])

     Kidney disease

     Liver dysfunction

     History of GI ulcer or inflammatory bowel disease

     Blood dyscrasias, especially clotting disorders or anemia

     Thyroid disease

     Children with viral infections (danger of Reye's syndrome with salicylates)

     GERD

     Older adults, pregnancy, lactation

     Those with aspirin and NSAID hypersensitivity

     Those with sulfonamide hypersensitivity *should not* take Celebrex

These medications should be given with meals or milk to reduce GI side effects. Enteric-coated, timed-release capsules or buffered aspirin are sometimes also recommended to reduce gastric irritation.

Interactions of NSAIDs (especially salicylates) are many, but the most important clinically occur with:

     Alcohol, which potentiates possibility of GI bleeding

     Anticoagulants, which potentiate possibility of bleeding (also true of vitamin E)

     Sulfonylureas (oral hypoglycemics), which potentiate hypoglycemia

Corticosteroids, which increase GI effects with prolonged administration of NSAIDs

Aspirin + NSAIDs—increased adverse GI effects (diminish GI risk-reducing effects of COX-2s)

Antihypertensives (attenuated response)

Lithium (decreased clearance)

Methotrexate, with potentiation and increased risk of methotrexate toxicity

Uricosurics (Benemid or Anturane), whose action is antagonized by salicylates

See Table 21-2 for a summary of the nonsteroidal anti-inflammatory drugs.

Table 21-2 Nonsteroidal Anti-inflammatory Drugs and Gout Medication

GENERIC NAME	TRADE NAME	DOSAGE
Nonselective (Traditional) NSAIDs		
diclofenac	Voltaren	PO 150–225 mg daily in div. doses
	Voltaren XR	PO 100 mg 1–2×/day
ibuprofen	Motrin, Advil (OTC)	200–800 mg 4×/day
indomethacin	Indocin	PO up to 200 mg daily in div. doses
	Indocin SR	PO 75 mg 1–2×/day
ketorolac	Toradol	PO 20 mg ×1, then 10 mg q4–6hrs (5 days max)
		IM/IV 15–30 mg q6h (5 days max)
naproxen	Naprosyn, Anaprox, Aleve (OTC)	220–550 mg BID (q12h)
oxaprozin	Daypro	PO 600–1200 mg once daily
sulindac	Clinoril	PO 150–200 mg BID
Partially Selective NSAIDs		
etodolac	Lodine	PO 600–1200 mg daily in div. doses
	Lodine XL	PO 400–1000 mg daily
meloxicam	Mobic	PO 7.5–15 mg daily
nambutone	Relafen	PO 1,000–2,000 mg daily
Selective COX-2 Inhibitor		
celecoxib	Celebrex	PO 100–200 mg BID
Combinations		
diclofenac/misoprostol	Arthrotec	PO 50 mg 3–4×/day; 75 mg BID
lansoprazole/naproxen	Prevacid NapraPAC	PO dose varies
Gout Medication		
colchicine		PO 0.5–1.8 mg daily in div. doses

Note: Other NSAIDs are available. This is a representative list.

Gout Medications

Gout is a metabolic disorder characterized by accumulation of uric acid crystals in various joints, especially the big toe, ankle, knee, and elbow, with resultant pain and swelling. Colchicine is a specific drug that is used to *relieve inflammation in acute gouty arthritis*. It is also used as a prophylaxis in persons prone to this condition.

Side effects of gout medications can include:

Rash

GI upset, diarrhea

Blood disorders

Always encourage large fluid intake to facilitate excretion of uric acid crystals.

Other medications for chronic gout are discussed in Chapter 15. They act in a different way and are not effective against inflammation in acute cases of gout or gouty arthritis.

Patient Education

Patients taking NSAIDs should be instructed regarding:

Administration with food to reduce gastric irritation

Caution with dosage (follow physician's directions carefully regarding amount of drug to reduce chance of overdose)

Discontinuing drug and reporting to physician any sign of abnormal bleeding (gums, stool, urine, and bruising), epigastric pain or nausea, ringing in the ears or hearing loss, visual disturbances, weight gain or edema, and skin rash

Avoiding taking any other drugs, either prescribed or OTC, without checking first with a physician or pharmacist regarding possible interactions

When taking gout medications (e.g., colchicine), always taking large amounts of fluids

Avoiding taking large amounts of aspirin or other NSAID with kidney, liver, or heart disease or with history of GI ulcer (with these conditions, take only under medical supervision). Patients with asthma may manifest sensitivity to aspirin and other NSAIDs.

The danger that GI ulceration and bleeding can occur without previous warning signs or symptoms

Discontinuing NSAIDs 10–14 days before elective surgery or dental procedures to reduce the risk of serious bleeding

Not taking Celebrex if allergic to sulfa

OSTEOPOROSIS THERAPY

Osteoporosis (porous bone) is a disease characterized by low bone mass and deterioration of bone tissue, leading to bone fragility and increased susceptibility to fracture, especially of the hip, spine, and wrist. It most commonly affects older populations, primarily postmenopausal women. **Osteoporosis therapy** includes several prescription medications currently approved for the prevention and/or treatment of osteoporosis.

Estrogens

As discussed in Chapter 24, hormone replacement therapy (HRT)—estrogen with or without progestin—is recommended for postmenopausal osteoporosis prevention (secondary to estrogen deficiency) *only* when unable to take other agents, and benefits outweigh risks. If started soon after menopause, estrogen prevents the accelerated phase of bone loss that occurs in the first five years after the onset of menopause.

Selective Estrogen-Receptor Modifiers (SERMs)

Raloxifene (Evista) is a selective estrogen receptor *modifier* with estrogen agonist activity on bone and lipids and estrogen antagonist activity on breast and uterine tissue. These properties result in increased bone mineral density and reduced fracture risk without promoting breast or endometrial cancer.

The incidence of vaginal bleeding and breast tenderness is lower with raloxifene than with HRT. However, in contrast to HRT, raloxifene can cause hot flashes and muscle cramps in the legs. Raloxifene is contraindicated in pregnancy and women with a history of thromboembolic disorders.

Calcitonin-Salmon

A synthetic form of the hormone calcitonin is available as a nasal spray (Miacalcin) for the treatment of postmenopausal osteoporosis in women who are more than five years past menopause. It increases spinal bone density and provides an analgesic effect in acute vertebral fractures. Calcitonin is reserved for women who refuse or cannot tolerate HRT or in whom HRT is contraindicated. Local nasal effects (e.g., irritation, redness, rhinitis, and epistaxis) are the most common adverse effects from the nasal spray.

Store the unopened bottle of calcitonin in the refrigerator. Once the pump has been activated, store at room temperature in an upright position. Discard all unrefrigerated bottles after 30 days.

Bisphosphonates

Bisphosphonates are nonhormonal agents that act directly to inhibit bone resorption, thereby increasing bone mineral density at the spine and hip, as well as decreasing the incidence of first and future fractures. Alendronate (Fosamax) and risedronate (Actonel) have been approved for both the prevention and treatment of osteoporosis and are considered first-line therapy. The bisphosphonates are also indicated for management of Paget's disease of the bone, a chronic disorder characterized by fractures, skeletal abnormalities, and significant bone pain.

Side effects of bisphosphonates, rare and mild, can include:

✳ GI distress (nausea, dyspepsia, esophagitis)

Abdominal and chest pain

Caution with bisphosphonates and active upper GI problems, for example, dysphagia, GERD, gastritis, or ulcers

Contraindications for bisphosphonates with:

Renal insufficiency, hypocalcemia

Inability to sit upright for 30 min after taking drug

See Table 21-3 for a summary of osteoporosis therapy.

Patient Education

Patients taking Fosamax or Actonel should be instructed regarding:

The importance of taking the medicine with a full glass of water (6–8 oz) at least 30 min before the first food, beverage, or medication of the day

Not lying down for at least 30 min to speed delivery to the stomach and avoid esophageal irritation

Taking supplemental calcium and vitamin D

Weight-bearing exercises

Modification of cigarette smoking and alcohol consumption, if these factors exist

Table 21-3 Agents for Osteoporosis Prevention and Therapy

GENERIC NAME	TRADE NAME	PREVENTION DOSE	TREATMENT DOSE	COMMENTS
Selective Estrogen *Receptor Modifier*				
raloxifene	Evista	PO 60 mg daily	PO 60 mg daily	Can be given without regard to meals
Calcitonin-Salmon				
calcitonin-salmon	Miacalcin	Not indicated	Intranasally 200 units (one activation) daily	Alternate nares
Bisphosphonates				
alendronate	Fosamax	PO 5 mg daily ac PO 35 mg qwk ac	PO 10 mg daily ac PO 70 mg qwk ac	See Patient Education
ibandronate	Boniva		PO 150 mg gmo	
risedronate	Actonel	PO 5 mg daily ac PO 35 mg qwk ac	PO 5 mg daily ac PO 35 mg qwk ac PO 30 mg daily ac × 2 mo	See Patient Education For Paget's disease

WORKSHEET FOR CHAPTER 21
MUSCULOSKELETAL AND ANTI-INFLAMMATORY DRUGS

Note the drugs listed and complete all columns.
Learn generic or trade names as specified by instructor.

Classifications and Drugs	Purpose	Side Effects	Contraindications or Cautions	Patient Education
Skeletal Muscle Relaxants 1. Flexeril 2. Valium 3. Robaxin 4. Soma				
NSAIDs 1. Ibuprofen OTC 2. Indocin 3. Naprosyn 4. Toradol 5. Daypro 6. Mobic 7. Relafen				
Gout Medication (Anti-inflammatory)				
Osteoporosis Therapy 1. Fosamax 2. Actonel 3. Calcitonin 4. Evista				

A. Case Study for Musculoskeletal Drugs

Truly Hardy, a 35-year-old construction worker, is diagnosed with muscle strain of the lumbar spine. Valium 5 mg q4h PRN is prescribed. His discharge instructions should contain the following information.

1. Muscle relaxants are only appropriate for which condition?
   - a. Chronic pain
   - b. Muscle weakness
   - c. As prophylactic
   - d. Acute muscle spasm

2. Muscle relaxants are *contraindicated* in some cases. Which one below would be appropriate for use?
   - a. Muscular dystrophy
   - b. Myasthenia gravis
   - c. Acute back pain
   - d. For children

3. Caution must be used with all of the conditions below EXCEPT
   - a. COPD
   - b. Diabetes
   - c. Nephritis
   - d. Cirrhosis

4. All of the following side effects are possible EXCEPT
   - a. Dizziness
   - b. Insomnia
   - c. Urinary retention
   - d. Blurred vision

5. Interactions with possible potentiation of effect can occur with all of the following EXCEPT
   - a. Alcohol
   - b. Analgesics
   - c. Antihistamines
   - d. Antacids

B. Case Study for Anti-inflammatory Drugs

Rita Robbins, age 65, comes into the physician's office with complaints of knee pain. The physician prescribes naproxen 500 mg q12h for arthritis. She should be given the following information.

1. How should the drug be administered?
   - a. Before meals
   - b. With fruit juice
   - c. With meals
   - d. With alcohol

2. Which of the following statements is true of NSAIDs?
   - a. Rapidly effective
   - b. Cure arthritis
   - c. Contraindicated with older adults
   - d. May be used long term

3. Side effects of NSAIDs can include all of the following EXCEPT
   - a. Gastric bleeding
   - b. Blurred vision
   - c. Anxiety
   - d. Heartburn

4. NSAIDs are contraindicated in all of the following conditions EXCEPT
   - a. COPD
   - b. Spondylitis
   - c. Gastroesophageal reflux
   - d. Inflammatory bowel disease

5. There are possible serious side effects from interactions of NSAIDs with all of the following EXCEPT
   - a. Alcohol
   - b. Antacids
   - c. Anticoagulants
   - d. Oral hypoglycemics

CHAPTER REVIEW QUIZ

Match the medication in the first column with the appropriate classification in the second column. Classifications may be used more than once.

Medication	Classifications
1. _____ Dantrolene	**A.** Combination NSAID
2. _____ Arthrotec	**B.** Osteoporosis Therapy
3. _____ Mobic	**C.** Muscle relaxant for multiple sclerosis
4. _____ Colchicine	**D.** Muscle relaxant for acute muscle strain
5. _____ Actonel	**E.** Partially selective NSAID
6. _____ Voltaren	**F.** Nonselective NSAID
7. _____ Flexeril	**G.** Gout medication
8. _____ Relafen	**H.** COX-2 inhibitor
9. _____ Evista	
10. _____ Celebrex	

Choose the correct answer.

11. Which muscle relaxant would <u>not</u> be used to treat acute muscle strain?
    a. Valium
    b. Succinylcholine
    c. Soma
    d. Robaxin

12. The following statements are true for skeletal muscle relaxants EXCEPT:
    a. Affect the brain
    b. Alter pain perception
    c. Reduce spasm
    d. Used long term

13. Which is not a side effect of skeletal muscle relaxants?
    a. Dry mouth
    b. Hypertension
    c. Confusion
    d. Tremor

14. Those at greater risk of adverse effects from NSAIDs include individuals with the following EXCEPT:
    a. Gallbladder disease
    b. Children with flu
    c. Renal dysfunction
    d. Clotting disorders

15. Side effects of nonselective NSAIDs can include all of the following EXCEPT:

    a. Liver toxicity

    b. Faster clotting

    c. Tinnitus

    d. Hematuria

16. Which is NOT true of colchicine therapy?

    a. Gout prophylaxis

    b. Fluids encouraged

    c. Take ac

    d. For gouty arthritis

17. Which is NOT true of Evista?

    a. Can cause hot flashes

    b. Can cause breast cancer

    c. Increases bone density

    d. Estrogen antagonist

18. Which is NOT true of Miacalcin?

    a. Increases bone density

    b. Can cause epistaxis

    c. Estrogen modifier

    d. Nasal spray

19. Which is NOT true of Fosamax?

    a. Osteoporosis treatment

    b. Take with juice

    c. Take ac

    d. Remain upright after taking

20. Celebrex is contraindicated for those individuals allergic to which of the following?

    a. Penicillin

    b. Aspirin

    c. Sulfa

    d. Quinolones

Chapter 22
Anticonvulsants, Antiparkinsonian Drugs, and Agents for Alzheimer's Disease

Objectives

Upon completion of this chapter, the learner should be able to

1. Define the Key Terms
2. Compare and contrast different types of seizures
3. List the medications used for each type of epilepsy and common side effects
4. List the drugs used for parkinsonism and common side effects
5. Describe the patient education appropriate for those receiving anticonvulsants and antiparkinsonian drugs
6. Describe the drugs for treatment of Alzheimer's disease

Key Terms

Absence epilepsy

Alzheimer's disease

Anticholinergics

Anticonvulsants

Antiparkinsonian drugs

Epilepsy

Grand mal

Mixed seizure

Parkinson's disease

Psychomotor epilepsy

Temporal lobe seizures

Unilateral seizures

ANTICONVULSANTS

Anticonvulsants are used to reduce the number and/or severity of seizures in patients with epilepsy. **Epilepsy** is defined as a *recurrent* paroxysmal disorder of brain function characterized by sudden attacks of altered consciousness, motor activity, or sensory impairment. Treatment is based on type, severity, and cause of seizures. Although most epilepsy is idiopathic (unknown cause), it may sometimes be associated with cerebrovascular disease, cerebral trauma, intracranial infection or fever, brain tumor, intoxication, or chemical imbalance. Sometimes the underlying disorder can be corrected, for example, fever, hypoglycemia, or electrolyte imbalance, and anticonvulsive medicine is not indicated.

The International Classification of Epilepsies and Epileptic Syndromes currently classifies seizure disorders into three main categories:

1. *Generalized* seizures—bilaterally symmetrical and without local onset
2. *Partial* seizures—complex symptomatology (temporal lobe or psychomotor seizures)
3. *Unclassified*—insufficient data to classify

Generalized Seizures

Generalized seizures include *grand mal (tonic-clonic)* and *absence (formerly petit mal)* seizures. They are bilaterally symmetrical and without local onset.

Grand mal seizures are characterized by loss of consciousness, falling, and generalized tonic, followed by clonic, contractions of the muscles. The attack usually lasts two to five minutes, and urinary and fecal incontinence may occur.

Initial treatment consists *only* of preventing injury by removing any objects that could cause trauma, cushioning the head and turning it to the side, and loosening tight clothing, especially collars and belts. Do not try to open the mouth or force anything between the teeth.

If seizures are so frequent that the patient does not regain consciousness between seizures, the condition is known as status epilepticus. The treatment of choice is IV diazepam (Valium) administered slowly. Sometimes IV phenytoin is also given.

DRUGS FOR ABSENCE EPILEPSY

Absence epilepsy, previously called petit mal, is so called because of the absence of convulsions. It is characterized by a 10–30-second loss of consciousness with no falling and usually occurs initially in children.

The drug of choice for management of absence epilepsy is ethosuximide (Zarontin), which is effective only for this type of epilepsy. Other drugs sometimes used in the treatment of absence seizures, when Zarontin is ineffective, include clonazepam (Klonopin) and valproic acid (Depakene).

Side effects of the drugs for absence epilepsy can include:

* Sedation, dizziness, or irritability
* Gastrointestinal (GI) distress including anorexia, nausea, vomiting, diarrhea
* Rash, leukopenia

Extreme caution with drugs for absence epilepsy applies to:

Hepatic or renal disease

Pregnancy and lactation

Pancreatitis (with valproate)

Contraindications with drugs for absence epilepsy include:

Medications should never be stopped abruptly

DRUGS FOR GRAND MAL AND PSYCHOMOTOR EPILEPSY

Psychomotor epilepsy (or **temporal lobe seizures**) are also called *partial seizures with complex symptomology*. They are caused by a lesion in the temporal lobe of the brain. Complex symptoms can include confusion, impaired understanding and judgment, staggering, purposeless movements, bizarre behavior, and unintelligible sounds, but no convulsions.

Unilateral seizures affect only one side of the body. Some patients may have **mixed seizure** patterns combining more than one type. It is important to observe and report type and length of seizures and general responsiveness to medications.

Prophylactic treatment of *grand mal* and *psychomotor* epilepsy usually consists of phenytoin (Dilantin), frequently combined with phenobarbital or valproic acid, administered orally. The aim of therapy is to prevent seizures without oversedation, and the dosage is adjusted according to the individual patient's response.

Side effects of phenytoin (Dilantin), which frequently decrease with continued treatment, can include:

- Sedation, ataxia, dizziness, and headache
- Blurred vision, nystagmus, and diplopia
- Gingivitis (inflamed gums)
- GI distress, including nausea, vomiting, anorexia, constipation, or diarrhea
- Rash and dermatitis, Stevens-Johnson syndrome

Megaloblastic anemia (treated with folic acid)

Osteomalacia (bone softening, treated with vitamin D)

Contraindications or extreme caution with Dilantin applies to:

Kidney or liver disease

Diabetes

Congestive heart failure, bradycardia, heart block, and hypotension

Pregnancy and lactation

Hematological disease

Abrupt discontinuation

Another medicine sometimes used for partial, generalized, or mixed seizures is carbamazepine (Tegretol).

Side effects of carbamazepine (Tegretol) can include:

- Cardiac, hematological, kidney, and liver complications

Interaction of Tegretol with grapefruit juice potentiates action and can increase risk of serious adverse effects. Do *not* take carbamazepine with grapefruit juice.

Febrile convulsions in children are frequently treated with phenobarbital alone. However, long-term use of phenobarbital in prophylaxis alone, when the child is afebrile, is controversial because of cognitive impairment. There is increasing evidence that anticonvulsant therapy may have adverse effects on behavior and cognition in children, especially phenobarbital, phenytoin, and carbamazepine. Close observation and monitoring of children in this area is essential, as is reporting of adverse changes to the physician for possible dosage reduction or substitution of an alternative anticonvulsant.

Alternative formulations of traditional anticonvulsants have been developed, for example, carbamazepine (Tegretol XR—extended release), diazepam (Diastat—rectal), fosphenytoin (Cerebyx—IM/IV), valproate (Depacon—IV; Depakote ER—extended release). The primary advantage of these newer formulations is related to an increased ease in administration and increased tolerability compared to their counterparts.

Second-generation anticonvulsants include gabapentin (Neurontin), lamotrigine (Lamictal), and topiramate (Topamax), which are indicated for adjuvant treatment of partial (psychomotor) seizures. These agents usually do not require laboratory monitoring of therapeutic levels. Second-generation anticonvulsants have fewer overall adverse effects (including effects on cognition), and fewer drug interactions than first-generation anticonvulsants. These agents require a *slow titration period* to avoid central nervous system (CNS) adverse effects. Second-generation anticonvulsants are contraindicated in pregnancy and lactation and should not be abruptly discontinued.

See Table 22-1 for a summary of the anticonvulsants. (Refer to Chapter 19 for a discussion on phenobarbital, and Chapter 20 for a discussion on diazepam.)

Patient Education

Patients taking any anticonvulsant medication should be instructed regarding:

Caution with driving or operating machinery until regulated with the medication, because of drowsiness or dizziness

Reporting of any side effects, such as rash or eye problems, staggering, slurred speech, and any other symptoms

Careful oral hygiene until tenderness of the gums subsides as treatment progresses

Always taking medication on time and *never* omitting dosage (abrupt withdrawal of medication can lead to status epilepticus)

Wearing Medic-Alert tag or bracelet at all times in case of accident or injury

Taking medication with food or milk to lessen stomach upset

Not taking grapefruit juice while on carbamazepine (Tegretol) because of potentiation of effect

Parents and teachers should be cautioned to observe and report changes in cognitive function, mood, and behavior in children receiving anticonvulsants

Table 22-1 Anticonvulsants

GENERIC NAME	TRADE NAME	DOSAGE	COMMENTS
First Generation			
carbamazepine	Tegretol	PO 400 mg–1.2 g daily in div. doses, susp, tabs	For psychomotor (partial or mixed seizures)
	Tegretol XR	PO 200–600 mg BID	Extended release; do not crush/chew
clonazepam	Klonopin	PO, dose varies	For absence seizures
fosphenytoin	Cerebyx	IV, IM, varies	Caution—do not confuse with Celexa (antidepressant) or Celebrex (for arthritis)
phenytoin	Dilantin	PO 300–600 mg daily in div. doses, IV varies, no IM	For grand mal, psychomotor, or focal seizures; frequently combined with phenobarb
ethosuximide	Zarontin	PO 250 mg–1.5 g daily in div. doses	For absence seizures
Valproic acid	Depakene, Depakote	PO 15–60 mg/kg daily, div. doses	For absence, partial, and tonic-clonic seizures
	Depakote ER	8%–20% higher than daily dose	One dose/day Do not crush/chew
	Depacon	IV 15–60 mg/kg daily, div. doses	
Second Generation			
gabapentin	Neurontin	PO 300–600 mg TID	For partial seizures, minimal drug interactions Decrease dose with renal dysfunction
lamotrigine	Lamictal	PO 100–300 mg BID	For partial seizures, monitor liver function Caution—do not confuse with Lamisil (antifungal)
topiramate	Topamax	PO 50–200 mg daily–BID	For partial seizures; may affect cognitive function at high doses

ANTIPARKINSONIAN DRUGS

Antiparkinsonian drugs are usually given for **Parkinson's disease,** a chronic neurological disorder characterized by fine, slowly spreading muscle tremors, rigidity and weakness of muscles, and shuffling gait. As the disease advances, patients develop dementia, confusion, psychosis, sleep disturbances, and declining cognitive function. There is no cure for Parkinson's disease, and the treatment goal is to relieve symptoms and maintain mobility.

Dopamine Replacement

Carbidopa-Levodopa

Levodopa crosses the blood-brain barrier, where it is converted to dopamine. Carbidopa augments the penetration of levodopa into the brain, increasing the therapeutic effect of dopamine in the CNS and reducing its adverse reactions. Sinemet (a combination of levodopa and carbidopa) is most often used for long-term treatment and is recommended as initial drug treatment for those over 70 years of age and those with dementia.

Side effects of Sinemet, which are numerous and frequent, can include:

* Dyskinesias (involuntary movements of many parts of the body)
* Nausea, vomiting, and anorexia
* Behavioral changes, anxiety, agitation, confusion, depression, psychosis
* Hypotension, dizziness, syncope

> *Note:* Side effects may be severe, requiring dosage reduction or withdrawal of the drug.

Contraindications for Sinemet include:

Discontinuing abruptly

Bronchial asthma or emphysema

Cardiac disease or hypotension

Active peptic ulcer

Diabetes, renal or hepatic disease

Glaucoma

Psychoses

Pregnant, postpartum, or nursing women

Interactions of Sinemet may occur with:

Antihypertensives, which may potentiate hypotensive effect

Phenytoin, which antagonizes levodopa

Iron salts that reduce bioavailability

Foods high in protein that reduce absorption

Monoamine oxidase inhibitors (MAOIs), which may cause hypertensive crisis

Patients receiving Sinemet for prolonged periods of time may develop a tolerance, resulting in ineffectiveness of the drug, called "wearing off." Sometimes, changing the timing of doses, changing to a controlled release preparation, or adding another agent (such as selegilene, entacapone, or a dopamine agonist), may bring the symptoms back under control.

Dopamine Agonists

The dopamine agonists bromocriptine (Parlodel), pramipexole (Mirapex), and ropinirole (Requip) are commonly used in conjunction with levodopa to delay the onset of levodopa-caused motor complications. Dopamine agonists may reduce the required dose of levodopa for patients with advanced Parkinson's. Bromocriptine is not generally used alone in treatment due to a high incidence of adverse side effects.

Pramipexole (Mirapex) and ropinirole (Requip) are recommended for initial monotherapy in patients less than 70 years old. These agents have a greater specificity for dopamine receptors and may have a neuroprotective effect, which leads to less dyskinesia, may delay the *wearing off* effect, and can postpone the need for Sinemet by several years.

Side effects of dopamine agonists can include:

* Psychosis, hallucinations, confusion, and somnolence
* Hypotension, syncopy
* Nausea, and vomiting

Interactions of dopamine agonists may occur with:

Antidopamine agents (i.e., antipsychotics, phenothiazines, metoclopramide) may decrease efficacy

Hypnotic and sedative agents may increase risk of somnolence

Other Drugs

Selegiline

Selegiline (Eldepryl), an MAO type-B inhibitor, is another drug sometimes prescribed after levodopa has been used for several years and begins to "wear off," or become less effective. Sinemet and selegiline are used *concurrently,* and the sinemet dosage is then reduced by 10%–30% to lessen the chance of additive side effects. Selegiline is not given alone.

Contraindicated with the following drugs, which can interact resulting in *severe* CNS toxicity, hyperpyrexia, hypertensive crisis, and even death. Do *not* use selegiline with:

Meperidine (Demerol)

Tricyclic antidepressants

Selective serotonin reuptake inhibitors (SSRIs)

Sympathomimetics (e.g., epinephrine, ephedrine, isoproterenol)

Abrupt discontinuation

When given at the recommended dosage of 10 mg daily in divided doses, there is minimal danger of hypertensive crisis associated with interactions of other MAOIs and certain foods (the "cheese reaction"). See Chapter 20 for a description of this reaction, which can occur if the recommended dosage is exceeded. No dietary restrictions are recommended for selegiline at the recommended dose.

Anticholinergic Agents

Drugs with anticholinergic and antihistaminic actions were the first to be used for parkinsonism and are still useful in mild forms of the disease and for drug-induced parkinsonism. The **anticholinergics** include synthetic atropine-like drugs, such as benztropine (Cogentin) and trihexyphenidyl (Artane), which are used to treat parkinson-like tremors associated with long-term use of the major tranquilizers or for other forms of parkinsonian syndrome. (See Chapter 13, Cholinergic Blockers.)

Side effects of the anticholinergic agents are:

* Dry mouth
* Dizziness and drowsiness
* Blurred vision
  Constipation or urinary retention
* Confusion
  Depression
  Nausea
* Tachycardia

Contraindications for anticholinergics apply to:

Older patients, who should not be treated with anticholinergics because of the risk of mental dysfunction. Those with benign prostatic hypertrophy (BPH) are also at risk for urinary retention.

Amantadine

Another drug unrelated to the other antiparkinsonian agents is amantadine (Symmetrel). It is used to treat parkinsonism (extrapyramidal reactions) associated with prolonged use of phenothiazines, carbon monoxide poisoning, or cerebral arteriosclerosis in the older adult.

Side effects of Symmetrel, usually dose related and reversible, can include:

* CNS disturbances including depression, confusion, hallucinations, anxiety, irritability, nervousness, and dizziness
  Headache, weakness, and insomnia
* Congestive heart failure, edema, and hypotension
* GI distress, constipation, and urinary retention

Contraindications or extreme caution with Symmetrel applies to:

Liver and kidney disease

Cardiac disorders

Psychosis, neurosis, and mental depression

Epilepsy

Patients taking CNS drugs

COMT Inhibitors

Catechol-*O*-methyl-transferase (COMT) inhibitors, such as entacapone (Comtan), block the enzyme responsible for metabolizing levodopa. COMT inhibitors increase the plasma concentration of levodopa, which enhances the amount of levodopa crossing the blood-brain barrier. This allows the patient's dose of levodopa to be lowered and results in a decrease in the incidence or severity of levodopa dose-related side effects (e.g., dyskinesias, nausea, etc.). COMT inhibitors increase the clinical response time to levodopa (*on* time), while decreasing the *off* time.

Side effects of entacapone can include:

* Orthostatic hypotension
* Hallucinations
* Dyskinesia
* Nausea/vomiting
* Diarrhea (can be severe)
* Orange discoloration of the urine

Drug interactions: Patients taking entacapone should not receive *nonselective* MAOIs (phenelzine or tranylcypromine), but can take a *selective* MAOI such as selegiline. Concomitant use of CNS depressants should be avoided to prevent additive sedation.

Patient Education

Patients taking antiparkinsonian drugs should be instructed regarding:

Administration on a regular schedule as prescribed, with food to lessen GI distress

Avoiding abrupt withdrawal of medication, which may greatly increase parkinsonian symptoms

Several weeks sometimes required before benefit is apparent

Caution with CNS drugs, alcohol, or antihypertensives (not taking other medicines including vitamins, without physician approval)

Caution with driving or operation of machinery; drugs may cause drowsiness, dizziness, or lightheadedness

Reporting adverse side effects to the physician (e.g., involuntary movements, blurred vision, constipation, urinary retention, GI symptoms, palpitations, and mental changes)

Reporting any signs that the drug is no longer effective after prolonged use (sometimes after months or years the dosage may need to be increased or another drug substituted by the physician); avoiding any dosage changes without medical supervision

Maintaining physical activity, self-care, and social interaction, an essential part of therapy for Parkinson's disease

Rising slowly

See Table 22-2 for a summary of the antiparkinsonian drugs.

Table 22-2 Antiparkinsonian Drugs

GENERIC NAME	TRADE NAME	DOSAGE	COMMENTS
Dopamine Replacement			
carbidopa and levodopa	Sinemet	PO 10/100–200/2,000 mg in 3–6 div. doses pc	
	Sinemet CR	PO 25/100–400/2,000 mg in 2–4 div. doses pc	Separate doses by at least 6 h
Dopamine Agonists			
bromocriptine	Parlodel	PO 1.25 mg BID with meals	Used with Sinemet; dosage gradually increased to optimum maintenance dose (up to 40 mg/day)
pramipexole	Mirapex	PO 0.125 mg TID	Increase to a max daily dose of 4.5 mg for desired effect balanced against side effects
ropinirole	Requip	PO 0.25 mg TID	Increase to a max daily dose of 24 mg for desired effect balanced against side effects
Anticholinergics			
benztropine	Cogentin	PO, IM, or IV 1–6 mg daily in one or div. doses	Not for the older adult For drug-induced parkinsonism and other forms of parkinsonian syndrome
trihexyphenidyl	Artane	PO 1–15 mg daily in div. doses	For drug-induced parkinsonism and other forms of parkinsonian syndrome
COMT Inhibitor			
entacapone	Comtan	200 mg–1,600 mg with each Sinemet	Use only with Sinemet
Other Drugs			
amantadine	Symmetrel	PO 100–300 mg daily div. doses	Also for viral upper respiratory infection and drug-induced parkinsonism
selegiline	Eldepryl	PO 5 mg BID (second dose no later than 2 P.M.)	Used when levodopa wears off, levodopa dosage can be decreased

AGENTS FOR ALZHEIMER'S DISEASE

Alzheimer's disease, or dementia of the Alzheimer's type, is characterized by a devastating, progressive decline in cognitive function, having a gradual onset, usually beginning between 60 and 90 years of age, followed by increasingly severe impairment in social and occupational functioning. Although the precise etiology of Alzheimer's disease is uncertain, cholinergic systems appear to be most clearly compromised and are frequently the target of drug treatment.

Cholinesterase Inhibitors

The first class of agents shown to be efficacious for symptom delay in Alzheimer's disease are the cholinesterase inhibitors. These agents prevent the breakdown of acetylcholine in the synaptic cleft, thereby improving cognitive function, but do not treat the underlying pathology of the disease. They may slow the progression, but do not cure the disease.

Tacrine (Cognex) was the first drug approved in this class, but is associated with significant hepatotoxicity and a frequent dosing schedule. Donepezil (Aricept) and rivastigmine (Exelon) are not associated with hepatotoxicity but do exhibit cholinergic side effects and dizziness. All drugs in this class cause GI upset (nausea, vomiting, anorexia), requiring slow dose titration to improve patient tolerance.

Interactions of cholinesterase inhibitors include:

Anticholinergics may decrease effectiveness—avoid using together

Cholinergics (bethanechol, succinylcholine)—may have a synergistic effect—monitor patient closely

Contraindications/Cautions of cholinesterase inhibitors:

GI bleeding

Jaundice, renal disease

Pregnancy, lactation

NMDA Receptor Antagonist

Memantine (Namenda) is the first *N*-methyl-*D*-aspartate (NMDA) antagonist approved for the treatment of moderate-to-severe dementia of the Alzheimer's type. Memantine is thought to selectively block the excitotoxic effects with abnormal transmission of glutamate while allowing for the physiological transmission associated with normal cell functioning. It can be used as monotherapy or in combination therapy with the cholinesterase inhibitor, donepezil (Aricept). Memantine may be efficacious in the earlier stages of Alzheimer's disease as well.

Side effects of memantine involve the CNS, are dose-dependent, and include:

Confusion, cerebrovascular disorder, falls, and agitation

Dizziness, headache, constipation

Contraindications/cautions include pregnancy, lactation, use in children, and renal disease

Drug interactions with other NMDA antagonists (amantadine, ketamine, and dextromethorphan)

See Table 22-3 for a summary of Alzheimer's drugs.

Table 22-3 Agents for Alzheimer's Disease

GENERIC NAME	TRADE NAME	DOSAGE	COMMENTS
Cholinesterase Inhibitors			
donepezil	Aricept	PO 5–10 mg at bedtime	May be taken with or without food
rivastigmine	Exelon	PO 1.5 mg BID with food	Increase to 3–6 mg BID (higher doses may be more beneficial)
tacrine	Cognex	PO 10–40 mg 4 ×/day on empty stomach	Monitor serum transaminase levels frequently
galantamine	Reminyl	PO 4–12 mg BID with food	Caution with hepatic/renal disease
NMDA Receptor Antagonist			
memantine	Namenda	PO 5 mg/day initially titrate to 10 mg BID	Can be used as monotherapy or in combo with donepezil CNS side effects, especially agitation

WORKSHEET 1 FOR CHAPTER 22
ANTICONVULSANTS AND ANTICHOLINERGICS

List the drugs according to category and complete all columns.

Classifications and Drugs	Purpose	Side Effects	Contraindications or Cautions	Patient Education
Anticonvulsants 1. Tegretol				
2. Klonapin				
3. Cerebyx				
4. Dilantin				
5. Zarontin				
6. Neurontin				
7. Depakote				
Anticholinergics for Parkinson's 1. 2.				

Classifications and Drugs	Purpose	Side Effects	Contraindications or Cautions	Patient Education
Antiparkinsonian Drugs 1. Sinemet 2. Parlodel 3. Mirapex 4. Requip 5. Entacapone (Comtan)				
Other Drugs for Parkinson's 1. Symmetrel 2. Eldepryl				
Alzheimer's Drugs 1. Aricept 2. Cognex 3. Exelon 4. Reminyl 5. Namenda				

A. Case Study for Anticonvulsants

Sandy, age 5, has been diagnosed with epilepsy. She has been placed on Dilantin and phenobarbital elixir. Her mother will need all of the following information.

1. Phenytoin (Dilantin) can have all of the following side effects EXCEPT
   a. Sore gums   c. Insomnia
   b. Headache   d. Nausea

2. All of the following should be reported to the physician EXCEPT
   a. Dizziness   c. Rash
   b. Increased appetite   d. Double vision

3. Sandy's teachers should be alerted to watch for and report all of the following EXCEPT
   a. Behavior changes   c. Hyperactivity
   b. Drowsiness   d. Inattention

4. The mother should do all of the following EXCEPT
   a. Give medicine with food   c. Stress oral hygiene
   b. Give medicine on time   d. Stop medicine if no seizures

5. Which of the following statements is NOT true?
   a. Doctor may reduce dosage   c. Side effects often subside
   b. Children outgrow epilepsy   d. Other drugs sometimes used

B. Case Study for Antiparkinsonian Drugs

Sam Snow, age 80, has Parkinson's disease and has been taking Sinemet for 10 years. He wants to discontinue the drug because he says it's not helping him anymore. He needs the following information.

1. He should be told the following EXCEPT
   a. Tolerance can develop   c. M.D. may change medicine
   b. He can increase the dose   d. Withdrawal increases symptoms

2. When Sinemet loses effectiveness, other drugs can be combined with it for better effect. Which is *not* a drug combined with Sinemet?
   a. Requip   c. Tegretol
   b. Mirapex   d. Parlodel

3. All of the following can be side effects of Sinemet EXCEPT
   a. Dizziness   c. Involuntary movements
   b. Constipation   d. Agitated confusion

4. All of the following may antagonize Sinemet or potentiate side effects EXCEPT
   a. Antihypertensives   c. Phenytoin
   b. Iron   d. Aspirin

5. Selegiline (Eldepryl) is sometimes combined with Sinemet. There are serious interactions with selegiline and the following medications EXCEPT
   a. Meperidine   c. Tricyclics
   b. Amantadine   d. SSRIs

CHAPTER REVIEW QUIZ

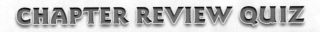

Match the medication in the first column with the condition in the second column that it is used to treat. Conditions may be used more than once.

Medication	**Condition**
1. _____ Aricept	**A.** Seizures
2. _____ Entacapone	**B.** Absence epilepsy
3. _____ Neurontin	**C.** Parkinson's
4. _____ Lamictal	**D.** Extrapyramidal reactions
5. _____ Zarontin	**E.** Alzheimer's
6. _____ Amantadine	
7. _____ Depakote	
8. _____ Cognex	
9. _____ Topamax	
10. _____ Reminyl	

Choose the correct answer.

11. Side effects of memantine (Namenda), used to treat Alzheimer's, can include all of the following EXCEPT:
    a. Dizziness   c. Headache
    b. Diarrhea   d. Confusion

12. All of the following statements are true of Mirapex used to treat Parkinson's EXCEPT:
    a. For patients less than 70   c. Less dyskinesia
    b. Slows "wearing off" effect   d. For monotherapy only

13. Which of the following can interact with carbamazepine (Tegretol), potentiating risk of side effects?
    a. Dairy products   c. Aspirin
    b. Grapefruit juice   d. Iron

14. Anticholinergic agents for Parkinsonism, for example Artane and Cogentin, are contraindicated in the following patients EXCEPT:
    a. With bradycardia   c. Depressed
    b. With BPH   d. Older adults

15. The following statements are true of the drugs for Alzheimer's EXCEPT
    a. Delay symptoms   c. Cause dizziness
    b. Improve cognition   d. Cure the disease

Chapter 23
Endocrine System Drugs

Objectives

Upon completion of this chapter, the learner should be able to

1. Define the Key Terms
2. Identify the hormones secreted by these four endocrine glands: pituitary, adrenals, thyroid, and islets of Langerhans
3. Describe at least five conditions that can be treated with corticosteroids
4. Explain administration practice important to corticosteroid therapy
5. List at least four serious, potential side effects of long-term steroid therapy
6. Compare and contrast medications given for hypothyroidism and hyperthyroidism
7. Describe side effects of thyroid and antithyroid agents
8. Explain uses and side effects of oral antidiabetics
9. Compare and contrast insulins according to action (rapid, intermediate, and long acting), naming onset, peak, and duration of each category
10. Identify the symptoms of hypoglycemia and hyperglycemia, and appropriate interventions
11. Explain appropriate patient education for those receiving endocrine system drugs

Key Terms

Antidiabetic

Antithyroid

Corticosteroids

Endocrine

Hyperglycemia

Hypoglycemia

Hypothyroidism

Immunosuppressant

Sulfonylurea

Endocrine refers to an internal secretion (*hormone*) produced by a ductless gland that secretes directly into the bloodstream. Endocrine system drugs include natural hormones secreted by the ductless glands or synthetic substitutes. Hormones that affect the reproductive system are discussed in Chapter 24. This chapter covers four categories: pituitary hormones, adrenal corticosteroids, thyroid agents, and antidiabetic agents.

PITUITARY HORMONES

The pituitary gland, located at the base of the brain, is called the master gland because it regulates the function of the other glands. It secretes four hormones: somatotropin, adrenocorticotropic hormone (ACTH), thyroid-stimulating hormone (TSH), and gonadotropic hormones (FSH, LH, and LTH; see Chapter 24). The two pituitary hormones discussed in this chapter are somatotropin and ACTH.

The anterior pituitary lobe hormone, somatotropin, is called human growth hormone (HGH). It regulates growth. Insufficient production of HGH will result in growth abnormalities, which should be treated only by an endocrinologist.

Adrenocorticotropic hormone (ACTH) is available only for parenteral use as corticotropin. Cosyntropin (Cortrosyn), a synthetic peptide of ACTH, is used mainly for diagnosis of adrenocortical insufficiency. Treatment of associated disorders is usually reserved for the corticosteroids in which dosage is more easily regulated and which are available in oral form as well.

ADRENAL CORTICOSTEROIDS

The adrenal glands, located adjacent to the kidneys, secrete hormones called **corticosteroids,** which act on the immune system to *suppress the body's response to infection or trauma.* They *relieve inflammation, reduce swelling,* and *suppress symptoms* in acute conditions. Corticosteroid use can be subdivided into two broad categories: (1) as replacement therapy when secretions of the pituitary or adrenal glands are deficient and (2) for their anti-inflammatory and **immunosuppressant** properties.

Corticosteroid therapy is *not curative,* but is used as *supportive therapy with other medications.* Some conditions treated with corticosteroids include:

Allergic reactions (e.g., to insect bites, poison plants, chemicals, or other medications) in which there are symptoms of rash, hives, or anaphylaxis

Acute flare-ups of rheumatic or collagen disorders, especially where only a few inflamed joints can be injected with corticosteroids to decrease crippling, or in life-threatening situations, such as rheumatic carditis or lupus

Acute flare-ups of severe skin conditions that do not respond to conservative therapy; topical applications are preferable to systemic therapy, when possible, to minimize side effects

Acute respiratory disorders such as status asthmaticus (oral inhalations preferable) and sarcoidosis, or to prevent hyaline membrane disease in prematures by administering IM to mother at least 24 h before delivery

Malignancies (e.g., leukemia, lymphoma, and Hodgkin's disease), in which corticosteroids (e.g., prednisone) are used with other antineoplastic drugs as part of the chemotherapy regimen; treatment of nausea and vomiting associated with chemotherapy (e.g., dexamethasone)

Cerebral edema associated with brain tumor or neurosurgery

Organ transplant, in which corticosteroids are used with other immunosuppressive drugs to prevent rejection of transplanted organs

Life-threatening shock due to adrenocortical insufficiency; treatment of other forms of shock is controversial

Acute flare-ups of ulcerative colitis; short-term only to avoid hemorrhage

Prolonged administration of corticosteroids can cause suppression of the pituitary gland with adrenocortical atrophy, and the body no longer produces its own hormone. To minimize this effect, corticosteroids are given by alternate-day therapy when they are required for extended time periods. Withdrawal of corticosteroids following long-term therapy should always be gradual with step-down (i.e., tapering) dosage. Abrupt withdrawal can lead to acute adrenal insufficiency, shock, and even death.

Because of potentially serious side effects, corticosteroids are administered for as short a time as possible and *locally if possible* to reduce systemic effects (e.g., in ointment, intra-articular injections, ophthalmic drops, and respiratory aerosol inhalants).

For *acute* episodes, some oral corticosteroids are available in *dose packs* (e.g., Medrol Dosepak, Sterapred UniPack, DexPak Taperpak) to facilitate dose tapering.

Side effects of the corticosteroids used for longer than very brief periods can be quite serious and possibly include:

Adrenocortical insufficiency, adrenocortical atrophy

Delayed wound healing and *increased susceptibility to infection*

Fluid and electrolyte imbalance, possibly resulting in edema, potassium loss, hypertension, and congestive heart failure

Muscle pain or weakness

Osteoporosis with fractures, especially in older women

Stunting of growth in children (premature closure of bone ends)

Increased intraocular pressure or cataracts

Endocrine disorders, including cushingoid state, amenorrhea, and *hyperglycemia*

Nausea, vomiting, diarrhea, or constipation

Gastric or esophageal irritation, ulceration, or hemorrhage

CNS effects including headache, vertigo, insomnia, euphoria, psychosis, or anxiety

Petechiae, easy bruising, skin thinning and tearing

Contraindications or extreme caution applies to:

Long-term use (regulated carefully); avoid abrupt discontinuation

Viral or bacterial infections (used only in life-threatening situations along with appropriate anti-infectives)

Fungal infections (only if specific therapy concurrent)

Hypothyroidism or cirrhosis (exaggerated response to corticosteroids)

Hypertension or congestive heart failure

Psychotic patients or emotional instability

Diabetes (drugs increase hyperglycemia)

Glaucoma (drugs may increase intraocular pressure)

History of gastric or esophageal irritation (may precipitate ulcers)

Children (drugs may retard growth)

Pregnancy and lactation

History of thromboembolic disorders or seizures

Interactions may occur with:

Barbiturates, phenytoin (Dilantin), and rifampin—require dosage adjustment

Estrogen and oral contraceptives may potentiate corticosteroids

Nonsteroidal anti-inflammatory agents (e.g., aspirin may increase risk of GI ulceration)

Diuretics, which potentiate potassium depletion, for example thiazides, furosemide

Vaccines and toxoids (corticosteroids inhibit antibody response)

Patient Education

Patients taking corticosteroids should be instructed regarding:

Following exact dosage and administration orders (never taking longer than indicated and *never stopping medicine abruptly*)

Notifying physician of any signs of infection or trauma *while taking corticosteroids or within 12 months after long-term therapy is discontinued* and similarly notifying surgeon, dentist, or anesthesiologist if required

Taking oral corticosteroids during or immediately after meals to decrease gastric irritation. Take single daily or alternate-day doses prior to 9 A.M. Take multiple doses at evenly spaced intervals throughout the day, but not near bedtime.

Avoiding any other drugs at same time (including OTC drugs, e.g., aspirin) without physician's approval. Antacids or other antiulcer drugs are sometimes prescribed

Side effects to expect with long-term therapy (e.g., fluid retention and edema)

Dangers of infection, delayed wound healing, osteoporosis, mental disorders

Reporting any side effects to physician immediately

See Table 23-1 for a summary of the pituitary and adrenal corticosteroids.

Table 23-1 Pituitary and Adrenal Corticosteroid Drugs

GENERIC NAME	TRADE NAME	DOSAGE[a]
Pituitary Drug		
corticotropin (ACTH) *(deficiency)*	H. P. Acthar	IM, sub Q repository gel for injection
cosyntropin	Cortrosyn	IM, IV, sub Q for adrenocortical insufficiency
Adrenal Corticosteroids[a]		
cortisone	Cortone	PO, IM for replacement
dexamethasone	Decadron	PO, IV, IM, inhalation
fludrocortisone	Florinef	PO, for orthostatic hypotension
hydrocortisone	Cortef or Solu-Cortef	PO, IV, deep IM, sub Q intraarticular
methylprednisolone	Depo-Medrol, Medrol or Solu-Medrol	PO, IV, deep IM, intra-articular
prednisone	Deltasone, Sterapred	PO tab or sol; do not confuse with prednisolone
triamcinolone	Aristocort, Kenalog	PO, IM

Note: Many other products available. Representative list only. Topical products are discussed in Chapter 12 and oral and nasal inhalation products in Chapter 26.

[a]Dosage varies greatly depending on the condition treated; large doses may be given for acute conditions on a short-term basis; long-term therapy is usually alternate-day, and dosage is reduced gradually.

THYROID AGENTS

Thyroid agents can be natural (thyroid) or synthetic (e.g., Synthroid). Thyroid preparations are used in replacement therapy for **hypothyroidism** caused by diminished or absent thyroid function. Synthetic agents, such as levothyroxine (Levoxyl), are generally preferred because their hormonal content is standardized and their effects are therefore predictable. Hypothyroid conditions requiring replacement therapy include *cretinism* (congenital; requires immediate treatment to prevent mental retardation) and *myxedema* or adult hypothyroidism due to simple goiter, Hashimoto's thyroiditis or other thyroid disorders, pituitary disorders, and thyroid destruction from surgery or radiation. Hypothyroidism causes slowed metabolism with symptoms ranging from fatigue, dry skin, weight gain, sensitivity to cold, and irregular menses to mental deterioration if untreated.

Hypothyroidism is diagnosed by blood tests (e.g., TSH and FT_4) before medication is given. The use of thyroid agents in weight reduction programs to increase metabolism when thyroid function is normal (euthyroid) is *contraindicated,* ineffective, and dangerous, leading to decrease in normal thyroid function and possibly life-threatening cardiac arrhythmias.

Transient hypothyroidism is rare, and thyroid replacement therapy for true hypothyroidism must be continued for life, although dosage adjustments may be required. Monitoring for toxic effects and periodic laboratory tests are recommended.

Note: When receiving orders for levothyroxine, caution is advised about decimal point placement (i.e., 0.025 mg vs. 0.25 mg) and dose conversions between *mg* and *mcg*, as medication errors have occurred.

Toxic effects are the result of overdosage of thyroid and are manifested in the signs of *hyperthyroidism:*

Palpitations, tachycardia, cardiac arrhythmias, and increased blood pressure

Nervousness, tremor, headache, and insomnia

Weight loss, diarrhea, and abdominal cramps

Intolerance to heat, fever, and excessive sweating

Menstrual irregularities

Contraindications or extreme caution with thyroid applies to:

Cardiovascular disease, including angina pectoris myocardial infarction and hypertension

Older adults (may precipitate dormant cardiac pathology)

Adrenal insufficiency—corticosteroids required first

Diabetes—close monitoring of blood glucose required

Euthyroid persons (normal thyroid function)

Interactions of thyroid may occur with:

Potentiation of oral anticoagulant effects if added after warfarin therapy stabilized

Insulin and oral hypoglycemics (dosage adjustment necessary)

Potentiation of adrenergic effect (e.g., epinephrine)—watch closely!

Estrogens and oral contraceptives (decreased thyroid response)

Soy products (decreased response)

Patient Education

Patients being treated with thyroid medication should be instructed regarding:

Importance of taking the prescribed dosage of thyroid medication consistently every day. It usually has to be taken for life. Take on empty stomach

Importance of reporting any symptoms of overdose (e.g., palpitations, nervousness, excessive sweating, and unexplained weight loss)

Periodic laboratory tests to determine effectiveness and proper dosage

Not changing from one brand to another or to a generic without physician approval

ANTITHYROID AGENTS

Antithyroid agents (e.g., Tapazole and propylthiouracil) are used *to relieve the symptoms of hyperthyroidism* in preparation for surgical or radioactive iodine therapy.

Side effects of antithyroid agents are rare and may include:

Rash, urticaria, and pruritus

Blood dyscrasias (especially agranulocytosis)

Contraindications or caution with antithyroid agents applies to:

Prolonged therapy (seldom used)

Patients older than 40 years old

Pregnancy and lactation

Hepatic disorders

Interactions with other drugs causing agranulocytosis are potentiated.

Patient Education

Patients being treated with antithyroid medication should be instructed to notify the physician immediately of signs of illness (e.g., chills, fever, rash, sore throat, malaise, and jaundice).

See Table 23-2 for a summary of thyroid and antithyroid agents.

Table 23-2 Thyroid and Antithyroid Agents

GENERIC NAME	TRADE NAME	DOSAGE
Thyroid Agents		
levothyroxine (Synthetic thyroid)	Synthroid, Levothroid, Levoxyl	25–200 mcg daily
thyroid	Armour Thyroid (real thyroid)	60–180 mg daily
Antithyroid Agents used for Graves Disease		
methimazole	Tapazole	Tabs, 5–30 mg daily, divided doses
propylthiouracil	PTU	Tabs, 100–150 mg daily, divided doses
potassium iodide	Iostat, Thyro-Block	Tabs, 130 mg daily for treatment of radiation emergencies

ANTIDIABETIC AGENTS

Antidiabetic agents are administered to *lower blood glucose levels* in those with impaired metabolism of carbohydrates, fats, and proteins. Diabetes mellitus is classified as insulin dependent (type 1) or non–insulin dependent (type 2). Type 1 diabetes was formerly described as maturity-onset diabetes because it was usually found in adults over 40 years of age. However, adults can also develop type 1 diabetes and require insulin.

There is also an increase in children and young adults with type 2 due to an increase in obesity at an earlier age.

Insulin

Insulin is required as replacement therapy for type 1 diabetics with insufficient production of insulin from the islets of Langerhans in the pancreas. Insulin is also required in patients with type 2 who have failed to maintain satisfactory concentrations of blood glucose with therapy including dietary regulation and oral antidiabetic agents. Insulin is also indicated for stable type 2 at the time of surgery, fever, severe trauma, infection, serious renal or hepatic dysfunction, endocrine dysfunction, gangrene, or pregnancy. Insulin (regular) is used in the emergency treatment of diabetic ketoacidosis or coma.

Insulin must be administered parenterally because it is destroyed in the GI tract. A new *inhaled* form of insulin, Exubera, became available in mid 2006. Because of possible respiratory side effects, it is contraindicated for smokers and those with COPD and asthma. All *injected* insulin products currently marketed are one of four types: pork, beef-pork, biosynthetic human, or analog. Both pork and beef-pork insulins are capable of causing antigenic reactions, and they are rarely used today. Biosynthetic insulins are referred to as "human" because their amino acid structure is identical to naturally occurring human insulin. Analog insulin (aspart, glargine, lispro) differs from human insulin only by substitution or position changes in the human insulin molecule, which mimics normal insulin secretion better than traditional insulins. Biosynthetic and analog insulins are created using recombinant DNA technology.

Most of the insulin used today is U-100, which means that there are 100 units of insulin in each milliliter. The insulin syringe *must be marked U-100* to match the insulin used. Remember that on the 100 unit (1 ml) insulin syringe each line represents 2 units. If a smaller 50 unit (1/2 ml) syringe is used, each line represents 1 unit of insulin (see Chapters 4 and 9 for details). *Always have someone else compare the insulin in the syringe with the dosage ordered to prevent errors,* which could have serious consequences.

Insulin preparations differ mainly in their onset, peak, and duration of action (Table 23-3). Aspart and lispro insulins are *rapid acting* and have a *very short duration* of action. *Regular* insulin is *rapid acting* and of *short duration*. *Regular* insulin is the *only* type that may be given intravenously as well as subcutaneously. All other insulins can *only* be given sub Q. Aspart and lispro are clear and rapid acting (onset in approximately 15 min). They peak in ½ to 1 h and last approximately 3 h. They can only be given subcutaneously. *Isophane* (NPH) and Lente are intermediate acting; and glargine and ultralente are long acting.

Regular insulin is sometimes combined with isophane or zinc insulin in the same syringe. When two insulins are ordered at the same time, the *regular insulin should be drawn into the syringe first*. Combinations of NPH and regular insulin are also available, for example, Humulin 70/30, or Novolin 70/30. This combination provides rapid onset with a duration of up to 24 h. Insulin *glargine* is not compatible with any of the other available types of insulin.

Table 23-3 Insulins

ACTION	PREPARATION	TRADE NAME	ONSET (H)	PEAK (H)	DURATION (H)
Rapid	Aspart	Novolog	1/4	½–1 *duration* 3	
	Lispro	Humalog			
Short	Regular	Humulin Reg.	½–1	2–5	5–8 (4-6)
		Novolin R eg.			
		Reg.Iletin II			
Intermediate	Isophane (NPH)	Humulin N,	1–2.5	6–12 *duration* 16–24	
	BID w/meals, QNH	Novolin N,			
		NPH Iletin II			
	Lente	Humulin L,			
		Novolin L,			
		Lente Iletin II			
Long	Glargine	Lantus	2	No peak	>24
	Ultralente	Humulin U	4–6	10–18	24–28
Mixtures	NPH/Reg	Humulin/Novolin	–	7–12	16–24
	% 70/30, 50/50				
	NPL/Lispro	Humalog Mix 75/25	5 min	7–12	1–24

Note: This is a representative list. Other insulin products are also available. Dosage varies. Before giving insulin, always check expiration date on the vial and be sure that regular, aspart, and lispro insulins are clear, and isophane and zinc insulins are cloudy. *Only regular insulins may be administered IV.* Isophane and zinc insulins are administered only sub Q, never IV. Opened vials may be stored at room temperature without loss of potency for one month.

Regular insulin is sometimes ordered on a *sliding scale*. This means that the blood is tested for glucose and a specific amount of regular insulin is administered sub Q based on the glucose level shown by the test. For example, the physician might write an order to give regular insulin sub Q according to the following blood glucose levels with this sliding scale:

Blood Glucose	Dosage of Regular Insulin
> 350	Call physician for dosage
301–350	12 units
251–300	8 units
200–250	5 units
< 200	No insulin

Remember, this is only a *sample* sliding scale. *Always check the physician's order carefully to determine the exact dosage of insulin, which varies with the individual.* Verification of insulin dosage with another caregiver is very important to prevent one of the most common and most dangerous of medication errors.

There are many different types of insulins available, many of which have names or packages that look or sound alike. There has been confusion between "Lente" and "Lantus" and "Humulin" and "Humalog." Confusion is also possible with the premixed products "Humulin 50/50 or 70/30," "Humalog Mix 75/25," "Novolog Mix 70/30," and "Novolin 70/30." *Be extremely careful to give the right insulin and the right dose! If in doubt, consult the pharmacist.*

Hyperglycemia

Hyperglycemia, or elevated blood glucose, may result from:

> Undiagnosed diabetes
> Insulin dose insufficient
> Infections
> Surgical or other trauma
> Emotional stress
> Other endocrine disorders
> Pregnancy

Symptoms of hyperglycemia may include:

> Dehydration and excessive thirst
> Anorexia and unexplained weight loss in persons under 40 years old
> Polyuria (frequent urination)
> Fruity breath
> Lethargy, weakness, flu symptoms, and coma if untreated
> Vision problems
> Ketoacidosis—can be determined by testing urine for acetone

Treatment of acute hyperglycemia includes:

> IV fluids to correct electrolyte imbalance
> *Regular* insulin added to IV fluids

Interactions: Insulin action is antagonized by corticosteroids or epinephrine, necessitating increased insulin dosage. Oral contraceptives and estrogen may also increase insulin requirements. Propranolol with insulin poses risks of hypoglycemia or hyperglycemia.

Interactions of insulin with *potentiation* of *hypoglycemic* effect include:

> Alcohol
> Monoamine oxidase inhibitors (MAOIs)
> Salicylates
> Anabolic steroids

Hypoglycemia

Hypoglycemia, or lowered blood glucose, may result from:

> Overdose of insulin
> Delayed or insufficient food intake (e.g., dieting)

Excessive or unusual exercise

Change in type of insulin, for example, from pork to human insulin

Symptoms of hypoglycemia may develop suddenly, and are manifested usually at peak of insulin action, including:

Increased perspiration

Irritability, confusion, or bizarre behavior

Tremor, weakness, headache, or tingling of the fingers

Blurred or double vision

Loss of consciousness and convulsions if untreated

Hypoglycemic reactions in older diabetics may mimic a CVA (cerebrovascular accident)

Treatment of hypoglycemia includes:

If conscious, administration of 4 oz orange juice, candy, honey, or syrup (especially sublingual). After initial treatment, provide a protein snack, for example, peanut butter, cheese, or glass of milk. Then recheck blood glucose with fingerstick test.

If comatose, administration of 10–30 ml of 50% dextrose solution IV or administration of 0.5–1 unit of glucagon (1 mg) IM or IV—follow with carbohydrate snack when patient awakens to prevent secondary hypoglycemia

Avoid giving excessive amounts of sugar or frequent overdoses of insulin, which can result in rebound hyperglycemia (Somogyi effect) from an accelerated release of glucagon. Treatment of rebound hyperglycemia involves reduction of insulin dosage with continuous monitoring of blood glucose.

Oral Antidiabetic Agents

Patients with type 2, non–insulin-dependent diabetes may sometimes be treated with diet alone; that is, low calorie, low fat diet, avoiding simple sugars and alcohol, and substituting complex carbohydrates, such as whole grain bread and cereals, brown rice, and vegetables high in fiber. Frequently it is necessary to combine diet and oral antidiabetic agents (see Table 23-4). Oral antidiabetic agents may be administered as a single daily dose before breakfast, or two divided doses daily, before morning and evening meals. These medications are not a substitute for dietary management. Weight reduction and modified diet are still considered the principal therapy for the management of type 2 diabetes.

Symptoms of type II diabetes may include:

Excessive weight gain after age 40

Excessive thirst (polydipsia)

Excessive urination (polyuria)

Excessive weakness, poor circulation, and slow healing

Visual problems

Oral antidiabetic agents are available in several pharmacological classes with differing mechanisms of action, offering different avenues for reducing glucose levels. Because they work at different sites, they are often synergistic; some may be used in combination with one another or with insulin.

Sulfonylureas

The oral hypoglycemic drugs known as **sulfonylureas** consist of first-generation agents (e.g., chlorpropamide, tolbutamide) and second-generation agents (e.g., glipizide, glyburide). The second-generation agents have mostly replaced the first-generation agents because of higher potency, better tolerance, and fewer drug interactions. The sulfonylureas work by increasing insulin production from the pancreas and by improving peripheral insulin activity.

Side effects of sulfonylureas may include:

* Gastrointestinal (GI) distress (may subside with dosage regulation)
  Dermatological effects, including pruritus, rash, urticaria, or photosensitivity
  Hepatic dysfunction, including jaundice (rare)
* Weakness, fatigue, lethargy, vertigo, and headache
  Blood dyscrasias, including anemia
* Hypoglycemia
  Possible increased risk of cardiovascular death—controversial
  Weight gain

Contraindications or extreme caution with sulfonylureas applies to:

Debilitated or malnourished patients

Impaired liver and kidney function

Unstable diabetes or type I diabetes

Major surgery, severe infection, and severe trauma

Contraindicated with the older adults—Diabinese, which has a longer half-life, greater chance of hypoglycemia, and also a risk of inappropriate antidiuretic hormone secretion (water intoxication)

Interactions of sulfonylureas with *potentiation* of hypoglycemic effect can include:

Beta-blockers, MAOIs, or probenecid

Alcohol with facial flushing (disulfiram-like reaction)

Cimetidine, miconazole, fluconazole, or sulfonamides

Salicylates and other nonsteroidal anti-inflammatory drugs (NSAIDs)

Interactions with antagonistic action (larger dose may be required)

Thyroid hormones

Thiazide and nonthiazide diuretics

Corticosteroids and phenothiazines

Estrogens and oral contraceptives

Calcium channel blockers

Rifampin and isoniazid

When these agents are administered or discontinued in patients receiving sulfonylureas, the patient should be observed closely for loss of diabetic control.

Alpha-Glucosidase Inhibitors

Alpha-glucosidase inhibitors such as acarbose (Precose) delay digestion of complex carbohydrates (e.g., starch) and subsequent absorption of glucose, resulting in a smaller rise in blood glucose concentrations following meals. Acarbose is often used as part of a combination regimen that includes an oral sulfonylurea.

Side effects of alpha-glucosidase inhibitors may include:

* GI effects (flatulence, abdominal distention/pain, loose stools), which tend to diminish with time or a reduction in dose; take at the start (with the first bite) of main meals

  Elevated liver enzymes, which are dose-related, generally asymptomatic, and reversible

Contraindications or extreme caution with alpha-glucosidase inhibitors applies to:

Impaired liver and kidney function

Patients with inflammatory bowel disease or intestinal obstruction

Pregnancy, lactation, use in children

Drug interactions with alpha-glucosidase inhibitors include:

Digestive enzymes (effect of acarbose reduced)

Digoxin (reduced serum digoxin concentrations)

Estrogens and oral contraceptives (impaired glucose tolerance)

Biguanides

The biguanides, for example metformin (Glucophage), work by decreasing hepatic glucose output and enhancing insulin sensitivity in muscle. Metformin can be used as initial monotherapy or in combination with sulfonylureas.

Side effects of biguanides may include:

* GI effects (diarrhea, nausea, vomiting, bloating, flatulence, anorexia), which are generally mild and resolve during treatment; can take with food to minimize epigastric discomfort

  Lactic acidosis (a rare, but serious metabolic complication) in patients with history of ketoacidosis, severe dehydration, cardiorespiratory insufficiency, renal dysfunction, and chronic alcoholism with liver damage

✳ Hypoglycemia

Contraindications or extreme caution with biguanides applies to:

Impaired liver and kidney function

Patients with congestive heart failure

Administration of radiocontrast dye (could result in acute alteration of renal function); withhold metformin prior to tests with radioactive dye

Pregnancy, lactation, children, and the elderly

Drug interactions with biguanides include:

Increased metformin effect seen with alcohol, calcium channel blockers, cimetidine, furosemide, digoxin, morphine, procainamide, quinidine, ranitidine, triamterene, trimethoprim, vancomycin, amiloride

Radiopaque contrast media (hold metformin the day of and at least 48 h after administration)

Meglitinides

Nateglinide (Starlix) and repaglinide (Prandin) stimulate beta cells of the pancreas to produce insulin. Repaglinide can be used as monotherapy or in combination with metformin.

Side effects of meglitinides may include:

✳ GI effects (nausea/vomiting, diarrhea, constipation, dyspepsia)
✳ Hypoglycemia
✳ Upper respiratory infection (URI), sinusitis, arthralgia, headache

Contraindications or extreme caution with meglitinides applies to:

Diabetic ketoacidosis

Impaired liver function

Pregnancy, lactation, use in children

Drug interactions with meglitinides include:

Refer to listing under sulfonylureas

Administer repaglinide before meals to maximize absorption

Gemfibrozil (Lopid) may enhance or prolong effects

Thiazolidinediones

Pioglitazone (Actos) and Rosiglitazone (Avandia) lower blood glucose by decreasing insulin resistance/improving sensitivity to insulin in muscle and adipose tissue. They can be used as monotherapy or concomitantly with a sulfonylurea, insulin, or metformin.

Side effects of thiazolidinediones may include:

- Weight gain, fluid retention, edema (Report weight gain over 6.6 lb, sudden onset of edema, or shortness of breath.)
- URI, sinusitis, pharyngitis, headache
- Myalgia

  Anemia
- Hypoglycemia (in combination with insulin or oral hypoglycemics)

Contraindications or extreme caution with thiazolidinediones applies to:

Chronic renal insufficiency

Impaired liver function

Congestive heart failure (causes edema)

May cause resumption of ovulation in premenopausal patients, increasing risk for pregnancy

Pregnancy, lactation, use in children

Drug interactions with thiazolidinediones include:

Pioglitazone with oral contraceptives (reduced effectiveness of the contraceptive)

Pioglitazone with ketoconazole, itraconazole (potentiation of hypoglycemic effect)

Rosiglitazone does not inhibit any of the major cytochrome enzymes responsible for drug metabolism/drug interactions seen with the other oral antidiabetic agents. To date, rosiglitazone does not interfere with the activity of a number of drugs in common usage.

See Table 23-4 for a summary of the oral hypoglycemics.

Patient Education

Both types of diabetics should be instructed regarding:

The importance of control with proper drug and diet therapy and *never* skipping meals.

Early symptoms and treatment of hypoglycemia—carrying ready source of carbohydrate (e.g., lump sugar or candy); orange juice, 4 oz, is also appropriate

Properly balanced diet (i.e., restricted calories; avoidance of simple sugars, alcohol, and foods high on the Glycemic Index (e.g., white bread, white potatoes, and white rice). Substitute foods low on the Glycemic Index—complex carbohydrates, such as whole-grain breads and cereal, and brown rice. Reduce fats, increase fiber, and be sure to have an adequate fluid intake.

Regular exercise and maintenance of proper body weight; weight reduction if obese

Importance of reporting to a physician *immediately* if nausea, vomiting, diarrhea, or infections occur (IV fluids may be required to prevent dehydration and acidosis)

Good foot care to reduce chance of infections

Carrying identification card and wearing identification tag

Taking medication (oral or insulin) at approximately the same time each day

Check blood glucose as directed by the physician, especially with hypoglycemia or stress

For type I diabetics (those requiring insulin), the foregoing instructions are important, as well as these additional rules:

Rotate injection sites (Figure 23-1). Insulin is absorbed more rapidly in arm or thigh, especially with exercise. Inject insulin into abdomen if possible for most consistent absorption.

Maintain aseptic technique with injections.

Have someone check the amount of insulin in the syringe before injection, especially with older adults or those with vision impairment (retinal problems are common in diabetics).

Check all insulin for expiration date.

Check regular insulin for clearness; do *not* give if cloudy or discolored.

Rotate isophane and zinc insulin vials to mix contents; do *not* give if solution is clear or clumped in appearance after rotation; do not shake the vial; rotate gently between hands (Figure 23-2).

If regular insulin is to be mixed with NPH or Lente, draw regular insulin into syringe first.

Unopened vials of insulin should be stored at 2–8°C and should not be subjected to freezing. The vial in use may be stored at room temperature without loss of potency for one month. Avoid exposure of insulin to extremes in temperature or direct sunlight. Do not put vial in glove compartment, trunk, or suitcase.

Regular insulin is sometimes administered on a sliding scale as ordered by the physician.

Notify physician of illness, increased stress, or trauma. *More* insulin may be required under these circumstances.

Notify physician if you increase your exercise significantly, or if you are taking less than the usual amount of food. *Less* insulin may be required under these circumstances.

Never omit insulin!

Table 23-4 Oral Antidiabetic Agents

GENERIC NAME	TRADE NAME	USUAL DOSAGE
First-Generation Sulfonylureas ~~not used any more~~		
acetohexamide	Dymelor	250–1500 mg/day ac or divided
chlorpropamide	Diabinese	100–500 mg/day w/meal (do not use for older adults)
tolazamide	Tolinase	100–1000 mg/day or divided ac
tolbutamide	Orinase	250–3000 mg/day or divided
Second-Generation Sulfonylureas		
glimepride	Amaryl	1–8 mg/day w/meal
glipizide	Glucotrol	2.5–40 mg/day ac or divided
	Glucotrol XL	5–20 mg/day w/meal
glyburide	Diabeta, Micronase	1.25–20 mg/day or divided w/meal
	Glynase	1.5–12 mg/day w/meal
Alpha-Glucosidase Inhibitors not used (in Digestive System, block glucose production)		
acarbose	Precose	25–100 mg TID, w/first bite of meal
miglitol	Glyset	*prevent absorption of sugar*
Biguanides		
metformin	Glucophage	500–2,550 mg/day divided w/meals
	Glucophage XR	500–2,000 mg/day w/meal or divided
Meglitinides		
nateglinide	Starlix	60–120 mg TID w/meals
repaglinide	Prandin	0.5–4 mg BID 2–4×/day
Thiazolidinediones		
pioglitazone	Actos	15–45 mg/day
rosiglitazone	Avandia	4 mg/day or BID divided
Combinations		
glyburide/metformin	Glucovance	1.25/250–10/2,000 mg/day BID w/meals
rosiglitazone/metformin	Avandamet	2/500–8/2,000/day w/meals or divided

Note: In older adults, start with the lowest dose possible and titrate upward to desired glycemic control.

[Byetta– Incretin mimetic
works on intestinal Incretin Hormones]

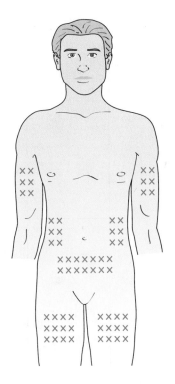

Figure 23-1 Common sites for insulin injection. Sites should be rotated and the site recorded each time on the medication record.

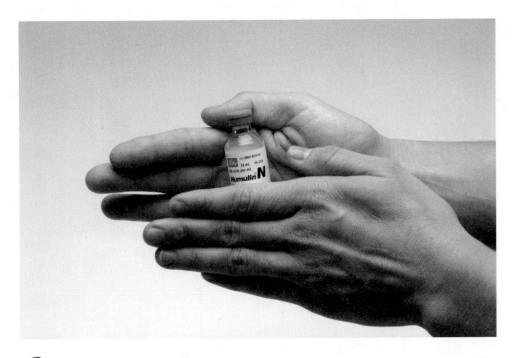

Figure 23-2 Rotate isophane and zinc insulin vials gently to mix contents. Do not shake.

WORKSHEET 1 FOR CHAPTER 23
ENDOCRINE SYSTEM DRUGS

List the drugs according to category and complete all columns.
Learn generic or trade names as specified by instructor.

Classifications and Drugs	Purpose	Side Effects	Contraindications or Cautions	Patient Education
Corticosteroids 1. Decadron 2. Solu-Medrol 3. Prednisone 4. Hydrocortisone				
Thyroid Agents 1. Synthroid 2. Levoxyl				
Antithyroid Agents 1. Tapazole 2. Propylthiouracil				
Oral Antidiabetic Agents 1. Diabinese 2. Dymelor 3. Glucotrol 4. Glucophage 5. Prandin 6. Avandia				

WORKSHEET 2 FOR CHAPTER 23
INSULINS

Fill in the blanks and complete all columns.

Action	Preparation	Trade Name	Onset (h)	Peak (h)	Duration (h)
Rapid	Aspart	Novolog			
	Lispro	Humalog			
Short	Regular	Humulin R			
		Novolin R			
		Reg. Iletin II			
Intermediate	Isophane (NPH)	Humulin N,			
		Novolin N,			
		NPH Iletin II			
	Lente	Humulin L			
		Novolin L			
		Lente Iletin II			
Long	Glargine	Lantus			
	Ultralente	Humulin U			
Mixtures	NPH/Reg 70/30, 50/50	Humulin/Novolin			
	NPL/Lispro	Humalog Mix 75/25			

NPL, neutral protamine lispro.

(continued)

WORKSHEET 2 FOR CHAPTER 23
INSULINS

Fill in the blanks and complete all columns.

Hyperglycemia	Causes	Symptoms	Treatment

Hypoglycemia	Causes	Symptoms	Treatment

A. Case Study for Endocrine System Drugs

Lois Pal, a 65-year-old patient with glaucoma, asks the physician for prednisone tablets to take long term for osteoarthritis in her knees. She needs the following information.

1. Corticosteroids for severe flare-ups of joint pain are usually administered
   - a. By mouth
   - b. Topically
   - c. Intramuscularly
   - d. Intra-articularly

2. The *usual* type of administration of corticosteroids include any of the following EXCEPT
   - a. Step-down
   - b. Ongoing
   - c. Alternate-day
   - d. Short-term

3. The following are possible long-term corticosteroid side effects EXCEPT
   - a. Osteoporosis
   - b. Decreased intraocular pressure
   - c. Fluid retention
   - d. Gastric bleeding

4. Other side effects can include all of the following EXCEPT
   - a. Headache
   - b. Anxiety
   - c. Sedation
   - d. Slow healing

5. Corticosteroids can be used to treat all of the following EXCEPT
   - a. Asthma attack
   - b. Poison ivy
   - c. Organ transplant
   - d. Fungal infection

B. Case Study for Antidiabetic Agents

Hope Moore, a 70-year-old type II diabetic, has been taking Orinase for 6 years. Her blood glucose is now elevated, and the physician plans to start her on insulin. She will need the following information.

1. The following is true of NPH insulin EXCEPT
   - a. Peaks in 6–12 hours
   - b. Can be Humulin N
   - c. Used for sliding scale
   - d. Acts in 1–2.5 hours

2. Signs of hypoglycemia can include the following EXCEPT
   - a. Tremor
   - b. Dehydration
   - c. Confusion
   - d. Blurred vision

3. Treatment of hypoglycemia could include any of the following EXCEPT
   - a. 4 oz orange juice
   - b. Candy
   - c. Diet cola
   - d. Glucagon IM

4. If vomiting and diarrhea occur, the following might be necessary EXCEPT
   - a. Decrease insulin
   - b. IV fluids
   - c. Regular insulin IV
   - d. NPH insulin subcu

5. The following is true of regular and NPH insulins EXCEPT
   - a. Can be mixed
   - b. Rotate injection sites
   - c. Keep at room temperature
   - d. Both are cloudy

CHAPTER REVIEW QUIZ

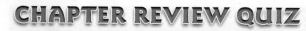

Match the medication in the first column with the appropriate classification in the second column. Classifications may be used more than once.

Medication	Classification
1. _____ Glucophage	**A.** Thyroid agent
2. _____ Prednisone	**B.** Antithyroid
3. _____ Humulin R	**C.** Oral Antidiabetic agent
4. _____ Synthroid	**D.** Corticosteroid
5. _____ Avandia	**E.** Insulin–Rapid acting
6. _____ Tapazole	**F.** Insulin–Short acting
7. _____ Lente	**G.** Insulin–Intermediate acting
8. _____ Prandin	**H.** Insulin–Long acting
9. _____ Lantus	
10. _____ Humalog	

Choose the correct answer.

11. Which is NOT a side effect of long-term corticosteroid use?
    a. Skin thinning
    b. Easy bruising
    c. Insomnia
    d. Hypoglycemia
12. *Corticosteroids are contraindicated* for patients with a history of all of the following conditions EXCEPT:
    a. Congestive heart failure
    b. Gastric ulcers
    c. Asthma
    d. Psychosis
13. Thyroid medication would be prescribed for all of the following EXCEPT:
    a. After thyroidectomy
    b. Weight reduction
    c. Cretinism
    d. Goiter
14. Which is NOT true of treatment with thyroid medication?
    a. Monitored with blood tests
    b. Overdose causes tachycardia
    c. Short-term use
    d. Insulin interactions
15. Which is NOT true of treatment with antithyroid medication?
    a. Before surgery
    b. Used for older adults
    c. Short-term use
    d. Rash possible
16. Which is NOT true of regular insulin?
    a. Combines with NPH
    b. Given IV
    c. Short action
    d. Cloudy

17. Which is NOT true of Aspart and Lispro insulins?
   a. Rapid acting
   b. Short duration
   c. Given IV
   d. Clear

18. Which is NOT true of NPH insulin?
   a. Used for sliding scale
   b. Combines with Regular
   c. Intermediate action
   d. Cloudy

19. Which is NOT part of first-line treatment for patients with type II diabetes?
   a. Low-calorie diet
   b. Oral antidiabetic agents
   c. High-fiber diet
   d. Insulin

20. Which oral antidiabetic agent is contraindicated for the older adults?
   a. Glucophage
   b. Diabinese
   c. Prandin
   d. Avandia

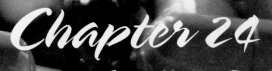

Chapter 24
Reproductive System Drugs

Key Terms

Androgens

Contraceptives

Estrogen

Follicle-stimulating
hormone (FSH)

Luteinizing hormone
(LH)

Luteotropic hormone
(LTH)

Oxytocin

Progesterone

Progestins

Testosterone

Objectives

Upon completion of this chapter, the learner should be able to

1. Define the Key Terms
2. Identify the uses, side effects, and precautions for the androgens
3. List the uses, side effects, and contraindications for the estrogens and progestins
4. Compare and contrast contraceptives
5. Describe the use of oxytocics and the precautions to be observed
6. Explain the uses of Brethine, Prostaglandin, and magnesium sulfate
7. Describe the uses of GnRH analogs
8. Explain drug therapy for infertility and impotence
9. Present appropriate patient education for all drugs in this section

Hormones that regulate the functions of the reproductive systems include *endogenous* chemical substances, which originate within different areas of the body. For the purpose of simplification, we will divide the reproductive hormones into four main categories: gonadotropic, androgens, estrogens, and progestins.

The pituitary gland is located at the base of the brain. The anterior lobe secretes four hormones. Those affecting growth, thyroid function, and adrenocorticosteroid production are discussed in Chapter 23. This chapter includes the gonadotropic hormones, which are secreted by the anterior and posterior pituitary lobes.

The gonadotropic hormones include (1) **follicle-stimulating hormone (FSH),** which stimulates development of ovarian follicles in the female and sperm production in the testes of the male; (2) **luteinizing hormone (LH),** which works in conjunction with FSH to induce secretion of estrogen, ovulation, and development of corpus luteum; and (3) **luteotropic hormone (LTH),** which stimulates the secretion of progesterone by the corpus luteum and secretion of milk by the mammary gland, hence the term *lactogenic hormone.*

ANDROGENS

Androgens, the male hormones, are secreted mainly in the interstitial tissue of the testes in the male and secondarily in the adrenal glands of both sexes. Androgens, which stimulate the development of male characteristics (masculinization), include **testosterone** and andosterone. Inadequate production of androgens in the male may be due to pituitary malfunction or to atrophy, injury to, or removal of the testicles (castration), resulting in eunuchism or eunuchoidism. Eunuchoid characteristics include retarded development of sex organs, absence of beard and body hair, high-pitched voice, and lack of muscular development. Hypogonadism may also result in impotence or deficient sperm production (oligospermia).

Uses of androgens include:

Replacement in cases of diminished testicular hormone with testosterone (e.g., impotence, oligospermia, or andropause ["male menopause"])

Congenital hypogonadism (e.g., cryptorchidism or undescended testicles) or delayed puberty in the male

Acquired hypogonadism (e.g., orchitis, trauma, tumor, radiation, surgery of the testicles, or drug-induced)

Palliative treatment of females with advanced metastatic (skeletal) carcinoma of the breast, for example, methyltestosterone

Endometriosis and fibrocystic breast disease, for example, danazol

Side effects of androgens can include:

✳ Edema (diuretics may be indicated)

✳ Acne, increased oiliness of skin and hair, or alopecia

Oligospermia (deficient sperm production resulting in sterility)

Increased or decreased sexual stimulation or libido, impotence

Gynecomastia in males (enlarged breast tissue)

Hirsutism, deepening of voice, and amenorrhea in females

✳ Jaundice and hepatitis

Nausea and vomiting

✳ Premature closure of bone ends in adolescents, with stunting of growth

✴ Anxiety, depression, headache

Increased low-density lipoprotein (LDL), decreased high-density lipoprotein (HDL), and insulin resistance

Contraindications or caution with androgens applies to:

Cardiac, renal, and liver dysfunction (edema common)

Geriatric males (may increase risk of prostatic hypertrophy and carcinoma or overstimulation sexually)

Prepubertal males who have not reached their full growth potential (may stunt growth by premature closure of bone ends)

Diabetes, obesity, or dyslipidemia (abnormal lipid profile)

Interactions of androgens may occur with:

Oral anticoagulants (potentiation may cause bleeding)

Decreased blood glucose and decreased insulin requirements in diabetics

Antiandrogens (dutasteride, finasteride)

Dangers of illegal use of anabolic steroids: Health care personnel have a responsibility to caution athletes, especially adolescents, regarding the hazards of taking illegal synthetic testosterone products to build muscle power or physique. Besides the *potentially serious adverse side effects* just
✴ mentioned, another risk is *the development of psychosis* with delusions, paranoia, depression, mania, and aggression with violence.

The FDA warned 23 companies to stop manufacturing, marketing, and distributing androstenedione (Andro, Androstene) and similar products in March 2004, due to increased cancer risk. These products were not Food and Drug Administration (FDA) approved, but were sometimes available in stores selling herbal remedies.

All agents in this class are classified as a controlled substance (C-III) by the DEA due to abuse potential.

See Table 24-1 for a summary of the androgens and impotence agents.

Patient Education

Patients on androgen therapy should be instructed regarding:

Taking only prescribed drugs according to directions

Side effects to report, especially edema, jaundice, nausea, or vomiting

Sexual effects for males to report, such as decreased ejaculatory volume and excessive sexual stimulation, especially in geriatric patients beyond cardiovascular capacity

Sexual effects for females to expect (e.g., hirsutism and voice deepening)

Possibility of stunted growth when administered to adolescent boys before puberty

IMPOTENCE AGENTS

Phosphodiesterase (PDE) inhibitors are a class of drugs given orally for the treatment of male erectile dysfunction (ED), also referred to as impotence. This represents a significant advance as other therapies require direct injection into the penis or insertion of a urethral suppository. Sildenafil (Viagra) was the first PDE inhibitor approved to treat ED, followed by vardenafil (Levitra) and tadalafil (Cialis).

Side effects of PDE inhibitors can include:

* Headache, flushing, abnormal vision, dizziness

  Dyspepsia, nasal congestion, rhinitis, diarrhea, rash

* Cardiovascular events (less than 2% of patients) including angina, syncope, tachycardia, palpitation, and hypotension

Contraindications with PDE inhibitors applies to:

Concurrent use of nitrates or alpha-blockers (e.g., Flomax, Hytrin) with PDE inhibitors potentiates the hypotensive effects

In the event of an erection persisting >4 h, advise patient to seek medical assistance immediately (tissue damage and permanent loss of potency may result)

Older adults and patients with preexisting cardiovascular risk factors

Hepatic/renal function impairment

Interactions with PDE inhibitors include:

Nitrates, antiretroviral protease inhibitors, macrolides, some antifungals (potentiate/prolong hypotensive effect)

Grapefruit juice—do not take concurrently (potentiates hypotensive effect)

See Table 24-1 for details regarding impotence agents.

ESTROGENS

Estrogens, the female sex hormones, are produced mainly by the ovary and secondarily by the adrenal glands. Estrogens are responsible for the development of female secondary sexual characteristics, including breast enlargement, and during the menstrual cycle they act on the female genitalia to produce an environment suitable for fertilization, implantation, and nutrition of the early embryo. Estrogens also affect the secretion of the hormones FSH and LH from the anterior pituitary gland in a complex way. This results in inhibition of lactation and inhibition of ovulation, the latter process utilized in contraceptive therapy.

Estrogen in combination with testosterone is sometimes used in the management of severe menopausal symptoms that do not respond to estrogen alone.

* Estrogen therapy (ET), that is, estrogen alone, has been associated with an *increased risk of endometrial carcinoma* in women with an intact

Table 24-1 Androgens and Impotence Agents

GENERIC NAME	TRADE NAME	DOSAGE	USES
Androgens			
danazol	Danocrine	PO 100–400 mg BID	Endometriosis, fibrocystic breast disease
methyltestosterone	Android, Testred	PO 10–50 mg/day Buccal 25–100 mg/day	Advanced breast cancer
nandrolone		50–200 mg q1–4 wk	Anemia of renal disease
oxandrolone	Oxandrin	PO 2.5–20 mg/day div doses	Treatment of cachexia
testosterone	Depo-Testosterone Testoderm, Androderm, AndroGel	Deep IM, pellet implant, buccal; dose varies Patch transdermal gel	Hypogonadism, advanced breast cancer
testosterone in combination with estrogen	Estratest	PO dose varies	Menopausal symptoms if estrogen alone insufficient
Impotence Agents			
sildenafil	Viagra	50 mg PO 1 h before sexual activity (max freq once daily)	Treatment of erectile dysfunction (has no effect in the absence of sexual stimulation)
tadalafil	Cialis	10 mg PO before sexual activity (max freq q48h)	Onset of action is 30–45 min; duration is up to 36 h
vardenafil	Levitra	10 mg PO 1 h before sexual activity (max freq once daily)	

uterus. When progestin is combined with estrogen (*combined hormone therapy [HT]*), the risk of endometrial cancer is substantially reduced.

In 2002, the results of the Women's Health Initiative (WHI) study were released. The main thrust of the WHI study was to determine the exact degree to which hormone therapies (HTs) presumably protected the heart and to investigate the degree to which some of the known and potential risks of HTs, such as breast cancer and blood clots, cancelled out any benefits. The WHI also explored whether HTs prevented fractures, colon cancer, and dementia, including Alzheimer's disease.

The WHI study authors announced not only that the risks of *combined HT* outweighed its benefits when used to prevent certain diseases, but it could actually *increase the risk* of certain conditions it was previously believed to prevent, such as heart attack. The American College of Obstetricians and Gynecologists (ACOG) have issued the following recommendations regarding HT:

1. *Combined HT should not be used* for prevention of diseases such as cardiovascular disease, due to the small but significant *increased risk of conditions such as breast cancer, heart attack, stroke, and blood clots;*

2. *Estrogen-alone therapy* used for women who have had a hysterectomy *should not be used for the prevention of diseases, due to the in-*

creased risks of blood clots and stroke. Although ET carries fewer risks than combined HT, women with a uterus should not use estrogen alone due to their increased risk of uterine cancer;

3. HTs are still the most effective therapies and are appropriate for the relief of vasomotor symptoms, so long as a woman has weighed the risks and benefits with her doctor; and

4. Women on combined HT or ET should take the *smallest effective dose for the shortest possible time and annually review the decisions to take hormones.*

Although further study is needed, preliminary evidence suggests that risks for blood clots *may* be lower in women at risk for such problems using *patches* rather than pills. One reason may be that pills are broken down in the liver, where proteins involved in the formation of blood clots are activated. The estrogens in skin patches are released directly into the blood stream, bypassing the liver completely. Research is ongoing, and the American College of Obstetricians and Gynecologists (ACOG) recommendations may change. Please refer to their Web site (www.acog.org) for updated information.

Uses of estrogen therapy include:

Contraceptives (combined with progestin)—these combination products are also used to treat menstrual irregularities and dysmenorrhea

Menopausal vasomotor symptom relief (use for mild to moderate depression only if unable to or unwilling to take selective serotonin reuptake inhibitors [SSRI])

Female hypogonadism due to ovarian pathology or oophorectomy

Postmenopausal prevention of osteoporosis (secondary to estrogen deficiency) *only* if unable to take other agents, and benefits outweigh the risks

Postmenopausal estrogen replacement may reduce cardiovascular heart disease and elevate the HDL levels in women. (Conflicting studies)

Atrophic vaginitis from decreased secretions—low-dose vaginal cream biweekly

Postcoital use after rape or incest (within 24–48 h) of a single large dose to prevent, not terminate, pregnancy.

Palliative treatment for males with advanced, inoperable prostate cancer

Side effects of estrogen therapy, especially with high doses, can include:

Increased risk of thromboembolic disorders, hypertension, myocardial infarction, and stroke

GI effects, including vomiting, abdominal cramps, bloating, diarrhea or constipation, and weight gain

Skin discolorations (acne may decrease or occasionally increase)

Fluid retention and edema

Increased serum triglyceride levels

Severe hypercalcemia in cancer patients with large doses

Folic acid deficiency (may require folic acid supplements)

Liver function abnormalities, including jaundice, anorexia, and pruritus

Breakthrough or irregular vaginal bleeding

Increased risk of cervical erosion and *Candida* vaginitis

✳ Headache, especially migraine, and depression

Visual disturbances

Breast tenderness, enlargement, and secretion

✳ Increased risk of gallbladder disease

✳ Cancer of the uterus with estrogen alone. Therefore, progesterone is recommended with estrogen. (See Women's Health Initiative study and recommendations at beginning of this section.)

Contraindications and cautions exist because the use of estrogens, especially in large doses, may be associated with increased risk of several serious conditions. Before estrogen therapy is begun, a complete history and physical examination are essential, and yearly physicals, including Pap test and mammogram, during therapy are important. Estrogens are *contraindicated* for anyone with a history of the following conditions, and estrogen therapy should be *discontinued with signs of these conditions:*

Thromboembolus, stroke, and myocardial infarction

Liver dysfunction and gallbladder disease

Breast cancer (except for palliative treatment)

Visual disturbances, severe headaches, and migraine

Shortness of breath, chest or calf pain

Seizure, asthma, and kidney disorders

Surgery (estrogens should be discontinued 4 weeks before if possible)

Other contraindications for estrogens include the following:

Prolonged, continued use of high-dose estrogens in postmenopausal women, which has shown an increased risk of endometrial cancer in some studies; therefore, cyclic administration at the *lowest* possible dose, is recommended with progesterone. Regular physical examinations, including a Pap test every year are also recommended.

Pregnancy, in which estrogens can cause serious fetal toxicity, congenital anomalies, and vaginal or cervical cancer for the offspring in later life. Estrogens should *never* be used to treat threatened abortions or if there is any possibility of pregnancy. A pregnancy test should be done before initiating therapy.

Nursing mothers should avoid estrogen.

Caution with diabetes and with heavy smokers

Interactions of estrogen include the following:

Rifampin and isoniazid decrease estrogenic activity, and therefore other forms of contraception should be used with patients receiving rifampin or isoniazid.

Corticosteroid effects are potentiated by estrogen.

Laboratory test interference includes endocrine function tests, decreased glucose tolerance, and thyroid function tests.

Anti-infectives may decrease contraceptive action.

Oral anticoagulant, anticonvulsant, and hypoglycemic actions may be decreased with estrogen.

Sunscreens with estradiol topical emulsion (increases absorption)

PROGESTINS

Progesterone is a hormone secreted by the corpus luteum and adrenal glands. It is responsible for changes in uterine endometrium in the second half of the menstrual cycle in preparation for implantation of the fertilized ovum, development of maternal placenta after implantation, and development of mammary glands. Synthetic drugs that exert progesterone-like activity are called **progestins.**

Uses of synthetic progestins include:

Treatment of amenorrhea and abnormal uterine bleeding caused by hormonal imbalance.

Contraception, either combined with estrogen or used alone.

Postmenopausal—sometimes combined with estrogen in replacement cyclical therapy. (Note the risks.)

Adjunctive and palliative therapy for advanced and metastatic endometrial or breast cancer (Megace). Megace is also used for the anorexia, weight loss, and cachexia associated with acquired immunodeficiency syndrome (AIDS).

Depo-Provera, 100–500 mg IM weekly to monthly has been used in the management of paraphilia (sexual deviancy in males), especially for pedophilia and sexual sadism. The drug has been shown to decrease erotic cravings, but sexual deviance usually returns following discontinuance of the drug.

Side effects of continuous progestin use can include:

Menstrual irregularity and amenorrhea, breakthrough bleeding, and spotting

Edema and weight gain

Nausea

Breast tenderness, enlargement, and secretion

Jaundice, rash, and pruritus

Headache and migraine

Mental depression

✦ Thromboembolic disorders

Vision disorders

Possible decrease in bone density with prolonged use

Contraindications with progestin (similar to cautions with estrogen) apply to:

Any condition that might be aggravated by fluid retention (e.g., asthma, seizures, migraine, and cardiac or renal dysfunction)

History of mental depression

History of thromboembolic disorders, especially with tobacco smoking

History of cerebrovascular accident

Liver disorders

Undiagnosed vaginal bleeding

Pregnancy (progestins are no longer used to treat threatened abortion because of the potential adverse effects to the fetus)

Breast, cervical, uterine, vaginal cancers (except for palliative treatment)

See Table 24-2 for a summary of the estrogens and progestins. Several different estrogen-progestin combinations are commercially available. Refer to the discussion of each individual agent.

Table 24-2 Estrogens, Progestins, and Contraceptive Agents

GENERIC NAME	TRADE NAME[A]	DOSAGE	USES
Estrogens			
estradiol	Estrace	PO, intravaginal	Menopause, prostate cancer, breast cancer, dysfunctional uterine bleeding
	Estrasorb, EstroGel	Topical, emulsion, gel	Only for menopausal symptoms
	Estraderm, Vivelle, Depo-Estradiol	Transdermal, IM, dose varies	
conjugated estrogens	Premarin	PO, vaginal cream parenteral; dose varies with condition symptoms	Female hypogonadism, breast engorgement, prostate cancer, menopausal sx.
esterified estrogens	Estratab, Ogen	PO, vaginal cream dose varies with condition	Female hypogonadism, prostate cancer, menopausal symptoms; dysfunctional uterine bleeding
Progestins			
medroxyprogesterone	Provera	PO tabs	Abnormal uterine bleeding, menopausal symptoms, contraception
	Depo-Provera	IM, dose varies	
megestrol acetate	Megace	PO 160–800 mg daily, div. doses	Endometrial and breast cancer, anorexia, and cachexia of AIDS

Table 24-2 Estrogens, Progestins, and Contraceptive Agents (continued)

GENERIC NAME	TRADE NAME[A]	DOSAGE	USES
Estrogen-Progestin Combinations			
conjugated estrogens/ medroxyprogesterone	Premphase, Prempro	PO, dose varies	For menopausal symptoms For female hypogonadism, menopausal symptoms
estradiol/norethindrone	CombiPatch	Transdermal, 1 patch 2×/wk (q3–4 days)	
Contraceptive Agents[a]			
Monophasic Preparations			
50 mcg estrogen	Ovral Ovcon-50	PO	Contain the same proportion of estrogen and progesterone in each tablet
35 mcg estrogen	Norinyl 1/50 Norinyl 1/35 Brevicon Ortho-Cyclen	PO	
30 mcg estrogen	Lo-Ovral Loestrin Yasmin	PO	
20 mcg estrogen	Loestrin	PO	
	Ortho Evra	Transdermal	1 patch q7days for 3 wk/cycle
Biphasic Preparation—2 sequences progestin/1 part estrogen			
35 mcg estrogen	Ortho-Novum 10/11 Neocon 10/11	PO	
Triphasic Preparations—3 sequences progestin/1 part estrogen			
	Seasonale/Triphasil Ortho-Novum 7/7/7 Tri-Cyclen	PO, dose varies	
Progestin-Only Preparations			
	Micronor/Ovrette	PO	
	Depo-Provera	IM, 150 mg q3m	
	Mirena	Intrauterine device (IUD)	
Postcoital Contraception			
	Ovral	PO, 2 tabs q12h for total of 4 tabs (must be administered within 72 h)	
estrogen/progestin	Preven	Dosage, see Ovral	Emergency contraceptive kit
mifepristone RU486	Mifeprex	PO 600 mg one time then 2 days later PO misoprostol 400 mg	***Follow protocol carefully!***

Note: Because of adverse side effects, estrogen and progestin products should be administered at the lowest possible dose for effectiveness.

[a]List of trade names is not all-inclusive as the number of available oral contraceptives are too numerous to mention.

Contraceptive Agents

The use of estrogen-progestin combined hormones as a safe and effective method of birth control has been well established. They act by suppressing release of the pituitary hormones, follicle-stimulating hormone (FSH), and luteinizing hormone (LH), thus resulting in the prevention of ovulation. Additional methods of action have been suggested; that is, changes in the cervical mucus to prevent sperm penetration and changes in the endometrium or lining to the uterus to discourage implantation and cell growth.

The *progestin-only* **contraceptives** prevent pregnancy by inhibiting ovulation, changing the amount or thickness of cervical mucus, thus inhibiting sperm transport, and creating a thin, atrophic endometrium not conducive to sustaining the fertilized ovum. The progestin-only preparations may be indicated for women who cannot tolerate estrogenic side effects or for whom estrogen is contraindicated. Examples would be estrogen-related headaches, or hypertension. Other indications include breast-feeding women, since *progestin has no effect on lactation or nursing infants.* Young women who have a history of noncompliance on oral contraceptives might benefit from injections or intrauterine devices (IUDs). The failure rate for progestin-only preparations ranges from 0.1%–0.3% for injections and implants, and 2%–3% for IUDs.

Uses of *combined* or *progestin-only* contraceptives include:

Prevention of pregnancy.

Treatment and/or improvement of other medical conditions, such as endometriosis; painful, heavy periods; irregular cycles; and acne.

Other medical benefits of oral contraceptives include decreased incidence of ovarian cysts, ovarian or endometrial cancer, benign breast disease, and ectopic pregnancy. There is also a protective effect against pelvic inflammatory disease.

Minor side effects of contraceptives include:

Nausea

Increased breast size, tenderness

Fluid retention

Weight gain or loss

Bleeding between periods, breakthrough bleeding

Scanty menstrual flow (considered a benefit)

Changes in libido

Mood changes

Facial discoloration

Serious side effects of estrogen can include:

Migraine headaches or headaches increasing in frequency and severity

Severe depression

Blurred vision or loss of vision

Absolute contraindications for estrogen products include:

> Thrombophlebitis or thromboembolic disorder or history thereof
>
> History of cerebrovascular accident
>
> Known or suspected history of breast cancer or other estrogen-dependent malignancy, or preexisting cervical cancer.
>
> Pregnancy
>
> History of liver disease or impaired liver function

In addition to the preceding contraindications, estrogen-progestin contraceptives should be used with caution in the following conditions:

> Women over 35 and currently smoking 15 or more cigarettes a day
>
> Migraine headaches that start after initiating oral contraceptives
>
> Hypertension with resting diastolic above 90 or systolic above 140
>
> Diabetes mellitus
>
> Undiagnosed vaginal bleeding
>
> Confirmed sickle cell disease
>
> Lactation
>
> Oral contraceptives may accelerate development of gallbladder disease in women already susceptible

Interactions of estrogen products may occur with:

> Many drugs may interact with oral contraceptives and alter the effectiveness, including pain relievers, alcohol, anticoagulants, antidepressants, tranquilizers or barbiturates, corticosteroids, antibiotics, asthma drugs, beta-blockers, anticonvulsants, oral hypoglycemic drugs, and vitamin C.

Patient Education

Women taking oral contraceptives should be instructed regarding the use of backup contraception for the first month on oral contraceptives, and for the first 2 weeks with Depo-Provera.

Taking the contraceptive at the same time every day. If oral contraceptives are missed, the general instruction is that the pill should be doubled up until the patient has caught up, using a backup method until period begins. If three pills or more are missed, the patient is instructed to throw away the pack until she starts her period, and then begin a new pack of pills. Stop oral contraceptives if pregnancy is suspected and stop smoking.

Use backup contraception when taking other medicines that may alter effectiveness (see Interactions).

Reporting the following symptoms to your health care provider should they occur while on oral contraceptives: chest pain, severe headache, dizziness, weakness, numbness, eye problems, or severe leg pains in the calf or thigh.

CHOICE OF CONTRACEPTIVES

Estrogen-progestin oral contraceptives are available in several formulations and varieties of chemical preparations. They are usually classified according to their estrogen content and formulation as follows:

1. Monophasic preparations contain the same proportion of estrogen and progestin in each tablet.

2. Biphasic preparations contain two sequences of progestin doses and less than 50 mcg estrogen.

3. Triphasic preparations contain three sequences of progestin doses and less than 50 mcg estrogen.

Choice of a particular contraceptive will be made after considering the patient's history, hormone-related side effects, prior use, and desired effect. In general, whenever possible the smallest dose of estrogen and progestin should be used that is compatible with a low failure rate and meets the individual needs of the woman. Broad categories are listed in Table 24-2. Individual oral contraceptives are too numerous to mention in their entirety; however, a few examples in each category are included.

Progestin-Only Contraceptives

These preparations are recommended for patients who do not tolerate estrogen or in whom it is contraindicated. Choice of method of delivery (i.e., oral tablets, injection, or IUD) should be made to appropriately accommodate the patient's needs and compliance.

Progestin-Containing Intrauterine Device (IUD)

Mirena contains a reservoir of levonorgestrel, a synthetic progestin. It releases small amounts of progesterone daily, providing five years of continuous contraception protection. The mechanism of action of the IUD is not fully understood but is generally thought to have an inhibitory effect on sperm migration, change in the ovum transport, and alteration of the endometrium. The progestin in the IUD is thought to offer support to all of these actions.

Cautions and side effects can include:

There are many considerations, contraindications, and side effects that must be addressed when considering the IUD as a method of contraception. These are too numerous to mention in this text. The purpose of including the IUD here is to inform the reader that it is one of several delivery systems in the use of progestin as a contraceptive drug.

Postcoital Contraception

While the use of combined estrogen-progestin contraceptive pills as a means of postcoital contraception is not without risk, it is an available option to women who are exposed to an unintentional risk of pregnancy.

This includes such circumstances as a broken condom, rape, defective barrier methods, lost or forgotten oral contraceptives, or any other method that is not available at the time that it is needed. When using post-coital or "morning after" contraception, it is essential that the woman's history is reviewed, that she is informed of the risks and benefits of post-coital contraception, and that she gives informed consent. It must be administered within 72 h of unprotected intercourse. Typical dosages for oral contraceptives in this instance would be Ovral, two tablets taken in two doses, 12 h apart, for a total of four tablets, or Lo\Ovral, Nordette, or Triphasil, four tablets taken in two doses, 12 h apart. Side effects, which include nausea and vomiting, headache, and breast tenderness, usually subside within one or two days after treatment. Again, it must be noted that postcoital contraception must be administered within 72 h of unprotected intercourse.

Emergency Contraceptive Kit

Preven is an emergency contraceptive kit containing a pregnancy test and 4 tablets of an estrogen/progestin combination. If the user is not pregnant, the kit instructs her to swallow a first dose of two pills as soon as possible but within 72 h after having unprotected sex. The second dose of 2 pills must be taken 12 h after the first dose. Taken within three days of sexual intercourse, this medication prevents ovulation, or if ovulation has already occurred, *blocks implantation of a fertilized egg*. It is not considered a form of abortion because it does not work if a fertilized egg has already implanted itself in the uterus, the scientific definition of pregnancy.

Mifepristone (RU-486)

Mifepristone (Mifeprex) is an antiprogesterone drug that is used to terminate an unwanted pregnancy. There are detailed requirements (including informed consent) to ensure that women fully understand the process. The drug is sold directly to trained doctors and is not available in pharmacies. Patient education (*Mifepristone Medication Guide*) is very important for the proper administration for this drug treatment.

Mifepristone is only for use very early in pregnancy—within 49 days from the beginning of a woman's last menstrual period. Mifepristone blocks the action of progesterone, a hormone essential for maintaining pregnancy. Without progesterone, the uterine lining thins, so the embryo cannot remain implanted and grow. It requires three visits to a qualified physician to complete the treatment:

1. At the first visit, the physician will determine the gestational status. If the woman qualifies for the procedure, she must sign an informed consent, agreeing to the necessary visits. She will then receive three mifepristone pills to be taken by mouth.

2. The second step requires the woman to swallow a second drug two days later to fully detach the embryo from the uterus and expel it. Misoprostol (Cytotec) causes uterine contractions with miscarriage-like cramping and bleeding.

3. The third step requires a follow-up visit to the physician within two weeks to make sure the abortion is complete. In case of

hemorrhage, it might be necessary to consult the physician sooner. Studies have shown that mifepristone is 77%–92% effective in terminating pregnancy. However, in some cases, a curettage of the uterine cavity is required to remove any remaining products of conception.

Side effects of mifepristone can include:

- Diarrhea, nausea
- Uterine hemorrhage in about 5% of patients
- Infection—if the embryo is not completely expelled
- A malformed child if the second and third steps are not completed

Contraindications of mifepristone include:

- Ectopic pregnancy
- Any time after 49 days from the beginning of the woman's last menstrual period
- Current long-term corticosteroid therapy
- Bleeding disorders
- Current anticoagulant therapy

See Table 24-2 for a summary of estrogens, progestins, and contraceptive agents.

Patient Education

Patients taking estrogen, progesterone, or combinations of the two should be instructed regarding:

Importance of following prescribed schedule with contraceptives

Taking with or after evening meal or at bedtime, same time every day

Minor adverse effects of contraceptives, for example, edema, weight gain, nausea

Possible serious side effects and the importance of reporting any signs of cardiovascular or kidney disorders, liver or gallbladder dysfunction, rash, jaundice, GI symptoms, visual disturbance, severe headache, breast lumps, irregular vaginal bleeding, shortness of breath, and chest or calf pain

Increased risk of stroke or myocardial infarction (MI) for smokers

Regular breast self-examination

Complete physical examination including Pap test at least yearly

Avoidance of all estrogen or progestin products if pregnant or nursing

DRUGS FOR LABOR AND DELIVERY

In addition to the hormones secreted by the anterior pituitary gland, there is also a hormone secreted by the posterior pituitary lobe: **oxytocin.** This hormone stimulates the uterus to contract, thus inducing childbirth. Oxytocin also acts on the mammary gland to stimulate the release of milk. Synthetic chemicals used to stimulate uterine contractions are called *oxytocics* and include *oxytocin* and prostaglandin E_1 and E_2.

Oxytocin

Uses of oxytocin (IV infusion of dilute solutions slowly and at a carefully monitored rate) include:

Induction of labor with at-term or near-term pregnancies associated with hypertension (e.g., preeclampsia, eclampsia, or cardiovascular-renal disease), maternal diabetes, or uterine fetal death at term

Stimulating uterine contractions during the first or second stages of labor if labor is prolonged or if dysfunctional uterine inertia occurs

Pelvic adequacy and other maternal and fetal conditions must be evaluated carefully prior to induction of labor. Cesarean section may be preferable and safer in some instances.

Side effects of oxytocin can be serious, resulting even in maternal or fetal death. *Extreme caution* with administration and *constant maternal* and *fetal monitoring* are required to prevent dangerous side effects such as:

* Tetanic contractions with risk of uterine rupture

  Cervical lacerations
* Abruptio placenta

  Impaired uterine blood flow

  Amniotic fluid embolism
* Fetal trauma, including intracranial hemorrhage or brain damage
* Fetal cardiac arrhythmias, including bradycardia, tachycardia, and premature ventricular contractions
* Fetal death due to asphyxia

  With large amounts of oxytocin, watch for:
* Severe hypotension
* Tachycardia and arrhythmias
* Postpartum hemorrhage

  Subarachnoid hemorrhage

  Hypertensive episodes

Contraindications for oxytocin include:

Elective induction of labor merely for physician or patient convenience, which is *not* a valid indication for oxytocin use

Cephalopelvic disproportion, unfavorable fetal position or presentation

Uterine or cervical scarring from major cervical or uterine surgery

Fetal distress when delivery is not imminent

Placenta previa, prolapsed cord, and multiparity

Prolonged use with eclampsia

Prostaglandins

Prostaglandins include dinoprostone or prostaglandin E_2 (Prostin E_2, Cervidil, Prepidil) and the oral synthetic prostaglandin E_1 analog, misoprostol (Cytotec).

Uses of dinoprostone intravaginal gel or vaginal insert include:

Cervical ripening

Uses of dinoprostone vaginal suppositories include:

Therapeutic abortion in the second trimester (beyond the 12th week)

Uterine evacuation in cases of intrauterine fetal death in late pregnancy, benign hydatidiform mole, or fetuses with acephaly, erythroblastosis fetalis, or other congenital abnormalities *incompatible with life*

Side effects of prostaglandins can be minimized by administration of a prior test dose and symptomatic treatment of such effects as:

 GI hypermotility, including nausea, vomiting, diarrhea—decreased by premedication with antiemetics and antidiarrhea agents

Bradycardia, hypotension, hypertension, and arrhythmias

Dizziness, syncope, flushing, and fever

Bronchospasm, including wheezing, dyspnea, chest constriction, and chest pain

Cervical laceration or uterine rupture (less common)

Retained placenta (less common)

Contraindications and precautions for prostaglandins include:

Use only by trained physicians in a hospital where intensive care and surgical facilities are available

Contraindicated with history of pelvic surgery, uterine fibroids, cervical stenosis, and acute pelvic inflammatory disease

Caution with asthma, hypertension, and cardiovascular or renal disease

Previous history of C-section

Methylergonovine

Use of this ergot alkaloid, Methergine, includes prevention and treatment of postpartum and postabortion hemorrhage.

Side effects of Methergine occur most commonly when administered IV undiluted or too rapidly, or in conjunction with regional anesthesia or vasoconstrictors, and can include:

✴ Nausea and vomiting

✴ Dizziness, headache, diaphoresis, palpitation, dyspnea, and arrhythmias

Hypertension (less common)

Numbness and coldness of extremities with overdose

Seizures with overdose

Contraindications of Methergine include:

When administered during third stage of labor, may lead to retained placenta

Contraindicated with cardiovascular disease, especially hypertension, and with hepatic and renal impairment

Patients with preeclampsia or eclampsia

Terbutaline

Terbutaline (Brethine), although classified as a bronchodilator drug primarily used for pulmonary disorders, is also used with careful monitoring in the management of preterm labor. Its sympathomimetic action inhibits uterine contractions by smooth muscle relaxation. Although the manufacturer does not recommend its use for preterm labor at this time, it is widely used for this purpose with careful monitoring, both in the hospital setting and with home uterine monitoring. It is available for oral or subcutaneous administration.

Side effects of terbutaline include:

✴ Nervousness, tremors, increased heart rate, headache, nausea, vomiting, heart palpitations. Side effects tend to be less severe with a subcutaneous pump, rather than PO.

Caution with terbutaline applies to:

Watching patient closely for signs of pulmonary edema. Should not be used in patients with hypertension, cardiac disease, hyperthyroidism, diabetes, or history of seizures.

Note: At this time, the manufacturer does not recommend that terbutaline be used for tocolysis in preterm labor. The safety of use of this drug for this purpose has not been adequately established. Therefore, the expected therapeutic benefit must be weighed against its possible hazards to mother and fetus.

Magnesium Sulfate

Treatment of severe preeclampsia or eclampsia consists of magnesium sulfate injection for prevention and control of seizures. Magnesium sulfate acts by depressing the CNS and blocking neuromuscular transmission, thus producing anticonvulsant effects. Magnesium sulfate has also been used in the management of uterine tetany associated with the use of oxytocic agents. Magnesium sulfate also acts peripherally, producing vasodilation and lowering the blood pressure. Patients receiving this drug must be monitored closely for vital signs and reflexes.

Side effects of magnesium sulfate, which can be serious and even fatal, can include:

* Flaccid paralysis and CNS depression
* Circulatory collapse, cardiac depression, and hypotension
* Fatal respiratory paralysis

Flushing and sweating

The antidote for overdose of magnesium sulfate (e.g., respiratory depression or heart block) is IV administration of calcium gluconate.

Contraindications or extreme caution when using magnesium sulfate applies to:

Impaired renal function

Heart block or myocardial damage

Use more than 24 h before delivery and within 2 h of delivery because of potential respiratory depression in the neonate

See Table 24-3 for a summary of drugs for labor, delivery.

Table 24-3 Drugs for Labor, Delivery, and Postpartum

GENERIC NAME	TRADE NAME	DOSAGE	COMMENTS
Oxytocics[a]			
methylergonovine	Methergine	PO, IM; dosage varies	For postpartum hemorrhage
oxytocin	Pitocin	IV, nasal spray	For induction of labor, postpartum hemorrhage
Prostaglandins			
dinoprostone	Prostin E$_2$	Vaginal supp. 20 mg	For therapeutic abortion
	Cervidil	Vaginal insert	For cervical ripening
	Prepidil	Intravaginal gel	For cervical ripening
misoprostol	Cytotec	Tablets	For pregnancy termination
Adrenergic[b]			
terbutaline	Brethine	IV, PO, dose varies	For premature labor
Treatment for Preeclampsia or Eclampsia			
magnesium sulfate		IM, IV; dosage varies	Watch for respiratory complications

[a]Stimulate uterine contractions.

[b]Inhibit uterine contractions in preterm labor.

OTHER GONADOTROPIC DRUGS

Drugs classified as analogs of *gonadotropin-releasing hormones* (GnRH) act in the pituitary to suppress ovarian and testicular hormone production and inhibit estrogen and androgen synthesis. Leuprolide (Lupron) has been used as an antineoplastic agent to inhibit the growth of hormone-dependent tumors. It has been used to reduce the size of the prostate and inhibit prostatic tumor growth. It has also been used following other therapies, for example mastectomy, radiation, and/or other antineoplastic drugs to treat breast cancer. Lupron is sometimes combined with the antiestrogen drug tamoxifen in the treatment of breast cancer (see Chapter 14 for dosage and side effects).

GnRH analogs that inhibit gonadotropin secretion, for example Lupron and Synarel, are used in the management of endometriosis. They inhibit ovulation and stop menstruation, thereby providing pain relief and a reduction in endometriotic lesions. Lupron is administered as a monthly IM injection. Synarel is administered as a nasal spray. Treatment with either is limited to six months. They appear to be better tolerated than the androgen, danazol, in the treatment of endometriosis.

Lupron is also the drug of choice for precocious puberty in children. Experimental studies indicate other potential uses for Lupron, for example as a male contraceptive agent, but the long-term safety and contraceptive efficacy of this therapy have not been determined.

Side effects of the GnRH agonists can include:

* Hot flashes
  Vaginal dryness
* Headache and insomnia
  Emotional or mood swings
  Weight gain or loss
  Nasal congestion
  Acne

Cautions and contraindications apply to:

Not to be considered effective as a contraceptive; patient should use a backup barrier method.

Not safe during pregnancy or lactation.

Prolonged use creates a hypoestrogenic state that may lead to an increased risk of loss of bone density.

Patients must be fully informed of the benefits and risks of the use of GnRH analog drugs and, generally speaking, the therapeutic values should outweigh any potential risks. Patient compliance is enhanced with adequate patient education, counseling, and support.

INFERTILITY DRUGS
Clomiphene Citrate (Clomid)

Clomiphene is an orally administered, nonsteroidal agent that may induce ovulation in selected anovulatory women. Its chief action is to stimulate the pituitary gland to release more FSH and LH, resulting in the maturation and release of mature follicles from the ovary.

Side effects of Clomid can include:

米 Ovarian enlargement, vasomotor flashes, breast tenderness, nausea and/or vomiting, nervousness, and insomnia. While the incidence of multiple pregnancies increases with use of clomiphene, 90% in one study were single pregnancies, 10% were twins, and less than 1% resulted in triplets.

Cautions with Clomid apply to:

Thorough evaluation to ensure that the patient is an appropriate candidate for clomiphene therapy is essential. The drug should not be given to women with a known ovarian cyst or known cancer of the endometrium, pregnant women, or women with undiagnosed vaginal bleeding or any liver, thyroid, adrenal, or intracranial disorder.

Menotropins for Injection (Repronex)

Repronex is a purified preparation of gonadotropin containing equal amounts of FSH and LH. It is injected IM to stimulate follicle development in the ovaries. In order to trigger ovulation, human chorionic gonadotropin (hCG) is given at the appropriate time to effect release of the mature follicles from the ovary. Repronex may also be given to men, along with hCG, to stimulate spermatogenesis.

Side effects of Repronex can include:

米 Ovarian enlargement with or without ovarian cysts

米 GI symptoms such as nausea, vomiting, or abdominal cramping

Dizziness

Cautions and contraindications of Repronex are:

Similar to clomiphene. Patients must be thoroughly and appropriately assessed and evaluated to ensure that they are candidates for treatment with Repronex and hCG.

Chorionic Gonadotropin (Profasi)

Chorionic gonadotropin (CG) is used to induce ovulation in women who have been appropriately treated with menotropins. This drug is given as a single IM dose one day following the course of therapy with Repronex.

Chorionic gonadotropin (CG) has also been used in the treatment of prepubertal cryptorchidism and hypogonadism resulting from pituitary deficiency. Treatment of such conditions should be managed by an endocrinologist.

Side effects of CG can include:

米 Headache, irritability, restlessness, depression, fatigue, and edema

Contraindications apply to:

Any known neoplasm or prior allergic reaction to CG

Urofollitropin for Injection (Bravelle)

Bravelle is a preparation containing FSH extracted from the urine of post-menopausal women. It has little or no LH activity. It is indicated for the induction of ovulation in women with polycystic ovarian disease who have an elevated LH level and a low to normal FSH level, and are unresponsive to clomiphene therapy. Like Repronex, ovulation is induced following the administration of Bravelle by using an injection of CG. It is administered IM for 7–12 days.

Side effects of Bravelle can include:

- Nausea, vomiting, or abdominal cramping
- Headache
- Breast tenderness
- Ovarian enlargement

Caution and contraindications apply to:

Bravelle should not be administered to patients who have demonstrated a hypersensitivity to gonadotropins, women with increased levels of FSH that would indicate ovarian failure, abnormal or undiagnosed bleeding, or pregnancy.

See Table 24-4 for a summary of other gonadotropin-associated drugs.

Table 24-4 Other Gonadotropin Associated Drugs

GENERIC NAME	TRADE NAME	DOSAGE	COMMENTS
nafarelin acetate	Synarel	Nasal spray, dose varies	For endometriosis, treatment not to exceed 6 months
leuprolide acetate	Lupron Depot	IM dose varies	For endometriosis, some cases of infertility, treatment not to exceed 6 months; also for prostate cancer (see Antineoplastics)
clomiphene citrate	Clomid, Seraphene	PO dose varies	For treatment of infertility, ovulation induction
menotropins	Repronex	IM daily for 7–12 days	Treatment of infertility, stimulates follicle development
chorionic gonadotropin (CG)	Profasi, Pregnyl	IM single dose, 5–10,000 units	For treatment of infertility, given 1 day after Repronex, to induce ovulation
urofollitropin	Bravelle	subQ, IM daily for 7–12 days	For induction of ovulation in women with polycystic ovaries followed with injections of CG

WORKSHEET FOR CHAPTER 24
REPRODUCTIVE SYSTEM DRUGS

List the drugs according to category and complete all columns.
Learn generic or trade names as specified by instructor.

Classifications and Drugs	Purpose	Side Effects	Contraindications or Cautions	Patient Education
Androgens 1. testosterone 2. danazol 3. Estratest				
Impotence Agents 1. Viagra 2. Cialis 3. Levitra				
Estrogens 1. Premarin 2. estradiol (Estrace) 3. Menest, Ogen				
Progestins 1. Provera/Depo-Provera 2. Megace				

Classifications and Drugs	Purpose	Side Effects	Contraindications or Cautions	Patient Education
Contraceptives 1. Estrogen-Progestin combinations 2. Progestin only Micronor/Ovrette PO Depo-Provera IM Mirena IUD 3. Postcoital Contraceptives Ovral Preven Mifeprex (RU 486)				
For Labor and Delivery 1. Oxytocics Pitocin 2. Prostaglandins Cervidil, Prepidill, Prostin E₂ Cytotec (misoprostol) 3. Andrenergics Brethine 4. Magnesium sulfate				
Other Gonadotropics GnRH analogs 1. Lupron 2. Synarel				
Ovulation Induction 1. Clomid 2. chorionic gonadotropin (CG) 3. Metrodin				

A. Case Study for Reproductive System Drugs

May B., age 38, visits her obstetrician's office for her 6-week postpartum checkup. She smokes. She has a history of thrombophlebitis. She plans to continue nursing her baby. She asks the doctor for a prescription for Ortho-Novum for birth control purposes. She needs all of the following information.

1. Which would be the only appropriate contraceptive type for her?
   a. Estrogen only
   b. Progestin only
   c. Estrogen-progestin combination
   d. Postcoital contraceptive

2. Contraceptives containing estrogen are not advised in which conditions?
   a. History of thrombophlebitis
   b. Coronary artery disease
   c. Lactation
   d. All of the above
   e. Only (a) and (c)

3. Progestin-only contraceptives are available in all of the following forms EXCEPT
   a. Tablets
   b. Suppository
   c. Intramuscular
   d. IUD

4. Side effects of estrogen products can include all of the following EXCEPT
   a. Severe headaches
   b. Depression
   c. Heavy menstrual flow
   d. Fluid retention
   e. Blurred vision

5. Those more at risk for complications with estrogen therapy include all of the following EXCEPT
   a. Diabetics
   b. Smokers
   c. With pernicious anemia
   d. With gallbladder problems

6. Those taking combination birth control pills would be wise to avoid all of the following EXCEPT
   a. Asthma drugs
   b. Antibiotics
   c. Antidepressants
   d. Tobacco
   e. Sex

B. Case Study for Reproductive System Drugs

I. M. Puny, a 16-year-old male weighing 100 pounds, asks the physician to prescribe some "steroids" to improve his physique and increase the size of his muscles. He needs to be given the following information about androgens.

1. Androgens are used in all of the following conditions EXCEPT
   a. Delayed puberty in male
   b. Endometriosis in female
   c. Testicular malfunction
   d. Impaired growth

2. Side effects of androgens can include all of the following EXCEPT
   a. Jaundice
   b. Impotence
   c. Growth spurts
   d. Fluid retention

3. The following statements are true of illegal anabolic steroids EXCEPT
   a. Can cause psychosis
   b. Can stunt growth
   c. Synthetic testosterone
   d. FDA approved

4. Androgens are generally contraindicated in all of the following
    EXCEPT
    a. Diabetics
    b. Cryptorchidism
    c. Geriatric males
    d. Prepubertal males

Note: Always explain medical information in terms the patient can understand.

CHAPTER REVIEW QUIZ

Match the mediation in the first column with the conditions they are used to treat. Conditions may be used more than once.

Medication	Condition
1. _____ Premarin	**A.** Endometriosis
2. _____ Megace	**B.** Menopausal symptoms
3. _____ Depo-Testosterone	**C.** Prostate cancer
4. _____ Danocrine	**D.** Impotence
5. _____ Estratest	**E.** Hypogonadism
6. _____ Terbutaline	**F.** Uterine inertia in labor
7. _____ Cialis	**G.** Infertility
8. _____ Levitra	**H.** Preterm labor
9. _____ Chorionic gonadotropin (CG)	**I.** Cachexia of AIDS
10. _____ Pitocin	

Choose the correct answer.

11. Androgens are used for all of the following EXCEPT:
   a. Advanced breast cancer   c. Muscle growth
   b. Fibrocystic breast disease   d. Cryptorchidism

12. Impotence agents, for example Viagra, can cause all of the following EXCEPT:
   a. Abnormal vision   c. Headache
   b. Hypertension   d. Flushing

13. Women with a uterus should not use estrogen-alone therapy because it puts them at risk for all of the following EXCEPT:
   a. Blood clots   c. Stroke
   b. Uterine cancer   d. Osteoporosis

14. Combined hormone therapy (estrogen/progestin), for example Prempro, can put posthysterectomy patients at risk for all of the following EXCEPT:
   a. Heart attack   c. Stroke
   b. Breast cancer   d. Uterine cancer

15. Estrogen uses include all of the following EXCEPT:
   a. Prostate cancer   c. Breast cancer
   b. Atrophic vaginitis   d. After rape

16. Uses of progestin-only products include all of the following EXCEPT:
   a. Cachexia of AIDS   c. Amenorrhea
   b. Threatened abortion d. Contraception

17. The following statements are true of RU486 therapy EXCEPT:

    a. For very early pregnancy   c. Blocks progesterone

    b. Available in pharmacies   d. Three-step procedure

18. Use of oxytocin for labor induction can have the following serious side effects EXCEPT:

    a. Prolapsed cord   c. Fetal trauma

    b. Cervical laceration   d. Abruptio placenta

19. Magnesium sulfate, used to treat eclampsia, can have the following serious side effects EXCEPT:

    a. CNS depression   c. Apnea

    b. Hypertensive crisis   d. Bradycardia

20. Methergine, used for postpartum hemorrhage, can have the following effects EXCEPT:

    a. Uterine contractions   c. Hypotension

    b. Dizziness   d. Diaphoresis

Chapter 25
Cardiovascular Drugs

Key Terms

Antiarrhythmic agents

Anticoagulants

Antihypertensives

Antilipemic agents

Bradycardia

Cardiac glycosides

Cardiotonic

Colony stimulating factors

Coronary vasodilators

Digitalization

Hypertension

Hypotension

Ischemia

Platelet inhibitors

Tachycardia

Thrombolytic agents

Vasoconstrictors

Objectives

Upon completion of this chapter, the learner should be able to

1. Define the Key Terms

2. Describe the action and effects of digitalis and toxic side effects that require reporting

3. Identify the different types of antiarrhythmics and the side effects of each

4. Identify the most commonly used antihypertensives and the usual side effects, as well as the exceptions to the rule

5. Describe the different types of coronary vasodilators with cautions and side effects

6. Name the five antilipemic agents and describe their action

7. Compare and contrast heparin and coumarin derivatives in terms of administration, action, and antidotes

8. Explain appropriate and important patient education for each of the nine categories of cardiovascular drugs

9. Describe platelet inhibitor therapy and appropriate patient education regarding it

Cardiovascular drugs include medications that affect the heart and blood vessels as well as the anticoagulants. The drugs described in this chapter are divided into nine categories: cardiac glycosides, antiarrhythmic agents, antilipemic agents, antihypertensives, vasodilators, vasoconstrictors, anticoagulants, platelet inhibitors, and thrombolytic agents. Some of the drugs described in this chapter fall into more than one category because of multiple actions and uses (e.g., propranolol, which is used to treat cardiac arrhythmias, hypertension, and angina). Diuretics, which also affect the blood vessels and reduce blood pressure, are discussed in Chapter 15. Autonomic Nervous System effects of these drugs are explained in Chapter 13.

CARDIAC GLYCOSIDES

Cardiac glycosides occur widely in nature or can be prepared synthetically. They have been called **cardiotonic** because they strengthen the heartbeat. These glycosides act directly on the myocardium to increase the force of myocardial contractions. Cardiac glycosides are used primarily in the treatment of congestive heart failure. They are sometimes also used in conjunction with antiarrhythmic agents to *slow* the heart rate in certain types of **tachycardia** or atrial fibrillation or flutter.

In patients with congestive heart failure, the heart fails to pump adequately to remove excess fluids from the pulmonary circulation, and pulmonary congestion results. The heart increases in size to compensate for the increased work load. Symptoms of congestive heart failure are dyspnea, cyanosis, increased heart rate, cough, and pitting edema.

In patients with congestive heart failure, the cardiac glycosides act by *increasing the force of the cardiac contractions* without increasing oxygen consumption, thereby increasing cardiac output. As a result of increased efficiency, the heart beats slowly, the heart size shrinks, and the diuretic action decreases edema.

The most commonly used cardiac glycosides are digitalis products. Of these, digoxin (Lanoxin) is used the most frequently because it can be administered orally and parenterally and has intermediate duration of action.

Digitalization is the process of establishing the correct therapeutic dose of digitalis for maintaining optimal functioning of the heart without toxic effects. There is a very narrow margin between effective therapy and dangerous toxicity. Careful monitoring of cardiac rate and rhythm with EKG (electrocardiogram), cardiac function, side effects, and blood digitalis level is required to determine the therapeutic maintenance dose. Checking the apical pulse before administering digitalis is an important part of this monitoring process. If the apical pulse rate is less than 60, digitalis should be withheld until the physician is consulted. The action taken should be documented.

Modification of dosage is based on individual requirements and response as determined by general condition, renal function, and cardiac function, monitored by EKG. When changing from tablets or IM therapy to liquid-filled capsules or IV therapy, digoxin dosage adjustments may be required.

Toxic side effects of digitalis, which should be reported to the physician immediately, can include:

* Anorexia, nausea, and vomiting (early signs of toxicity)
  Abdominal cramping, distention, and diarrhea

* Headache, fatigue, lethargy, and muscle weakness
* Vertigo, restlessness, irritability, tremors, and seizures
* Visual disturbances including blurring, diplopia, or halos
* Cardiac arrhythmias of all kinds, especially bradycardia (rate less than 60)
* Electrolyte imbalance
* Insomnia, confusion, and mental disorders, especially with older adults

Treatment of digitalis toxicity includes:

Discontinuing the drug immediately (usually sufficient)

Monitoring electrolytes for hyperkalemia and especially hypokalemia

Drugs such as atropine for severe bradycardia

Antiarrhythmics if indicated

Digoxin immune Fab as antidote in life-threatening toxicity

Contraindications or extreme caution applies to:

Severe pulmonary disease

Hypothyroidism

Acute myocardial infarction, acute myocarditis, severe heart failure

Impaired renal function

Arrhythmias not caused by heart failure

Pregnancy and lactation

High doses in older adults

Interactions of digitalis may occur with:

Antacids, cholestyramine, neomycin, and rifampin reduce absorption of digitalis (administer far apart).

Diuretics, calcium, verapamil, and corticosteroids can increase chance of arrhythmias.

Antiarrhythmics, *especially* quinidine, may potentiate digitalis toxicity.

Adrenergics (epinephrine, ephedrine, and isoproterenol) increase the risk of arrhythmias.

Phenobarbital or phenytoin reduces digitalis levels.

Patient Education

Patients taking digitalis should be instructed regarding:

Recognition and immediate reporting of side effects

Holding medication, if any side effects occur, until the physician can be consulted

Avoiding taking any other medication at the same time without physician approval

Avoiding all over-the-counter (OTC) medication, especially antacids and cold remedies

Avoiding abrupt withdrawal after prolonged use; must be reduced gradually under physician supervision

Checking heart rate (pulse) and blood pressure on a regular basis

Not changing the brand or dosage form being taken—other brands or dosage forms may act differently

ANTIARRHYTHMIC AGENTS

Antiarrhythmic agents include a variety of drugs that act in different ways to suppress various types of cardiac arrhythmias, including atrial or ventricular tachycardias, atrial fibrillation or flutter, and arrhythmias that occur with digitalis toxicity or during surgery and anesthesia. The choice of a particular antiarrhythmic agent is based on careful assessment of many factors, including the type of arrhythmia; frequency; cardiac, renal, or other pathological condition; and current signs and symptoms.

The role of the health care worker is vital in this area in accurate and timely reporting of vital signs and pertinent observations regarding effectiveness of medications and adverse side effects. Adequate knowledge of drug action and effects, along with good judgment are essential.

Side effects of the individual medications are discussed separately. However, keep in mind that most of the drugs given to counteract arrhythmias have the potential for lowering blood pressure and slowing heartbeat. Therefore, it is especially important to be alert for signs of **hypotension** and **bradycardia,** which could lead to cardiac arrest. Although the antiarrhythmics commonly slow the heart rate, there are exceptions (e.g., procainamide and quinidine, which may cause *tachycardia*). When other cardiac drugs are administered concomitantly, cardiac effects may be additive or antagonistic. Antiarrhythmic agents can worsen existing arrhythmias or cause new arrhythmias and *careful monitoring is essential.*

Arrhythmia detection and monitoring can include EKG rhythm strips and 24-h Holter monitoring as indicated. Electrolyte surveillance, especially for hyperkalemia, is very important for patients on antiarrhythmic agents.

Adrenergic Blockers

Beta-adrenergic blockers, for example, propranolol (Inderal), combat arrhythmias by inhibiting adrenergic (sympathetic) nerve receptors. The action is complex, and the results can include a membrane-stabilizing effect on the heart. Propranolol (Inderal), a nonselective beta-blocker, is effective in the management of some cardiac arrhythmias and less effective with others. It is also used in the treatment of hypertension and some forms of chronic angina. Low doses of atenolol (Tenormin), a selective beta-antagonist, may be used with caution in patients with lung conditions that cause bronchospasm. For *additional* use of beta-blockers, for example with migraine, see Chapter 13.

Side effects of propranolol, especially in patients over 60 years old and more commonly with IV administration of the drug, can include:

- Hypotension, with vertigo and syncope
- Bradycardia, with heart block and cardiac arrest
- CNS symptoms (usually with long-term treatment with high doses), including dizziness, irritability, confusion, nightmares, insomnia, visual disturbances, weakness, sleepiness, lassitude, or fatigue
- GI symptoms, including nausea, vomiting, and diarrhea or constipation
- Rash or hematological effects (rare or transient)
- Bronchospasm, especially with history of asthma
- Hypoglycemia
- Impotence reported rarely

Contraindications or extreme caution with the beta-blockers applies to:

- Withdrawal after prolonged use (should always be gradual)
- Major surgery (withdrawal before surgery is controversial)
- Diabetes—may cause hypoglycemia and mask the tachycardic response to hypoglycemia
- Renal and hepatic impairment
- Asthma and allergic rhinitis—may cause bronchospasm
- Bradycardia, heart block, and congestive heart failure (CHF)
- Pediatric use, pregnancy, and lactation
- Chronic obstructive pulmonary disease (COPD)

Interactions include *antagonism* of beta-blockers by:

- Adrenergics (e.g., epinephrine and isoproterenol)
- Anticholinergics
- Tricyclic antidepressants

Potentiation of the *hypotensive effect* of propranolol occurs with:

- Diuretics and other antihypertensives, for example, calcium channel blockers
- Phenothiazine and other tranquilizers
- Cimetidine (Tagamet), which slows metabolism of drug
- Other cardiac drugs (e.g., quinidine), which may potentiate toxic effects
- Alcohol, muscle relaxants, and sedatives, which may precipitate hypotension, dizziness, confusion, or sedation

Calcium Channel Blockers

Calcium channel blockers, such as verapamil (Isoptin), counteract arrhythmias by suppressing the action of calcium in contraction of the heart muscle, thereby reducing cardiac excitability and dilating the main coronary arteries. Calcium channel blockers are also used in the treatment of angina and hypertension.

Side effects of calcium channel blockers can include:

✳ Hypotension, with vertigo, *headache*

✳ Bradycardia, with heart block

✳ Edema

✳ *Constipation,* nausea, and abdominal discomfort

Contraindications or extreme caution with calcium channel blockers applies to:

> Heart block, heart failure, or angina
> Hepatic and renal impairment
> Pregnancy and lactation
> Children

Interactions of calcium channel blockers with other cardiac drugs, for example digoxin, can potentiate both good and adverse effects. It has antagonistic effects with:

> Barbiturates
> Salicylates
> Phenytoin, rifampin
> Lithium
> Hypotensive effect potentiated with diuretics, ACE (angiotensin-converting enzyme) inhibitors, beta-blockers, and quinidine

> *Note: Do not take grapefruit juice with calcium channel blockers; adverse effects potentiated.*

Contraindicated calcium channel blockers with:

> Hypotension and heart block
> Certain arrhythmias and severe heart failure

Disopyramide

Another antiarrhythmic, similar to procainamide and quinidine, is disopyramide (Norpace), a synthetic agent that decreases myocardial excitability, inhibits conduction, and may depress myocardial contractility. It has significant anticholinergic properties.

Side effects of Norpace can include:

✳ Hypotension, dizziness, and chest pain

✳ Edema and weight gain

✳ Anticholinergic effects, including dry mouth, blurred vision, constipation, and urinary retention

> Nausea, vomiting, bloating, and gas

Contraindications of Norpace with:

Heart block and congestive heart failure

Hepatic and renal disorders

Pregnancy and lactation

Older adults—may induce heart block

Interactions of disopyramide occur with potentiation of the effects of:

Other cardiac drugs

Oral anticoagulants

Anticholinergics, antiretroviral protease inhibitors, and tricyclic antidepressants

Lidocaine

Local anesthetics (e.g., lidocaine) are administered for their antiarrhythmic effects and membrane-stabilizing action. Although lidocaine has been historically used as a first-line antiarrhythmic agent for ventricular arrhythmias, it is now considered a second choice behind other alternative agents (e.g., IV amiodarone) for the treatment of ventricular arrhythmias.

Side effects of lidocaine are usually of short duration, are dose related, and can include:

 CNS symptoms, including tremors, seizures, dizziness, confusion, and blurred vision

Hypotension, bradycardia, and heart block

Dyspnea, respiratory depression, and arrest

EKG monitoring and availability of resuscitative equipment are necessary during IV administration of lidocaine.

Contraindications or extreme caution with lidocaine applies to:

Patients hypersensitive to local anesthetics of this type (amide type)

Heart block and respiratory depression

Pregnancy, lactation, and children

Interactions of lidocaine with other cardiac drugs may be additive or antagonistic and may potentiate adverse effects. Other interactions may be of minor clinical significance since lidocaine is usually titrated to response.

Procainamide

Procainamide (Pronestyl) is usually administered orally in antiarrhythmic therapy. It is used primarily as prophylactic therapy to maintain normal rhythm after conversion by other methods. Its action is similar to that of quinidine and disopyramide. It possesses anticholinergic properties.

Side effects of procainamide are numerous and can include:

✳ Hypotension

✳ *Tachycardia,* conduction defects, asystole

✳ Hypersensitivity reactions, including rash, fever, and weakness

Blood dyscrasias, especially eosinophilia and leukopenia

Nausea and vomiting or diarrhea—more common with large dose

Contraindications with procainamide include:

Heart block and CHF

Hypersensitivity to local anesthetics of this type (ester type)

Myasthenia gravis

Pregnancy

Renal and hepatic disease caution

Systemic lupus erythematosis (SLE)

Interactions of procainamide may occur with potentiation of:

Neuromuscular blockers

Anticholinergics and tricyclic antidepressants

Other cardiac drugs

Quinidine

Quinidine (Quinaglute, Cardioquin) is one of the oldest antiarrhythmic agents. It acts by decreasing myocardial excitability and may depress myocardial contractility. Quinidine, like procainamide and disopyramide, is used primarily as prophylactic therapy to maintain normal rhythm after conversion by other methods. It is commonly administered orally in regular or timed-release tablets. It has anticholinergic properties.

Side effects of quinidine are numerous and may necessitate cessation of treatment. They may include:

✳ Diarrhea, anorexia, nausea, and vomiting, which are common

✳ *Tachycardia* and syncope

✳ Severe hypotension

✳ Vascular collapse and respiratory arrest

✳ Headache, tinnitus, vertigo, fever, and tremor

✳ Confusion and apprehension

Vision abnormalities or hearing disturbances

Blood dyscrasias, including anemia, clotting deficiencies, and leukopenia

Hepatic disorders

Precipitation of asthmatic attacks

✳ Hypoglycemia

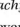

Contraindications or extreme caution with quinidine applies to:

Atrioventricular block and conduction defects

Electrolyte imbalance

Digitalis intoxication

Congestive heart failure and hypotension

Myasthenia gravis

Asthma and other respiratory disorders

Children, pregnancy, and lactation

Hepatic or renal disorders

Interactions with increased possibility of quinidine toxicity may occur with:

Muscle relaxants, neuromuscular blockers

Anticholinergics, tricyclic antidepressants, phenothiazines

Thiazide diuretics, antiretroviral protease inhibitors

Antacids or sodium bicarbonate

Anticonvulsants (e.g., phenytoin and phenobarbital) cause decreased serum levels

Other cardiac drugs, especially digitalis and antihypertensives

Anticoagulants, whose action can be potentiated by quinidine

Patient Education

Patients taking antiarrhythmics should be instructed regarding:

Immediate reporting of adverse side effects, especially palpitations, irregular or slow heartbeat, faintness, dizziness, weakness, respiratory distress, and visual disturbances

Holding medication, if there are side effects, until the physician is contacted

Rising slowly from reclining position

Modification of lifestyle to reduce stress

Mild exercise on a regular basis as approved by the physician

Not discontinuing medicine, even if the patient feels well

Taking proper dosage of medication on time, as prescribed, without skipping any dose

If medication is forgotten, not doubling the dose

Taking medication with a full glass of water on an empty stomach, one hour before or two hours after meals, so that it will be absorbed more efficiently (unless stomach upset occurs or the physician prescribes otherwise)

Avoiding taking any other medication, including OTC medicines, unless approved by the physician

Discarding expired medicines and renewing the prescription

Avoiding comparisons with other patients on similar drugs

Contacting the physician immediately with any concerns regarding medicines

See Table 25-1 for a summary of the cardiac glycoside and antiarrhythmics.

Table 25-1 Cardiac Glycoside and Antiarrhythmics

GENERIC NAME	TRADE NAME	DOSAGE	COMMENTS
Cardiac Glycoside			
digoxin	Lanoxin, Lanoxicaps	PO: tablets, liquid-filled capsules, elixir IV, dosage varies	Intermediate duration Maximum dose 0.125 mg (long term in the older adult)
Antiarrhythmics			
atenolol[a]	Tenormin	PO 50 mg daily IV 5–10 mg	Beta-blocker
propranolol[a]	Inderal	PO 10–30 mg 3–4×/day IV 0.5–3 mg	Beta-blocker
verapamil[a]	Isoptin, Calan	IV 2.5–10 mg PO 240–480 mg daily in div. doses	Calcium channel blocker
lidocaine	Xylocaine	IM or IV diluted	Local anesthetic-type **Check IV dilution directions**
☆ amiodarone	Cordarone	IV, PO, dose varies	Antiarrhythmic and vasodilator; for Medication Guide now required
☆ procainamide	Pronestyl, Procanbid	PO, dose varies IV or IM for emergency	Local anesthetic, anticholinergic
propafenone	Rythmol Rythmol SR	PO, 150–300 mg q8h PO, 225–425 mg q12h	Membrane stabilizer; for ventricular arrythmias
quinidine		PO tabs, ER, IV, IM dose varies	Myocardial depressant, anticholinergic
disopyramide	Norpace, Norpace CR	PO 150 mg q6h, or PO 300 mg q12h, extended release	Myocardial depressent, anticholinergic properties Not for older adults

☆ Sotalol

☆ antiarrythmic drugs ONLY-no other use

Note: Other antiarrhythmics are available. This is a representative sample.

[a]Has other cardiac uses. hypertension (?)

ANTIHYPERTENSIVES

Hypertension is a widespread epidemic that affects as many as one billion people worldwide. It is defined as systolic blood pressure (SBP) of 140 or greater or diastolic blood pressure (DBP) of 90 or greater. There is a strong, consistent relationship between blood pressure (BP) and the risk of cardiovascular disease (CVD). High blood pressure increases the risk of myocardial infarction, heart failure, stroke, and kidney disease and thus requires aggressive treatment.

Recently, a new category termed *prehypertension* (range of 130/80 to 139/89) was added to identify patients who are at higher cardiovascular risk based on BP and higher risk for developing sustained hypertension in later years. The purpose of this classification is to encourage patients to initiate or continue healthy lifestyle practices, rather than to begin antihypertensive drug therapy. Such practices include weight reduction (in overweight and obese patients), use of the *Dietary Approaches to Stop Hypertension* (DASH) eating plan, dietary sodium reduction, increased physical activity, modified alcohol use, and smoking cessation.

Antihypertensives (hypotensives) do not cure hypertension; they only control it. After withdrawal of the drug, BP will return to levels similar to those before treatment with medication, if all other factors remain the same. If antihypertensive therapy is to be terminated for some reason, the dosage should be gradually reduced, as abrupt withdrawal can cause rebound hypertension.

Drugs given to lower blood pressure act in various ways. The drug of choice varies according to the stage of hypertension (mild, moderate, or severe), other physical factors (especially other cardiac or renal complications), and effectiveness in individual cases. Frequently, antihypertensives are prescribed on a trial basis and then the dosage or medication is changed, and sometimes antihypertensives are combined for greater effectiveness and to reduce side effects. The health care worker must be observant of vital signs and side effects in order to assist the physician in the most effective treatment of hypertension on an individual basis.

Side effects of antihypertensives are common, and the health care worker must be observant of changes in vital signs and adverse side effects. The most common side effect of the antihypertensives is *hypotension,* especially postural hypotension. Another side effect common to many of the antihypertensives is *bradycardia.* Exceptions include hydralazine (Apresoline), which can cause tachycardia.

Thiazide Diuretics

Most patients meeting the criteria for drug therapy should be started on thiazide-type diuretics, either alone or in combination with a drug from one of the other drug classes: ACE inhibitors, angiotensin receptor blockers, beta-blockers, or calcium channel blockers. Thiazide diuretics appear to be as effective as other antihypertensive agents and, in addition, are the most cost-effective antihypertensives to date. See Chapter 15 for a detailed discussion of these agents, especially *Side effects, Contraindications or Cautions, and Interactions.*

Beta-Adrenergic and Calcium Channel Blockers

Like thiazide diuretics, beta-adrenergic blockers such as propranolol (Inderal) and atenolol (Tenormin) are generally well tolerated and are suitable for initial therapy in some patients. Beta-blockers can benefit hypertensive patients with angina, postmyocardial infarction, and certain arrythmias. Calcium channel blockers such as diltiazem (Cardizem) and nifedipine (Procardia) are an initial therapy option for hypertensive patients with diabetes or high coronary disease risk.

Refer to the discussion under Antiarrhythmic Agents earlier in this chapter for more information on these agents.

Angiotensin-Converting Enzyme (ACE) Inhibitors (ACEIs)

Another class of antihypertensives are the angiotensin-converting enzyme (ACE) inhibitors, for example, captopril or enalapril. Inhibition of ACE lowers blood pressure by *decreasing vasoconstriction*; there are not significant changes in heart rate or cardiac output. ACEIs are first- or second-line agents in the treatment of hypertension and are excellent alone, but also effective and synergistic in combination with other antihypertensives, including diuretics and calcium channel blockers.

ACEIs are especially good choices for patients who also have other serious conditions, including those with heart failure, diabetes, renal disease, and cerebrovascular disease. For example, ACEIs can be considered drugs of choice for hypertensive patients with nephropathy because they slow the progression of the renal disease.

Side effects of ACE inhibitors can include:

- Rash or photosensitivity
- Loss of taste perception
- Blood dyscrasias
- Renal impairment
- Severe hypotension
- Chronic dry cough or nasal congestion
- Hyperkalemia (monitor serum potassium levels periodically)

Contraindications or extreme caution with ACE inhibitors applies to:

- Collagen disease, for example, lupus or scleroderma
- Heart failure
- Angioedema
- Pregnancy, lactation, children

Interactions of ACE inhibitors apply to:

- Diuretics—potentiate hypotension; watch BP closely
- Vasodilators; watch BP closely
- Potassium-sparing diuretics and potassium supplements—hyperkalemia risk
- Nonsteroidal anti-inflammatory drugs (NSAIDs) and salicylates—antagonize effects of ACE inhibitors and increase deterioration of renal function

Antacids—decrease absorption

Digoxin—possible digitalis toxicity

Lithium—risk of lithium toxicity

Angiotensin Receptor Blockers (ARBs)

Angiotensin receptor blockers (ARBs) are similar to ACE inhibitors (ACEIs). Although they both block the hormone that causes vasoconstriction, they interrupt different sites. ARBs such as losartan (Cozaar) and valsartan (Diovan) block the effects of angiotensin II, decreasing blood pressure without a marked change in heart rate.

Compared to ACEIs, ARBs are associated with a lower incidence of drug-induced cough, rash, and/or taste disturbances and are used in those patients who cannot tolerate ACEIs. The addition of a low-dose thiazide diuretic to an ARB significantly improves hypertensive efficacy. ARBs are also good choices for patients with other serious conditions, including those with heart failure, diabetes, and renal disease.

Side effects are relatively uncommon in ARBs and include dizziness, upper respiratory tract infections and hyperkalemia.

Contraindications or extreme caution with ARBs applies to:

Renal impairment

Heart failure

Pregnancy, lactation, children

Interactions with ARBs are similar to those seen with ACEIs.

OTHER ANTIHYPERTENSIVES

Methyldopa

Another antihypertensive used for moderate to severe hypertension is methyldopa (Aldomet), a central-acting alpha-adrenergic agent. It is usually administered with a diuretic. It is the drug of choice for hypertension in pregnant women because of safety to the fetus.

Side effects of methyldopa can include:

 Hypotension and drowsiness

Anemia or leukopenia—rare

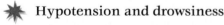 GI symptoms, including nausea, vomiting, diarrhea, constipation, and sore tongue

Sexual dysfunction

Liver disorders

Nasal congestion

Contraindications or extreme caution with methyldopa applies to:

Liver disorders

Dialysis patients

Blood dyscrasias

Older adults

Interactions of methyldopa may occur with:

Levodopa (can cause CNS effects and psychosis)

Lithium

NSAIDs, tricyclic antidepressants, sympathomimetics (leads to hypertension)

Hydralazine

Hydralazine, a peripheral vasodilator, is sometimes used in the treatment of moderate to severe hypertension, especially in patients with congestive heart failure, because it *increases* heart rate and cardiac output. The drug is generally used in conjunction with a diuretic and another hypotensive agent, for example, a beta-blocker.

Side effects of hydralazine can include:

* *Tachycardia* and palpitations

Headache and flushing

* Orthostatic hypotension

GI effects, including nausea, vomiting, diarrhea, and constipation

Blood abnormalities

* Edema and weight gain

Contraindications with hydralazine include:

Systematic lupus erythematous (SLE)

Renal disease

Coronary artery disease, rheumatic heart disease

Pregnancy, usually (however, many regard hydralazine as the antihypertensive of choice during preeclampsia)

Clonidine

Clonidine (Catapres) is a central-acting alpha-adrenergic agent, used mainly in the treatment of hypertension. It has also been used successfully in a variety of other conditions including nicotine/opiate withdrawal, vascular headaches, glaucoma, ulcerative colitis, Tourette's syndrome, and treatment of severe pain in cancer patients.

Prazosin

Prazosin (Minipres) is a *peripheral acting* alpha-adrenergic blocker used primarily to treat hypertension. Other agents in this class are used to treat (BPH) (see Chapter 15 for a discussion on the alpha-blockers).

See Table 25-2 for a summary of the antihypertensives.

Table 25-2 Antihypertensives

GENERIC NAME	TRADE NAME	DOSAGE
Beta-Adrenergic Blockers		
atenolol	Tenormin	25–100 mg PO daily
carvedilol	Coreg	6.25–25 mg PO BID w/food
metoprolol	Lopressor	100–450 mg PO daily in div. doses
	Toprol Xl[a]	50–100 mg PO daily (SR)
propranolol	Inderal	80–240 mg PO daily in 2–3 div. doses
Corgard	Inderal LA[a]	80–160 mg PO daily (SR)
Calcium Channel Blockers		
amiodipine	Norvasc	2.5–10 mg PO daily
diltiazem	Cardizem CD[a] *continued dose long-acting*	120–360 mg PO daily (SR)
	Cardizem LA[a]	
	Diltiazem SR[a] *sustained release*	120–180 mg PO BID (SR)
nifedipine	Procardia XL[a]	30–90 mg PO daily (SR)
	Adalat CC[a]	
verapamil *+antiarrythmic*	Calan SR[a], Isoptin SR[a]	120–240 mg PO 1–2×/day (SR)
ACE Inhibitors		
benazepril	Lotensin	10–20 mg 1–2×/day
captopril	Capoten	12.5–50 mg PO BID–TID
enalapril	Vasotec	5–20 mg PO BID
✶ lisinopril *no cough side effect*	Zestril	2.5–40 mg PO daily
ramipril	Altace	2.5–20 mg PO 1–2×/day
trandolapril	Mavik	1–4 mg PO daily
Angiotensin Receptor Blockers		
losartan	Cozaar	25–50 mg PO 1–2×/day
telmisartan	Micardis	20–80 mg PO daily
valsartan	Diovan	80–320 mg PO daily
Other Antihypertensives *- hydrochlorothiazides*		
clonidine *-alpha adrenergic*	Catapres - *short acting*	0.1–1.2 mg PO daily in div. doses
	Catapres TTS	Weekly patch (delivers 0.1–0.3 mg per 24 h)
hydralazine *alpha blocker → for end stage congestive heart failure last resort*		10–50 mg PO 4×/day; IV, IM dose varies
methyldopa	Aldomet	200–500 mg PO 2–4×/day
prazosin	Minipres	1–20 mg PO daily in 2–3 div. doses

[a]All extended release products (ER/SR) must be swallowed intact! Quick release of the medication can cause the blood pressure to drop suddenly, sending the patient into shock.

Note: This is only a representative list of the most commonly used drugs in this category. There are others.

Patient Education

For all antihypertensives, patients should be instructed regarding:

Immediate reporting of any adverse side effects, especially slow or irregular heartbeat, dizziness, weakness, breathing difficulty, gastric distress, and numbness or swelling of extremities

Taking medication on time as prescribed by the physician; *not* skipping a dose or doubling a dose; *not* discontinuing the medicine, even if the patient is feeling well, without consulting the physician first

Rising slowly from reclining position to reduce lightheaded feeling

Taking care in driving a car or operating machinery if medication causes drowsiness (ask the physician, nurse, or pharmacist about the specific medication, since medicines differ and individual reactions differ; older people are more susceptible to this effect)

Potentiation of adverse side effects by alcohol, especially dizziness, weakness, sleepiness, and confusion

Reduction or cessation of smoking to help lower blood pressure

Importance of diet in control of blood pressure; following the physician's instructions regarding appropriate diet for the individual, which may include a low-salt or low-sodium or weight-reduction diet if indicated

Avoiding hot tubs and hot showers, which may cause weakness or fainting

Mild exercise on a regular basis as approved by the physician

Always swallowing the extended-release products intact. Quick release of the medication into the system can cause the blood pressure to drop suddenly, causing loss of consciousness and possible shock.

Avoiding grapefruit juice while taking calcium channel blockers, which can increase the risk of hypotension and other adverse cardiac effects.

CORONARY VASODILATORS

Coronary vasodilators are used in the treatment of angina. When there is insufficient blood supply (**ischemia**) to a part, the result is acute pain. The most common form of angina is angina pectoris, chest pain resulting from decreased blood supply to the heart muscle. Obstruction or constriction of the coronary arteries results in angina pectoris. Vasodilators are administered to dilate these blood vessels and stop attacks of angina or reduce the frequency of angina when administered prophylactically.

Coronary vasodilators used in the treatment and prophylactic management of angina include nitrates, beta-blockers, and calcium channel blockers.

The nitrates used most commonly for relief of acute angina pectoris, as well as for long-term prophylactic management, are nitroglycerin and isosorbide (Isordil, Sorbitrate).

Nitroglycerin is available in several forms and can be administered in sublingual tablets allowed to dissolve under the tongue or a sublingual spray for relief of acute angina pectoris. If relief is not attained after a single dose during an acute attack, additional tablets may be administered at five-minute intervals, with *no more than three doses given in a 15-minute period.* If chest pain is not relieved after three doses, a physician should be contacted at once because unrelieved chest pain can indicate acute myocardial infarction.

Nitroglycerin is also available in timed-release capsules and tablets, and in a solution that must be diluted carefully according to the manufacturer's instructions for IV administration. Nitroglycerin tablets and capsules must be stored *only in glass containers* with tightly fitting metal screw tops away from heat. Plastic containers can absorb the medication, and air, heat, or moisture can cause loss of potency. Impaired potency of the SL tablets can be detected by the patient if there is an absence of the tingling sensation under the tongue common to this form of administration.

For long-term prophylactic management of angina pectoris, nitroglycerin is frequently applied topically as a transdermal system. One type of nitroglycerin that is absorbed through the skin is Nitro-Bid ointment, applied with an applicator-measuring (Appli-Ruler) paper. Usual dosage is 0.5–2 inches applied every eight hours. *Remove old patch first.* The ointment is spread lightly (not massaged or rubbed) over any non-hairy skin area, and the applicator paper is taped in place. Care must be taken to avoid touching the ointment when applying (accidental absorption through the skin of the fingers can cause headache). If nitroglycerin ointment is discontinued, the dose and frequency must be decreased gradually to prevent sudden withdrawal reactions. See Figure 9-1 in Chapter 9, Administration, for ointment application technique.

Another topical nitroglycerin product, which has longer action, is in transdermal form (e.g., Nitro-Dur or Transderm-Nitro). The skin patch is applied every 24 h (on in A.M./off 12 h later in the P.M.) to clean, dry, hairless areas of the upper arm or body. Do not apply below the elbow or knee. The sites should be rotated to avoid skin irritation and raw, scarred, or callused areas should be avoided. Dosage varies widely, from 2.5- to 19-mg patches. *Check prescribed dosage carefully. Remove old patch.*

Another nitrate used for acute relief of angina pectoris and for prophylactic long-term management is isosorbide. It is available in SL tablets, regular-release tablets, and timed-release capsules and tablets. When using long-acting nitrates, a 12–14 h *nitrate-free* interval between the last dose of the day and the first dose of the following day is recommended to lessen the risk of nitrate tolerance.

Side effects of the nitrates can include:

 Headache (usually diminishes over time)

 Postural hypotension, including dizziness, weakness, and syncope *(patients should be sitting during administration of fast-acting nitrates)*

Transient flushing

 Blurred vision and dry mouth (discontinue drug with these symptoms)

 Hypersensitivity reactions, enhanced by alcohol, including nausea, vomiting, diarrhea, cold sweats, tachycardia, and syncope

Contraindications or extreme caution with nitrates applies to:

Glaucoma

GI hypermotility or malabsorption (with timed-release forms)

Intracranial pressure

Severe anemia

Hypotension

Interactions of nitrates may occur with alcohol, which potentiates hypotensive effects. Phosphodiesterase (PDE) inhibitors such as sildenafil (Viagra), used for male erectile dysfunction, are contraindicated in men taking nitrates. The two drugs interact to cause a large, sudden, dangerous drop in blood pressure.

For long-term prophylactic treatment of angina pectoris, beta-blockers such as propranolol (Inderal), and calcium channel blockers, such as nifedipine (Procardia) and verapamil (Isoptin), are frequently used (see Antiarrhythmic Agents for information on side effects, etc.).

Patient Education

Patients receiving coronary vasodilators (nitrates) should be instructed regarding:

Administering fast-acting preparations (sublingual tablets or spray) while sitting down because the patient may become lightheaded

Rising slowly from a reclining position

Not drinking alcohol or taking PDE inhibitors while taking these medicines, which can cause serious drop in blood pressure

Using timed-release capsules or tablets to prevent attacks (they work too slowly to help once an attack has started)

Taking timed-release capsules or tablets on an empty stomach with a full glass of water

Allowing sublingual tablets, to dissolve under the tongue or in the cheek pouch and not chewing or swallowing them

Repeating sublingual, tablets, or spray in 5–10 min for a maximum of three tablets or sprays (if no relief of chest pain within 15–30 min, call the physician at once or report to the Emergency Room)

Not discontinuing medication suddenly if administered for several weeks (dosage must be reduced gradually under physician's supervision)

Sensations to be expected, including facial flushing, headache for a short time, lightheadedness upon rising too suddenly (if these symptoms persist or become more severe, or other symptoms occur, such as irregular heartbeat or blurred vision, notify the physician at once)

Preventing attacks of angina by administering a sublingual tablet or spray before physical exertion or emotional stress (it is preferable to avoid physical or emotional stress when possible)

See Chapter 9 for patient education regarding administration of nitroglycerin ointment or patch.

ANTILIPEMIC AGENTS

More than 100 million American adults have elevated total blood cholesterol levels above 200 mg/dl—a key risk factor for coronary heart disease (CHD). Cardiovascular disease (CHD) is the leading killer of men and women in the United States. High cholesterol can lead to arterial blockage, hardening of the arteries, blood clots, heart attack, or stroke and may even play a role in dementia.

Lipoproteins are responsible for transporting cholesterol and other fats through the blood stream. *Low-density lipoproteins* (LDLs) carry the largest amount of the cholesterol in the blood and are responsible for transporting and depositing it in arterial walls. *Very low-density lipoproteins* (VLDLs, triglycerides) are precursors of LDL and compose the largest proportion of lipids in the diet, adipose tissue, and the blood. *High-density lipoproteins* (HDLs; *good cholesterol*) help transport LDL cholesterol from the walls of the arteries through the bloodstream to the liver for excretion.

LDL cholesterol is the primary target of treatment in clinical lipid management. The use of therapeutic lifestyle changes (TLC), including LDL-lowering dietary management (e.g., restriction of saturated fat/cholesterol intake, including fiber and soy protein in diet), weight control, appropriate exercise, and smoking cessation will achieve the therapeutic goal (LDL below 100 mg/dl) in many persons. If these measures are inadequate, drug therapy may be added. Five **antilipemic agents** to lower blood cholesterol levels are available: HMG-CoA reductase inhibitors (the *statins*), bile acid sequestrants, nicotinic acid (niacin), fibric acid derivatives, and the cholesterol absorption inhibitor.

Statins

HMG-CoA reductase inhibitors (*statins*) inhibit the enzyme for cholesterol synthesis. These agents are the most potent lipid-lowering medications available for monotherapy and are considered to be the first choice in managing high cholesterol. Statins (e.g., atorvastatin—Lipitor, simvastatin—Zocor) have been shown to be very effective in lowering LDL levels and are modestly effective in reducing triglyceride levels and increasing HDL levels, thereby reducing cardiovascular morbidity and mortality. Statins are generally well tolerated.

Side effects of statins include:

Mild GI disturbances, headache, rash, fatigue

 Myalgia and muscle weakness

 Rarely, rhabdomyolysis (destruction of muscle tissue leading to renal failure)

 Elevated liver enzymes (periodic liver function tests are necessary)

Contraindications or extreme caution with statins applies to:

Hepatic or renal disease

Existing myalgia or muscle weakness

Pregnancy, breast-feeding, children

Interactions of statins with immunosuppressive drugs, erythromycins, some antifungals, antiretroviral protease inhibitors, *grapefruit juice,* or other antilipemic drugs increase risk of myopathy and renal failure.

Bile Acid Sequestrants

The resins cholestyramine (Questran) and colestipol (Colestid), which are not absorbed from the GI tract, bind bile acids in the intestine, interrupting the process by which bile acids are returned to the liver for reuse. Since bile acids are formed from cholesterol, sequestrants reduce total body cholesterol. Bile acid sequestrants can be used as monotherapy when moderate reductions in LDL are required or as add-on therapy to statins. They should not be used as a single agent in the presence of elevated triglycerides.

Side effects of bile acid sequestrants include:

✳ Constipation, heartburn, nausea, and bloating (occurs frequently and may affect compliance)

Contraindications for bile acid sequestrants include:

Biliary cirrhosis and obstruction

GI obstruction or fecal impaction

Interactions with bile acid sequestrants can reduce the absorption of many drugs, including antibiotics, cardiac glycosides, fat-soluble vitamins, thiazide diuretics, and thyroid hormones (administer at least one hour before or four hours after the bile acid sequestrants).

Nicotinic Acid (Niacin)

Nicotinic acid reduces hepatic synthesis of triglycerides and limits secretion of VLDLs by inhibiting the mobilization of free fatty acids from the peripheral tissues. It lowers serum total and LDL cholesterol and triglyceride levels and also raises HDL cholesterol levels. Niacin may be useful in combination with a statin in patients with diabetic dyslipidemia (abnormal levels of various blood lipid fractions).

Side effects of niacin can be troublesome and include:

✳ GI upset, blurred vision, fatigue

✳ *Skin flushing,* itching, and irritation (more common with immediate-release preparations; pretreatment with aspirin or ibuprofen can diminish cutaneous reactions)

Glucose intolerance and hyperuricemia (higher doses)

✳ Hepatotoxicity (especially with sustained-release products)

Note: The extended-release formulation (Niaspan) causes much less flushing and little hepatic toxicity in daily doses up to 2 g.

Contraindications of niacin include:

Hepatic or peptic ulcer disease, diabetes, or gout

Pregnancy and lactation (high doses); children (<10 years old)

Interactions of niacin with antihypertensives and vasodilators potentiates hypotensive effects; antidiabetic agents with loss of blood glucose control.

Fibric Acid Derivatives (Fibrates)

The fibrates fenofibrate (TriCor) and gemfibrozil (Lopid) possess minimal LDL reducing capacity but are especially effective in patients who have extremely high triglyceride levels and in patients with combined forms of hyperlipidemia. The mechanism by which fibrates reduce triglycerides is poorly understood. Fibrates may be used in combination with other antilipemics, since these agents appear to be additive in lowering LDLs and raising HDLs. Fibrates are generally well tolerated.

Side effects of fibrates can include:

✳ GI complaints (diarrhea, dyspepsia, nausea, and vomiting)

✳ Cholethiasis, jaundice, blood dyscrasias, myopathy

Hypersensitivity reactions, rarely

Contraindications of fibrates include:

Gallbladder, hepatic, renal disease, or peptic ulcer

Pregnancy, lactation, and use in children

Interactions of fibrates with oral anticoagulants and hypoglycemic agents (potentiate effects); with statins to increase risk of serious muscle problems (use together only in the lowest effective doses).

Cholesterol Absorption Inhibitor

Ezetimibe (Zetia) inhibits intestinal absorption of both dietary and biliary cholesterol, blocking its transport in the small intestine. It can be taken simultaneously with a statin, and the LDL-lowering effects of the two drugs are additive. Ezetimibe is generally well tolerated, with back pain and arthralgia being reported. Patients with moderate to severe hepatic insufficiency should not take it. Administer eztimibe at least one hour before or two hours after administering antacids.

See Table 25-3 for a summary of the coronary vasodilators and antilipemic agents.

Table 25-3 Coronary Vasodilators and Antilipemic Agents

GENERIC NAME	TRADE NAME	DOSAGE
Nitrates[2]		
nitroglycerin *fast acting*	Nitrostat tabs S.L.	1–3 tabs q5min × 3 max in 15 min PRN
	Nitrolingual spray	1–2 sprays (0.4–0.8 mg) SL q5min × 3 max in 15 min PRN
	Caps E.R.	2.5–9 mg PO q8–12h
	Nitro-Bid oint 2%	1–2 inches q8h (while awake and at bedtime)
	Nitro-Dur,	1 transdermal patch 2.5-19mg daily, rotate site;
On 12hrs/off 12 hrs.	Transderm-Nitro, others	on 12 h/off 12 h
	IV, premixed or sol for inj	IV dose varies
isorbide dinitrate	Tabs SL	2.5–5 mg × 3 max in 30 min
unstable angina	Tabs PO *to prevent angina*	Prophylactic 10–40 mg BID–TID ac
every 8hr/tid	Caps, tabs ER	PO 20–40 mg q6–12h
isosorbide mononitrate	Monoket, Ismo	10–20 mg PO BID, 7 h apart
	Imdur (SR)	30–60 mg PO 1–2×/day
Antilipemic Agents		
Statins		
atorvastatin	Lipitor	10–80 mg PO at bedtime
lovastatin	Mevacor	20–80 mg PO at bedtime
pravastatin	Pravachol	10–80 mg PO at bedtime
rosuvastatin	Crestor	5–40 mg PO at bedtime
simvastatin	Zocor	10–80 mg PO at bedtime
Bile Acid Sequestrants *not used much, side effects in GI tract*		
cholestyramine	Questran, Questran Light	4 g TID ac; mix powder with water, milk, or juice
colestipol	Colestid granules	5–20 g in 2–4 div. doses; mix with above fluids
	Colestid tabs	2–16 g PO in 2 div. doses with a full glass of water
Nicotinic Acid		
niacin	Niaspan, Slo-Niacin	Dose varies with response; take after meals or a snack
Fibric Acid Derivatives		
fenofibrate	Tricor	54–160 mg PO daily with food
gemfibrozil	Lopid	600 mg PO BID ac
Cholesterol Absorption Inhibitor		
ezetimibe	Zetia	10 mg PO daily
Combinations		
atorvastatin/amlodipine	Caduet *lipitor/norvasc*	PO daily dose varies with response
ezetimibe/simvastatin	Vytorin	PO daily evening dose varies with response
lovastatin/niacin	Advicor	PO daily bedtime dose varies with response

[a]For prevention and treatment of angina pectoris

Note: Beta-blockers and calcium channel blockers are also administered prophylactically for angina pectoris, and can be given concurrently with the nitrates.

Other antilipemic agents are available. Some reduce triglycerides as well.

Patient Education

Patients on antilipemic therapy should be instructed regarding:

Continuing diet (low-fat, low-cholesterol) and aerobic exercise

Taking medicine with meals to reduce GI upset

Reporting side effects to the physician immediately, *especially muscle pain, weakness, or bleeding*

With cholestyramine, high-fiber diet, and/or a stool softener, fat-soluble vitamin/folic acid supplements, and not taking other medication within four hours

Expecting facial flushing with niacin

Taking statins in the evening (the body synthesizes most cholesterol at night)

Avoiding grapefruit juice while taking statins; adverse effects potentiated, note other interactions

The importance of regular liver function tests

If all other factors remain the same, medication will probably need to be taken throughout the patient's lifetime. Sometimes diet and exercise will eliminate the need

VASOCONSTRICTORS

Vasoconstrictors are adrenergic in action (see Chapter 13). Drugs such as norepinephrine (Levophed) constrict blood vessels, resulting in increased systolic and diastolic BP. These drugs, administered IV, are used mainly in the treatment of shock, short term only.

Side effects of Levophed can include:

* Headache (may be a symptom of hypertension)

  Weakness, dizziness, tremor, and pallor

* Respiratory difficulty or apnea

  Pain in the cardiac area

* Palpitation, bradycardia, cardiac arrhythmias

  Necrosis of tissues

Cautions with Levophed include:

Close monitoring of IV site

Close monitoring of BP and other vital signs

ANTICOAGULANTS

Anticoagulants are divided into two general groups: coumarin derivatives and heparins. The action of these two classes is quite different. However, their purpose is the same: to prevent formation of clots or decrease the extension of existing clots in such conditions as venous thrombosis, pulmonary embolism, and coronary occlusion. Also, many patients with artificial heart valves, mitral valve disease, or chronic atrial fibrillation, or postsurgical patients (cardiac bypass, vascular surgery, and hip/knee replacement) receive anticoagulants to prevent embolism/thrombosis. Patients on anticoagulants, especially older patients, should be constantly observed for *bleeding complications,* such as cerebrovascular accidents (CVAs). The coumarin derivatives and heparin do not dissolve clots; they only interfere with the coagulation process as a prophylaxis.

Coumarin Derivatives

Coumarin derivatives (e.g., Coumadin) are administered *orally.* The coumarin derivatives alter the synthesis of blood coagulation factors in the liver by interfering with the action of vitamin K. The *antidote for serious bleeding complications during coumarin therapy is vitamin K.* In some cases, fresh, frozen plasma is also given for bleeding complications. The action of the coumarin derivatives is slower than that of heparin; therefore these drugs are generally used as follow-up for long-term anticoagulant therapy, although coumadin may be started at the same time as heparin. The most commonly used laboratory method of monitoring therapy with coumarin derivatives is the International Normalized Ratio (INR). The INR serves as a guide in determining dosage.

Interactions of coumarin derivatives with *many* drugs have been reported. Concurrent administration of any other drug should be investigated, and the following drugs should be *avoided* if possible. Some of the drugs that may *increase* response to coumarin derivatives include:

> Anabolic steroids
>
> Chloral hydrate and alcohol (acute intoxication)
>
> Disulfiram
>
> All NSAIDs, including aspirin
>
> Tricyclic antidepressants
>
> Thyroid drugs
>
> Amiodarone and quinidine
>
> Many anti-infective agents
>
> Acetaminophen (large daily doses or long duration)

Some of the drugs that may *decrease* response to coumarin derivatives include:

> Alcohol (chronic alcoholism)
>
> Barbiturates
>
> Estrogen (including oral contraceptives)
>
> Corticosteroids

There are many other interactions with coumarin derivatives. *Always check before administering any other medicine.*

Heparin

There are two types of heparin: the standard or unfractionated type (UFH) and the newer type, low molecular weight (LMW).

Heparin is not absorbed from the GI tract and the standard type (UFH) must be administered *intravenously* or *subcutaneously*. The LMW type is only administered subcutaneously. Heparin acts on thrombin, inhibiting the action of fibrin in clot formation. The *antidote for serious bleeding complications during heparin therapy is protamine sulfate.* When administered IV, the action of heparin is immediate. A dilute flushing solution of heparin is also used to maintain patency of indwelling venipuncture devices used to obtain blood specimens and of catheters used for arterial access (arterial lines). Be sure to check that it is a *dilute flushing* solution before injection, and not full-strength heparin. However, 0.9% sodium chloride (normal saline) injection alone is used to flush *peripheral* venipuncture devices, for example, PRN adapters. Heparin is *not* used to flush these devices because of possible drug incompatibilities and laboratory test interferences.

Low-molecular-weight heparins (LMWHs) include enoxaparin (Lovenox). Administered subcutaneously, enoxaparin and other LMWHs have a better bioavailability and produce a more predictable anticoagulant response than does UFH. At recommended doses, enoxaparin does not significantly affect platelet activity, INR, or activated partial thromboplastin time (aPTT). Monitoring of anticoagulant effect is not necessary, but periodic complete blood counts (CBCs), stool occult blood tests, and platelet counts are recommended during treatment.

Enoxaparin was the first LMWH to be approved in the United States. It is currently approved for prevention of deep vein thrombosis (DVT) in patients undergoing hip or knee replacement or abdominal surgery, for the treatment of unstable angina and non–Q-wave myocardial infarction, and for the inpatient treatment of acute pulmonary embolism (PE). It is also used in the outpatient treatment of acute DVT not associated with pulmonary embolism and is combined with warfarin.

When heparin is administered subcutaneously, especially if the patient is discharged and the medication will be administered at home, be sure to stress *patient education:*

1. Administer the heparin subcutaneously in the fat pad along the lower abdomen, at least two inches (approximately three fingers) below the umbilicus. Use 5/8- or 7/8-inch needle. Grasp the skin to form a fat pad, but do not pinch the tissues. Insert the needle with a dart-like motion at 90-degree angle. DO NOT ASPIRATE. Release fingers holding the fat pad and inject *slowly.*

2. *Rotate injection sites* and document site of injection.

3. Do *not* rub the site with an alcohol sponge. Merely hold the sponge on the site *gently* for approximately 10 seconds.

4. Be sure there is no bleeding from the site.

5. Review additional cautions in the following Patient Education box.

Measurement of the activated aPTT is the most common laboratory test for monitoring heparin therapy. When long-term anticoagulant therapy is begun with coumarin derivatives, there is a short-term overlap period in which both heparin and coumarin derivatives are administered concurrently.

Interactions of heparins with aspirin and other NSAIDs, or with thrombolytic agents, for example streptokinase or alteplase (TPA), may increase the risk of hemorrhage.

Side effects of all anticoagulants can include:

* Major hemorrhage
* Minor bleeding (e.g., petechiae, nosebleed, and bruising)
* Blood in urine (hematuria) or stools (melena)

Contraindications of anticoagulants include:

> GI disorders and ulceration of GI tract
>
> Hepatic and renal dysfunction
>
> Blood dyscrasias
>
> Pregnancy (heparin can be used with caution as it does not cross the placenta)
>
> After stroke may increase risk of fatal cerebral hemorrhage

See Table 25-4 for a summary of the Anticoagulants, Platelet Inhibitors, Thrombolytic Agents, and Colony Stimulating Factors.

Patient Education

It is *very important* that patients on anticoagulant therapy be instructed regarding:

Careful daily observation of skin, gums, urine, and stools, and *immediate* reporting of any signs of bleeding

Avoiding sports and activities that may cause bleeding

Immediate reporting to the physician of any falls, blows, or injuries (internal bleeding is always a possibility)

Special care with shaving (electric razor only) and with teeth brushing or dental floss

Wearing an identification tag or carrying a card indicating use of anticoagulant

Immediate reporting of severe or continued headache or backache, dizziness, joint pain or swelling, tarry stools, abdominal distention, vomiting of material resembling coffee grounds, or nosebleed

Avoiding other medications without the physician's approval, especially OTC aspirin, anti-inflammatory drugs, and antacids

Avoiding alcohol

Note: Patients receiving anticoagulant therapy should be consistent in the amount of vitamin K-rich foods they eat daily in order to keep prothrombin levels stable. Large amounts of vitamin K–rich foods can counteract the anticoagulant therapy. See Chapter 11, Vitamins and Minerals, for a list of foods containing vitamin K.

Table 25-4 Anticoagulants, Platelet Inhibitors, Thrombolytic Agents, and Colony Stimulating Factors

GENERIC NAME	TRADE NAME	DOSAGE
Anticoagulants		
Coumarin Derivatives		
warfarin	Coumadin	PO dose varies, based on PT/INR results
Unfractionated Heparin		
heparin		IV, subq dose varies
Low-Molecular-Weight Heparins		
dalteparin	Fragmin	subq, dose varies
enoxaparin	Lovenox	subq, dose varies
Platelet Inhibitors		
aspirin	Ecotrin, Ascriptin, others	81–325 mg PO daily
clopidogrel	Plavix	75 mg PO daily with or without food
dipyridamole	Persantine	75–100 mg PO 4×/day with warfarin
dipyridamole with aspirin	Aggrenox	I cap PO BID
Thrombolytic Agents		
alteplase, TPA	Activase	IV bolus, then IV infusion
reteplase, r-PA	Retavase	IV bolus × 2 (30 min apart)
streptokinase	Kabikinase	IV bolus, then IV infusion
Colony Stimulating Factors		
darbepoetin alfa	Aranesp	IV, subq dose varies
epoetin alfa	Epogen, Procrit	IV, subq dose varies
filgrastim, G-CSF	Neupogen	IV, subq dose varies

Note: Representative sample; many other products available.

PLATELET INHIBITOR THERAPY

Platelet inhibitors are given as prophylactic therapy to decrease platelet clumping in patients with a history of recent stroke, recent MI, or established peripheral vascular disease.

Dipyridamole (Persantine)

Persantine is a non-nitrate coronary vasodilator that inhibits platelet aggregation (clumping). It is used with coumarin anticoagulants in the prevention of postoperative thromboembolic complications of cardiac valve replacement.

Side effects of dipyridamole (Persantine), usually transient, can include:

Headache, dizziness, weakness

Nausea, vomiting, diarrhea

Flushing, rash

Caution with older adults.

A combination of aspirin with dipyridamole (Aggrenox) is approved for stroke prophylaxis.

Aspirin

Because of its ability to inhibit platelet aggregation (clumping), aspirin has been investigated extensively for use in the prevention of thrombosis. Patients with prosthetic heart valves usually receive aspirin or dipyridamole to reduce the incidences of thrombosis.

Aspirin therapy, usually 81–325 mg daily, has also been used after myocardial infarction or recurrent transient ischemic attacks (TIAs) to reduce the risk of recurrence of attacks. Aspirin has also been used to reduce the risk of myocardial infarction in patients with unstable angina. However, aspirin therapy is not recommended for those without clinical signs of coronary heart disease because of an increased risk of hemorrhagic stroke associated with long-term aspirin therapy. Patients should be instructed not to start aspirin therapy without consulting a physician first. Patient education should include instruction regarding measures to reduce risk factors for coronary heart disease and stroke; that is, abstinence from all forms of tobacco, weight control, low-fat and low-cholesterol diet, and aerobic exercise on a regular basis.

Because of *gastric irritation,* aspirin should be administered with food or milk. Film-coated tablets, enteric-coated tablets, and buffered aspirin preparations are available to reduce gastric irritation.

Aspirin is contraindicated for anyone with bleeding disorders. See Chapter 19 for a description of other side effects, contraindications, and interactions.

Clopidogrel (Plavix)

Clopidogrel (Plavix) is an oral antiplatelet agent used to reduce atherosclerotic events (myocardial infarction, stroke, and vascular death) in patients with a history of recent stroke, recent MI, or established peripheral vascular disease. Overall tolerability associated with use of clopidogrel appears to be similar to that of aspirin; however, GI bleeding may occur less often with clopidogrel. Conversely, clopidogrel appears to possess a slightly higher incidence of neutropenia than does aspirin, although severe neutropenia is rare with either drug. Clopidogrel should be considered in aspirin-intolerant or aspirin-failure patients.

THROMBOLYTIC AGENTS

The body maintains a process to dissolve clots (fibrinolysis) after they have formed. Thrombolytic drugs (e.g., streptokinase and alteplase) potentiate this process. **Thrombolytic agents,** given IV, reduce mortality when used in the first few hours (less than 6) after acute myocardial infarction (MI) or cerebral vascular accident (CVA).

Administered in an ER or ICU setting, close monitoring of hemodynamics and vital signs is generally considered standard with thrombolytic therapy, particularly during the initial 24–48 h.

Bleeding is the most serious complication of thrombolytic therapy and can manifest as minor bleeding or major internal bleeding. Bleeding occurs most commonly at access sites such as catheter insertion sites or venipuncture sites. Patients with preexisting coagulation problems are at the highest risk for developing bleeding complications during thrombolytic therapy.

Hemorrhage can result from concomitant therapy with heparin or other platelet-aggregation inhibitors. If severe bleeding occurs during therapy, the drug should be discontinued promptly. Rapid coronary lysis can result in the development of arrhythmias; however, they are generally transient in nature.

See Table 25-4 for a summary of platelet inhibitors and thrombolytic agents.

COLONY STIMULATING FACTORS (CSFS)

Colony stimulating factors such as epoetin alfa (Epogen or Procrit) are responsible for the regulation of the production and development of blood cells, normally in the bone marrow. All CSFs are products of recombinant technology. Epoetin alfa stimulates the bone marrow to produce more red blood cells and is approved for treatment of anemia in chronic renal failure, human immunodeficiency virus (HIV) infection, and anemia associated with chemotherapy. It also reduces the need for blood transfusions in anemic patients scheduled to undergo certain kinds of surgery. Darbepoetin alfa (Aranesp) is a *second-generation* agent that is dosed less frequently than epoetin alfa.

Side effects of epoetin alfa (Epogen) include:

Hypertension—especially in dialysis patients

Flu-like symptoms

GI effects

Rash

Chest pain

A granulocyte colony-stimulating factor, filgrastim (Neupogen), lessens the severity of myelosuppression in cancer patients and has allowed chemotherapy dose intensification or maintenance of dose intensity.

Side effects of filgrastim include:

Bone pain is common

Headache

Dermatological reactions

See Table 25-4 for a summary of anticoagulants, platelet inhibitors, thrombolytic agents, and colony stimulating factors.

WORKSHEET FOR CHAPTER 25
CARDIOVASCULAR DRUGS

Note the drugs listed according to category and complete all columns.
Learn generic trade names as specified by instructor.

Classifications and Drugs	Purpose	Side Effects	Contraindications or Cautions	Patient Education
Cardiac Glycosides 1. digoxin				
Antiarrhythmics 1. propranolol (a beta-adrenergic blocker with other uses) 2. verapamil (a calcium channel blocker with other uses) 3. lidocaine 4. procainamide 5. quinidine				
Antilipemic Agents 1. cholestyramine 2. niacin 3. statins 4. gemfibrozil 5. zetia				

(continued)

Classifications and Drugs	Purpose	Side Effects	Contraindications or Cautions	Patient Education
Antihypertensives (Hypotensives) (see previous page for beta-blockers and calcium channel blockers) 1. methyldopa 2. prazosin 3. hydralazine				
ACE inhibitors 1. captopril 2. enalapril				
Vasodilators (Coronary) 1. nitroglycerin Tabs SL Ointment Patch Spray 2. isosorbide (Isordil)				
Anticoagulants 1. coumarin derivatives 2. heparins				
Platelet Inhibitors 1. aspirin 2. dipyridamole (Persantine) 3. Plavix				

A. Case Study for Cardiovascular Drugs

Wilbur Worthington, a 65-year-old patient, has been treated in the hospital for cardiac arrhythmias with tachycardia. He will be discharged on Lanoxin and Calan and will need the following patient information.

1. Side effects of Lanoxin can include all of the following EXCEPT
    a. Double vision
    b. Appetite loss
    c. Diarrhea
    d. Palpitations

2. Older adults on Lanoxin are also more prone to the following EXCEPT
    a. Sedation
    b. Confusion
    c. Mental disorder
    d. Insomnia

3. The following drugs can increase risk of digitalis toxicity and arrhythmias EXCEPT
    a. Diuretics
    b. Antacids
    c. Quinidine
    d. Decongestants

4. Calan does all of the following EXCEPT
    a. Dilates coronary arteries
    b. Increases heart contractions
    c. Blocks calcium
    d. Lowers blood pressure

5. Calan can have all of the following side effects EXCEPT
    a. Diarrhea
    b. Postural hypotension
    c. Bradycardia
    d. Vertigo

B. Case Study for Cardiovascular Drugs

Homer Grange is diagnosed with hypertension and elevated cholesterol with increased LDL. The following information will be helpful.

1. The following antihypertensives can cause bradycardia EXCEPT
    a. Tenormin
    b. Procardia
    c. Apresoline
    d. Aldomet

2. The following advice would be appropriate EXCEPT
    a. Stop smoking
    b. Rise slowly
    c. Reduce salt intake
    d. Stop medicine when better

3. What medicine is often prescribed with antihypertensives?
    a. Antacids
    b. NSAIDs
    c. Diurectis
    d. Hypnotics

4. Lovastatin, an antilipemic, can cause all of the following EXCEPT
    a. Muscle cramps
    b. Edema
    c. Liver damage
    d. GI upset

5. Advice for patients taking statins should include all of the following EXCEPT
    a. Weight control
    b. Take medicine ac
    c. Low-fat diet
    d. Appropriate exercise

CHAPTER REVIEW QUIZ

Match the medication in the first column with the condition in the second column that it is used to treat. Conditions may be used more than once.

Medication   **Condition**

1. _____ Isorbide   **A.** Elevated cholesterol

2. _____ Zetia   **B.** Hypertension

3. _____ Lovenox   **C.** Angina

4. _____ Cardizem   **D.** Pulmonary emboli

5. _____ Zocor   **E.** Cardiac arrhythmia

6. _____ Plavix   **F.** Stroke prevention (platelet inhibitor)

7. _____ Crestor

8. _____ Apresoline

9. _____ Quinidine

10. _____ Pronestyl

Choose the correct answer.

11. Which one should be checked before administering digitalis?
    a. INR laboratory test   c. Apical pulse
    b. Blood pressure   d. Respirations

12. Which is not a toxic side effect of digitalis to be reported to the physician immediately?
    a. Nausea and vomiting   c. Confusion
    b. Visual disturbances   d. Tachycardia

13. Which is not a side effect of ACE inhibitors?
    a. Photosensitivity   c. Dry cough
    b. Hypokalemia   d. Hypotension

14. Which is not a side effect of beta-blockers, for example, Tenormin?
    a. Dizziness   c. Confusion
    b. Insomnia   d. Hyperglycemia

15. Which would not potentiate the hypotensive effect of beta-blockers, for example, Inderal?
    a. Isuprel   c. Lasix
    b. Alcohol   d. Tagamet

16. Which is not a side effect of calcium channel blockers, for example, Isoptin?
    a. Edema   c. Vertigo
    b. Headache   d. Tachycardia

17. Which is not a side effect of quinidine?
    a. Diarrhea   c. Hypotension
    b. Hypoglycemia   d. Bradycardia

18. Which is not an antihypertensive?
   a. Atenolol
   b. Hydrochlorothiazide
   c. Cholestyramine
   d. Verapamil

19. Which is not a side effect of nitrates?
   a. Postural hypotension
   b. Bradycardia
   c. Headache
   d. Flushing

20. Which is not a side effect of statins?
   a. Muscle pain
   b. Low liver enzymes
   c. GI distress
   d. Headache

21. Which drug, a fibrate, is the most effective single agent for lowering the triglyceride level?
   a. Questran
   b. Lipitor
   c. Lopid
   d. Zocor

22. Which is not a side effect of bile acid sequestrants, for example, Questran?
   a. Bloating
   b. Diarrhea
   c. Heartburn
   d. Nausea

23. Which is not a side effect of niacin?
   a. GI upset
   b. Low uric acid level
   c. Blurred vision
   d. Flushing

24. What is the antidote for bleeding problems with coumarin?
   a. Protamine
   b. Vitamin K
   c. Persantine
   d. Procrit

25. What is the antidote for bleeding problems with heparin?
   a. Streptokinase
   b. Vitamin K
   c. Plavix
   d. Protamine

Chapter 26
Respiratory System Drugs and Antihistamines

Objectives

Upon completion of this chapter, the learner should be able to

1. Describe uses of and precautions necessary with oxygen therapy
2. Explain the purpose of carbon dioxide inhalations
3. Define the Key Terms
4. Classify a list of respiratory system drugs according to action
5. List uses, side effects, and contraindications for bronchodilators and antitussives
6. Explain appropriate patient education for those receiving respiratory system drugs
7. Describe the action and uses of the antihistamines and decongestants
8. List the side effects, contraindications, and interactions of the antihistamines and decongestants

Therapeutic measures for respiratory distress include oxygen, respiratory stimulants, bronchodilators, corticosteroids, mucolytics, expectorants, and antitussives.

OXYGEN

Oxygen is used therapeutically for hypoxia (insufficient oxygen). Some of the conditions for which oxygen is indicated are heart and lung diseases, carbon monoxide poisoning, and some central nervous system (CNS) conditions with respiratory difficulty or failure. Oxygen may be administered by endotracheal intubation, nasal cannula, masks, tents, and hoods.

Side effects of oxygen delivered at too high a concentration or for prolonged periods of time can include:

Hypoventilation, particularly with COPD (chronic obstructive pulmonary disease), may cause CO_2 retention and acidosis

Confusion

Changes in the alveoli of the lungs

Blindness (in premature infants)

Cautions apply to:

Patients with COPD (high O_2 concentrations may cause hypoventilation or apnea).

Danger of fire when oxygen is used. Oxygen is not flammable but does support combustion. Smoking, matches, and electrical equipment that may spark (e.g., electric razors, hair dryers) are not allowed in rooms where oxygen is in use.

RESPIRATORY STIMULANTS

Respiratory stimulants include:

- Caffeine citrate in the treatment of neonatal apnea (see Chapter 20)
- Theophylline administered IV and orally to stimulate respiration in infants and patients with Cheyne-Stokes respiration
- Carbon dioxide (CO_2) inhalations to increase both depth and rate of respiration (e.g., in treatment of hyperventilation or hiccups)

BRONCHODILATORS

Bronchodilators act by relaxing the smooth muscles of the bronchial tree, thereby relieving bronchospasm and increasing the vital capacity of the lungs. Bronchodilators are used in the symptomatic treatment of acute respiratory conditions such as asthma, as well as many forms of COPD. Classifications of bronchodilators include the sympathomimetics (adrenergics), the parasympatholytics (anticholinergics), and the xanthine derivatives.

Review Chapter 13 for adrenergics and anticholinergics.

Sympathomimetics

Sympathomimetics (*adrenergics*) are potent bronchodilators that increase vital capacity and decrease airway resistance. The adrenergics work on the smooth muscle in the lungs to cause relaxation. However, they also can affect the entire sympathetic nervous system. The adrenergics may produce serious side effects, and manufacturer's directions should be followed carefully regarding dosage and administration. The inhalation route of administration is preferred to minimize systemic adverse effects. Examples include albuterol, epinephrine, terbutaline, and others.

Although *metered dose inhalers (MDIs)* remain popular due to ease of use, efficacy, and portability, the availability of this formulation is decreasing. In the past, all MDIs contained chlorofluorocarbon (CFC) as the propellant. Because of its detrimental effects on the ozone layer, the use of CFC is being phased out. Some manufacturers have reformulated their MDI to contain hydrofluoroalkane (HFA) as the propellant. Other manufacturers are discontinuing production of MDIs and utilizing dry-powder formulations instead.

Breath-actuated inhalers provide medication only under the pressure of inspiration, rather than through compression of the valve. This option is helpful for patients who are unable to coordinate inspiration with actuation of a conventional MDI. Unfortunately, the breath-actuated system, unlike the MDI, does not allow for use of a spacer.

See Table 26-1 for selected sympathomimetic products and dosages.

Side effects of the adrenergics include potentiation of theophylline effects with increased risk of toxicity, especially:

Gastrointestinal (GI)—nausea, vomiting, decreased appetite

CNS stimulation—nervousness, tremor, dizziness

Cardiac irregularities—tachycardia, palpitations, arrhythmias, angina

Levalbuterol (Xopenex), an isomer of albuterol, exhibits less cardiac stimulation than albuterol

Hypertension

Hyperglycemia

Cautions for the adrenergics apply to:

First administration, which should be observed by medical personnel for hypersensitivity reactions

Contacting physician if decreased effectiveness occurs

Close monitoring, if administering oral inhaled adrenergics with other oral inhaled bronchodilators, for cardiovascular effects.

Patients on beta-blocking drugs (Inderal) will have a significant decrease in the effectiveness of adrenergic drugs.

Patients with cardiovascular or kidney disorders, diabetes, seizure disorders, or hyperthyroidism.

Parasympatholytics

Parasympatholytics (*anticholinergics*), for example Atrovent, achieve bronchodilation by decreasing the chemical that promotes bronchospasm. Parasympatholytics block the parasympathetic nervous system and can cause drying of pulmonary secretions. Adequate hydration should be encouraged to avoid mucus plugging. See Table 26-1 for dosage and other product names.

Side effects of parasympatholytics can include:

✳ Cardiac effects—changes in heart rate, palpitations

✳ CNS stimulation—headache, drowsiness, dizziness, confusion, agitation

✳ Thickened secretions and mucus plugging

Cautions: Not indicated for patients with unstable cardiac status, history of heart attacks, glaucoma, drug sensitivity, or prostatic hypertrophy.

Tiotropium (Spiriva), which is structurally similar to ipratropium, is administered daily (vs. four times daily for ipratropium). It is more efficacious than ipratropium and may lead to a reduction in the use of sympathomimetics for maintenance or rescue therapy.

Xanthines

Xanthine derivatives, such as theophylline and aminophylline, listed in Table 26-1, cause bronchodilation. They are no longer a first-line treatment due to the need for serum monitoring, their adverse effects, and drug interactions. Because different individuals metabolize xanthines at different rates, appropriate dosage must be determined by carefully monitoring the patient's response, tolerance, and blood concentrations. For faster absorption, oral forms may be taken with a full glass of water on an empty stomach. To reduce gastric irritation, take with meals.

IM injection is contraindicated. When used, xanthines are usually administered with other respiratory system drugs such as adrenergics and parasympatholytics.

Side effects of theophyllines can be mild, or severe with acute toxicity including:

✳ GI distress—nausea, vomiting, epigastric pain, abdominal cramps, anorexia, or diarrhea

✳ CNS stimulation—nervousness, insomnia, irritability, headache, tremors, seizures (can be fatal)

✳ Cardiac effects—palpitation, tachycardia, arrhythmias, *especially with rapid IV administration*

  Urinary frequency (mild diuresis)

✳ Hyperglycemia

Caution when administering theophylline applies to:

  Cardiovascular, kidney, pulmonary, or liver dysfunction

  Diabetes, peptic ulcer, or glaucoma

  Children and older adults—more prone to toxicity

  IV injection—*must be done slowly*—see cardiac side effects

  Patients undergoing influenza immunization or who have influenza

  Pregnancy and lactation

Interactions occur with:

Cimetidine, allopurinol, erythromycin, oral contraceptives, calcium channel blockers, and beta-blockers, which increase theophylline levels

Smoking, barbiturates, phenytoin, and rifampin, which decrease theophylline effectiveness

See Table 26-1 for a summary of parasympatholytics and xanthines.

Patient Education

Patients taking bronchodilators (e.g., adrenergics, anticholinergics, or the xanthines) should be instructed regarding:

Following the written directions on the package very carefully regarding dosage and administration because of the danger of serious side effects

Watching closely for cardiac irregularities or CNS stimulation (e.g., nervousness, tremor, dizziness, confusion, headache), and reporting these symptoms to the physician immediately

Other side effects possible with adrenergics and xanthines, for example gastric distress, insomnia, or hyperglycemia

Drinking adequate fluids to prevent mucus plugging, especially with anticholinergics

Avoiding any new medications, including over-the-counter (OTC) drugs, without consulting the physician first, because of the danger of serious complications; many interactions are possible

Avoiding changing brands of medicine without consulting the physician or pharmacist

---

CORTICOSTEROIDS

Synthetic corticosteroids are used to relieve inflammation, reduce swelling, and suppress symptoms in acute and chronic reactive airway disease (asthma and some COPDs). Corticosteroids should be administered systemically (IV) in the acute or emergency setting. In the nonacute setting, corticosteroids may be administered by dry powder for inhalation, MDI, or aerosol. Inhaled corticosteroids have less systemic side effects than oral or IV administration.

Nasal corticosteroids are increasingly considered first-line therapy for most *noninfectious* types of rhinitis and should be started before symptoms occur and taken regularly throughout the period of exposure. Aerosol preparations seem to be more irritating to the nasal mucosa. Aqueous preparations may drip into the throat, resulting in reduced deposition of drug in the nasal mucosa.

Side effects of inhaled corticosteroids

Throat irritation and dry mouth

Hoarseness

Coughing

Oral fungal infections—patient should be encouraged to rinse mouth with water after administration

Contraindications and extreme caution with corticosteroids include:

Viral, bacterial, or fungal infections

Hypertension or congestive heart failure

Diabetes

Hypothyroidism or cirrhosis

Renal failure

See Chapter 23 for further information about corticosteroids and see Table 26-1 for summary of corticosteroids.

ASTHMA PROPHYLAXIS
Anti-Leukotrienes

Zafirlukast (Accolate) and montelukast (Singulair) are oral leukotriene receptor antagonists for asthma prophylaxis and treatment of chronic asthma. Leukotriene receptor antagonists primarily help to control the inflammatory process of asthma, thus helping to prevent asthma symptoms and acute attacks. Montelukast can be used in children as young as two years old and has fewer drug interactions compared to zafirlukast.

Side effects of Singulair include:

Headache

Dizziness

Nausea or dyspepsia

Pain

Fatigue

Respiratory infections and fever

Contraindications/precautions include:

Hepatotoxicity (zafirlukast)

Pregnancy or lactation

Children under age 12 (zafirlukast)

Do not use to treat acute episodes of asthma

Drug interactions occur with:

Aspirin (increased levels of zafirlukast)

Erythromycin and theophylline (decreased levels of zafirlukast)

Warfarin and zafirlukast (increased prothrombin time)

Phenobarbital and rifampin (decreased levels of montelukast)

Cromolyn

A prophylactic for asthma, cromolyn (Intal) is not classified with the other medications mentioned previously. It is described as a mast-cell stabilizer. Cromolyn has no value in the treatment of acute attacks of asthma. Patients with severe, perennial bronchial asthma are required to have a prior pulmonary function test to determine the probability of a satisfactory response to this therapy. Some patients are able to discontinue corticosteroids and have better response to bronchodilator drugs given concomitantly. Cromolyn has also been used in the prevention of exercise-induced bronchospasm. Some patients do not respond to this therapy. Cromolyn is available as an aerosol or solution for inhalation or a nasal solution (to treat seasonal allergic rhinitis). To be effective, the manufacturer's directions must be followed carefully.

Side effects of cromolyn can include:

- Throat irritation, cough, bronchospasm
- Nose burning, stinging, sneezing with nasal solution
- Nausea or headache

Caution applies to:

- Those with cardiovascular disorders
- Proper use on a regular schedule

See Table 26-1 for a summary of asthma prophylaxis.

Table 26-1 Bronchodilators, Corticosteroids, and Asthma Prophylaxis

GENERIC NAME	TRADE NAME	DOSAGE
Sympathomimetics		
albuterol sulfate *mild to moderate asthma*	Proventil, Proventil HFA	MDI 1–2 puffs q4–6h
		Inhal sol 0.5 ml 0.5% sol/3 ml NS
		Tabs 2–4 mg q6–8h
	Volmax	Tabs ER 4–8 mg q12h
epinephrine	Primatene, Adrenalin	MDI 1–2 puffs q3–4h
		IM/sub Q 1:100 sol 0.3–0.5 ml
		Watch dose carefully! *raises heart rate*
isoproterenol	Isuprel	MDI 1–2 puffs q4–6h
		IV 1:50,000 sol 0.5–1 ml
		Inhal sol 0.5 ml 0.5% sol/3 ml NS TID
levalbuterol *(mixed w/ albuterol sometimes)*	Xopenex	Inhal sol 0.63–1.25 mg q6–8h
metaproterenol sulfate	Alupent	Tabs 10–20 mg TID–4×/day
		Aerosol 0.3 ml 5% sol/3 ml NS TID–4×/day
		MDI 2–3 puffs q3–4h
salmeterol*	Serevent Diskus *(beta agonist)*	Powder for inhal, 1 puff q12h
terbutaline sulfate	Brethine	Sub Q 0.25 mg, repeat ×1 in 15–30 min
		Tabs 2.5–5mg q6h while awake

Table 26-1 continued

GENERIC NAME	TRADE NAME	DOSAGE
Parasympatholytics		
ipratropium bromide *anticholinergic COPD reduces*	↗ Atrovent	MDI 1–2 puffs 4×/day
		Aerosol 1 unit dose (500 mcg/2.5 ml NS) 4×/day
		Nasal sol 0.03–0.06% each nostril TID–4×/day
ipratropium/albuterol	Combivent	MDI 2 puffs 4×/day
	↗ DuoNeb	Neb sol 1 vial (3 ml) 4×/day
tiotropium *(COPD)*	↗ Spiriva	Powder for inhal, 18 mcg daily
Xanthines		
aminophylline		Dosage based on response and drug levels
		IV 25 mg/ml slowly
theophylline	Uniphyl	Tabs ER 100–600 mg daily
	Theo-24	Caps ER 100–300 mg daily
Corticosteroids (inhaled and intranasal)		
beclomethasone	QVAR	MDI 1–2 puffs BID
	Beconase AQ	Spray 1–2 inhal each nostril daily–BID
budesonide *Allergic Asthma*	Pulmicort Turbuhaler	Powder for inhal, 1–2 puffs (200–400 mcg) BID
	Pulmicort Respules	Neb susp 0.25 mg daily or BID
nasal spray	Rhinocort Aqua	Aerosol 1–2 inhal each nostril daily
fluticasone *asthma*	Flovent	MDI 2–4 puffs BID (88–880 mcg)
nasal	Flonase	Spray 2 inhal each nostril daily
w/salmeterol	Advair Diskus	Powder for inhal, 1 inhal q12h
flunisolide	Aerobid	MDI 2 puffs BID
	Nasalide, Nasarel	Spray 2 inhal each nostril BID–TID
nometasone	↗ Nasonex	Spray 2 inhal each nostril daily
triamcinolone	↗ Azmacort	MDI 2 puffs TID-4×/day
	Nasacort AQ	Inhaler, 2 inhal each nostril daily
Asthma Prophylaxis and Treatment of Chronic Asthma		
cromolyn sodium	Intal	Inhal sol 20 mg per treatment
		MDI 2 puffs 4×/day
	Nasalcrom	Inhaler, 1 spray each nostril TID–4×/day
montelukast *Cell stabilizer*	*Singulair (w/maintenance drug)*	Tabs 5–10 mg daily
zafirlukast	Accolate	Tabs 10–20 mg BID

*Note: Due to delayed onset of action, salmeterol should never be used to treat an acute attack. This is a representative list. Other products are available.

Patient Education

Patients treated with inhaled corticosteroids or the asthma prophylaxis agents should be instructed regarding:

Side effects to expect, such as throat irritation, dry mouth, and cough, and with products administered nasally, for example cromolyn, nose burning, stinging, or sneezing are possible

Complications of inhaled corticosteroids without proper precautions, for example, oral fungal infections. Patient should be encouraged to rinse mouth with water after treatment and to always rinse and air dry equipment after use

Administering bronchodilator before corticosteroid when the two inhaled medications are ordered at the same time

Reporting side effects to the physician, especially respiratory distress

The importance of not smoking

MUCOLYTICS AND EXPECTORANTS

Mucolytics, such as acetylcysteine (Mucomyst), liquefy pulmonary secretions. **Expectorants,** such as guaifenesin and others listed in Table 26-2, increase secretions, reduce viscosity, and help to expel sputum. Iodinated products were commonly used as a respiratory expectorant, but are no longer recommended for this purpose due to lack of evidence for clinical efficacy and the potential for thyroid dysfunction and other side effects. Adequate fluid intake also helps loosen and liquefy secretions. Guaifenesin is commonly combined in cough syrups for symptomatic management of coughs associated with upper respiratory tract infections, bronchitis, pharyngitis, influenza, measles, or coughs provoked by sinusitis. Expectorants should not be used for self-medication or persistent or chronic coughs such as that associated with smoking or COPD. A persistent cough may be indicative of a serious condition. If cough persists for more than a week or is recurrent, or accompanied by a fever, a physician should be consulted.

Side effects of the expectorants are infrequent, usually not serious at recommended doses, and can include:

Nausea and vomiting, diarrhea

Runny nose

Drowsiness, dizziness, and headache

Contraindications or caution with expectorants applies to:

Patients with persistent or chronic cough

Some asthmatics (prone to bronchospasm)

Cardiovascular disease and hypertension, especially with combination products

Pregnancy or lactation

See Table 26-2 for a summary of the mucolytics and expectorants.

Table 26-2 Mucolytics and Expectorants

GENERIC NAME	TRADE NAME	DOSAGE
Mucolytic acetylcysteine	Mucomyst *antedote for tylenol O.D.*	Aerosol 3–5 ml 10% sol adrenergic may be added for bronchospasm
Expectorants guaifenesin	Mucinex Robitussin	ER tabs 600–1200 mg, daily-bid Sol 1–2 tsp q3–4h

Note: Guaifenesin is frequently combined with other drugs, for example, antihistamines, decongestants, and antitussives in OTC cough syrups.

ANTITUSSIVES

Antitussives are medications to prevent coughing in patients not requiring a productive cough. Coughing, a reflex mechanism, helps eliminate secretions from the respiratory tract. A dry, nonproductive cough can cause fatigue, insomnia, and, in some cases, pain to the patient (e.g., pleurisy and fractured ribs). Narcotic antitussives may be used to relieve these patients but have limited use because of respiratory depressant action and bronchial constriction (e.g., morphine). Codeine, a narcotic with fewer side effects, is frequently used, but is addictive with long-term use. Codeine is added to some cough syrups, as is hydrocodone, another narcotic (e.g., Hycodan).

Many over-the-counter cough syrups are available that combine several drugs, for example, antitussives with expectorants, antihistamines, and decongestants. Patients should be cautioned to seek advice from a professional person familiar with each ingredient, such as a physician, pharmacist, nurse, or medical assistant. Some ingredients are contraindicated in certain conditions. For example, antitussives and antihistamines would make it more difficult to expel secretions and thereby worsen conditions such as COPD. Products containing decongestants can cause serious adverse side effects in those with cardiovascular or thyroid conditions.

Side effects of narcotic antitussives can include:

- Respiratory depression
- Constipation
- Urinary retention
- Sedation and dizziness
- Nausea and vomiting

Contraindications for narcotic antitussives apply to:

Addiction-prone patients

Asthma

COPD

Nonnarcotic antitussives (e.g., dextromethorphan) are more frequently used because they do not depress respirations, do not cause addiction, and have few side effects. Dextromethorphan is frequently combined with other drugs, such as antihistamines and decongestants, in cough syrups.

Contraindications for nonnarcotic antitussives include:

Asthma

COPD

Caution: with children—some CNS side effects reported, especially large doses:

Ester-type anesthetic (e.g., tetracaine) hypersensitivity with *benzonatate*

Interactions with dextromethorphan can include:

Triptans used for migraine headache

Monoamine oxidase inhibitors (MAOIs)

The SSRIs fluoxetene and paroxetine

Memantine (Namenda)

See Table 26-3 for a summary of the antitussives.

Table 26-3 Antitussives

GENERIC NAME	TRADE NAME	DOSAGE	COMMENTS
Narcotic			
codeine	Tussi-Organidin NR Robitussin AC	Sol or tabs 10–20 mg q4–6h	Any cough medicine containing a controlled
hydrocodone bitartrate	Hydromet Hycodan, Lorcet	Syrup or tabs 5–10 mg q4–6 h	substance is not for extended use; can develop physical dependence and tolerance; watch for side effects
Nonnarcotic			
benzonatate	Tessalon	Caps 100–200 mg tid	Swallow caps whole
dextromethorphan	Benylin, Robitussin DM	Sol 10–20 mg q4h Sol 30 mg q6–8h	Note interactions
diphenhydramine	★ Benadryl	Caps 25 mg q4–6h	Anticholinergic effects, especially drying

Patient Education

Patients taking antitussives should be instructed regarding:

Starting with a low dose of antitussive and increasing the dose only if cough supression does not occur

Caution with those operating machinery because of sedative effect

ANTIHISTAMINES

Antihistamines, such as diphenhydramine (Benadryl), competitively antagonize the histamine$_1$ receptor sites. Through this action, the antihistamines combat the increased capillary permeability and edema, inflammation, and itch caused by sudden histamine release.

Antihistamines are not curative, but provide *symptomatic relief of allergic symptoms caused by histamine release.* They are also used as adjunctive treatment of anaphylactic reactions *after* the acute symptoms (e.g., laryngeal edema and shock) have been controlled with epinephrine and corticosteroids.

Antihistamines are used to treat the symptoms of allergies (e.g., rhinitis, conjunctivitis, and rash). However, when antihistamines are used to reduce nasal secretions in the common cold, the consequent thickening of bronchial secretions may result in further airway obstruction, especially in those with COPD and asthma.

Some antihistamines are used in the symptomatic treatment of vertigo associated with pathology of the middle ear or in the prevention and treatment of motion sickness (see Chapter 16).

H_1-blockers are grouped into two categories: the first-generation agents and the newer second-generation agents.

Side effects of the first-generation antihistamines are *anticholinergic* in action and include:

★ Drying of secretions, especially of the eyes, ears, nose, and throat

★ Sedation, dizziness, and hypotension, especially in older adults

Muscular weakness and decreased coordination

Urinary retention and constipation

Visual disorders

★ Paradoxical excitement, insomnia, and tremors, especially in children

GI—nausea, vomiting, anorexia

Contraindications or extreme caution with first-generation antihistamines applies to:

COPD and asthma

Persons operating machinery or driving a car

Older adult patients (extended half life with sedation)

Cardiovascular disorders

Benign prostatic hypertrophy (BPH)

Infants, pregnancy, and lactation

Seizure disorders

Interactions of first-generation antihistamines may occur with:

Potentiation of CNS depression with tranquilizers, analgesics, hypnotics, alcohol, and muscle relaxants

Potentiation of anticholinergic effect with MAOIs

Phenothiazine antihistamines, which antagonize the vasopressor effect of epinephrine

Patient Education

Patients taking first-generation antihistamines should be instructed regarding:

Avoiding frequent or prolonged use of antihistamines, which may cause increased bronchial or nasal congestion and dry cough

No self-medication (check with the physician first) in those with COPD or cardiovascular disorders, BPH, older adults, and children

Caution with those operating machinery because of sedative effect

Not mixing with alcohol or any other CNS depressant drugs

The *second-generation antihistamines* include fexofenadine (Allegra) and loratadine (Claritin). These drugs are *selective* histamine receptor antagonists and have fewer CNS effects, for example, less sedation, and no anticholinergic effects compared to the first-generation antihistamines. Although these agents cause little or no sedation, it is important to note that the incidence of sedation is *not* zero. They are used to provide symptomatic relief of seasonal allergic rhinitis, for example, hay fever.

Side effects of second-generation antihistamines, usually mild, can include:

Headache

Dry mouth

Contraindications or caution with second-generation antihistamines apply to:

Asthma

Renal and hepatic impairment

Driving or operating machinery

Pregnancy or lactation, use in neonates

Patient Education

Patients taking second-generation antihistamines should be instructed regarding:

Avoiding any other drug, including OTC, without consulting physician first

Reporting symptoms such as fainting, dizziness, or palpitations to physician immediately

Using caution with driving or operating machinery

DECONGESTANTS

Several adrenergic drugs, for example, phenylephrine (Neosynephrine) or pseudoephedrine (Sudafed), act as **decongestants.** These drugs constrict blood vessels in the respiratory tract, resulting in shrinkage of swollen mucous membranes and helping to open nasal airway passages. However, these drugs, both oral and nasal, should be used only on a short-term basis because rebound congestion may occur within a few days. Decongestants are frequently combined with antihistamines, analgesics, caffeine, and/or antitussives. Many of these products are available over the counter and, by combining several drugs, the possibility of adverse side effects is increased, especially without adequate medical supervision.

Side effects of decongestants can include:

* Anxiety, nervousness, tremor, seizures
* Palpitations, hypertension, headache, cerebral hemorrhage
  Reduced cardiac output and reduced urine output

Contraindications or extreme caution with decongestants applies to:

Cardiovascular disorders

Hyperthyroid or diabetes

Older adults—especially those with glaucoma or BPH

Pregnancy or lactation

Interactions may occur with:

Potentiation of adverse side effects with other adrenergics, ergot, tricyclics, MAOIs

Patient Education

Patients taking decongestants should be instructed regarding:

Using decongestants for only a few days to avoid rebound congestion

Avoiding when cardiac or thyroid conditions or diabetes are present

Discontinuing with side effects such as nervousness, tremor, palpitations, or headache

Avoiding combining with any other medications without consulting physician

See Table 26-4 for a summary of the antihistamines and decongestants.

Table 26-4 Antihistamines and Decongestants

GENERIC NAME	TRADE NAME	DOSAGE
First Generation		
chlorpheniramine	Chlor-Trimeton, Aller-Chlor	Elix 2 mg/5 ml q4–6h
		Tabs 4 mg q4–6h
		ER Tabs 8–12 mg BID
clemastine	Tavist Allergy	Tabs 1.34–2.68 mg BID–TID
diphenydramine	Diphenhist	Elix 25–50 mg q4–6h
	Benadryl Allergy	Tabs 25–50 mg q4–6h
	Benadryl (in sleeping pills)	IM or IV 10–50 mg q4–6h
promethazine	Phenergan	Elix 6.25–25 mg/5 ml q4–6h
Second Generation		
certrizine	Zyrtec	Tabs 5–10 mg/day, syrup 5 mg/5 ml
desloratadine	Clarinex (changed molecule of Claritin)	Syrup, tabs 5 mg daily
fexofenadine	Allegra	Tabs 30–60 mg BID, 180 mg/day
loratadine	Claritin, Alavert (racemic mixture)	Syrup, tabs 5 mg daily
Decongestants		
oxymetazoline	Afrin, Allerest	Sol 0.025%–0.05% 2–3 sprays, drops q12h
phenylephrine	Neosynephrine, Nostril (hospital only)	Sol 0.125%–1% 1–3 drops/sprays q4h
pseudoephedrine	Sudafed, Efidac	Sol or tabs 30–60 mg q4–6h
		Tabs ER 120 mg q12h or 240 mg q24h

Note: This is a representative list. Many prescription and OTC drugs have combinations of antihistamines and decongestants. These combinations sometimes also include antitussives.

Patient Education

Patients taking respiratory system drugs should be instructed regarding:

Care in taking medications only as prescribed and required

Avoiding combining respiratory system drugs with other prescription or OTC drugs or alcohol, which could potentiate CNS stimulation or depression, resulting in serious adverse side effects

Avoiding self-medication when cardiac, thyroid, or CNS conditions are present

Liberal intake of fluids, which is encouraged to help liquefy secretions

Benefit from desensitization therapy and air-conditioned environmental control for patients with allergic conditions

Avoiding air pollution (e.g., smoke-filled rooms)

Exercises (e.g., swimming) that increase lung capacity and help reduce the necessity for medication

Proper use of inhalers when prescribed (see administration with inhalers in Chapter 9)

Not crushing, chewing, or breaking extended-release preparations; swallow whole

SMOKING CESSATION AIDS

Smoking cessation aids (Table 26-5), including Nicorette gum, the Nicoderm CQ patch, and the Nicotrol inhaler, are used to slowly lower the level of nicotine while the patient participates in a behavior modification program for smoking cessation.

Bupropion is an oral antidepressant drug (Wellbutrin) that is also prescribed as an aid to smoking cessation (Zyban). Zyban is also indicated for use in combination with nicotine patches for treating the symptoms of smoking cessation. (Refer to Chapter 20 for information on bupropion.)

Side effects of smoking cessation aids can include:

Mechanical problems with chewing gum, especially if patient has dentures

✸ Cardiac irritability

✸ Chewing too fast—may cause lightheadedness, nausea, vomiting, throat and mouth irritation

Cautions with smoking cessation aids apply to:

Patients with dental problems that might be exacerbated by chewing gum

Drug abuse and/or overdependence

Overdosage

Pregnancy and lactation

Severe cardiovascular disease

Patients should be warned not to smoke

Table 26-5 Smoking Cessation Aids

GENERIC NAME	TRADE NAME	DOSAGE
nicotine	Nicorette	1 piece of gum whenever urge to smoke
		Daily max of 2 mg pieces = 30
		Daily max of 4 mg pieces = 15
	Nicoderm CQ, Habitrol	lst dose 2l mg patch/day, 4–8 wk
		2nd dose l4 mg patch/day, 2–4wk
		3rd dose 7 mg patch/day, 2–4wk
	Nicotrol inhaler	24–64 mg (6–12 cartridges) daily up to 12 wk,
		then gradual reduction in dose up to 12 wk
bupropion	Zyban (wellbutrin)	Tabs, SR 150 mg daily × 3d, then 150 mg BID
	Chantix	for 7–12 wk

WORKSHEET FOR CHAPTER 26
RESPIRATORY DRUGS

Note the drugs listed according to category and complete all columns.
Learn generic trade names as specified by instructor.

Classifications and Drugs	Purpose	Side Effects	Contraindications or Cautions	Patient Education
Bronchodilators Xanthines 1. Aminophylline				
2. Theo-24				
Adrenergics 1. Epinephrine (Primatene, Adrenalin)				
2. Alupent				
3. Isuprel				
4. Serevent				
5. Terbutaline (Brethine)				
Anticholinergics 1. Atrovent				
2. Combivent				

(continued)

Classifications and Drugs	Purpose	Side Effects	Contraindications or Cautions	Patient Education
Corticosteroids 1. beclomethasone (Beconase) 2. fluticasone (Flonase) 3. triamcinolone (Azmacort)				
Asthma Prophylaxis 1. cromolyn (Intal) 2. Singulair 3. Accolate				
Mucolytics and Expectorants 1. Mucomyst 2. guaifenesin				
Antitussives 1. codeine 2. dextromethorphan (Robitussin DM) 3. Tessalon				
Antihistamines 1. Claritin/Allegra 2. Benadryl				
Decongestants 1. Neosynephrine 2. Sudafed 3. Afrin				

A. Case Study for Respiratory Medications

Fred Farmer, a 68-year-old man with a history of COPD, complains of increased shortness of breath and nasal congestion. His Theo-24 prescription ran out last week and was not refilled. He has been using an Alupent inhaler more frequently without relief, and also taking an OTC decongestant for a week.

1. Decongestants can cause all of the following EXCEPT
   a. Rebound congestion   c. Tremor
   b. Frequency   d. Nervousness

2. Side effects or Theo-24 can include the following EXCEPT
   a. GI distress   c. Sedation
   b. Nervousness   d. Frequency

3. The following statements are true of Alupent EXCEPT
   a. CNS stimulant   c. Dilates bronchioles
   b. Avoid with decongestants d. Can be used PRN q2h

4. Side effects of Alupent can include the following EXCEPT
   a. Palpitations   c. Sedation
   b. Dizziness   d. Tremor

5. Side effects of decongestants can include the following EXCEPT
   a. Anxiety   c. Headache
   b. Insomnia   d. Hypotension

B. Case Study for Respiratory Medications

Mae Wright, a 70-year-old asthmatic, began using a Flovent inhaler a week ago. Today, she complains of a thick white coating on her tongue. She has also been taking OTC Benadryl for a runny nose and fever.

1. Inhaled corticosteroids are used for all of the following EXCEPT:
   a. chronic asthma   c. some URI
   b. some COPD   d. acute asthma

2. Side effects of Beclovent can include the following EXCEPT
   a. Rash   c. Dry mouth
   b. Oral fungal infections   d. Hoarseness

3. What should Ms. Wright be reminded to do after using her Beclovent inhaler?
   a. Hold her breath for   c. Rest for several minutes
      one minute   d. Rinse mouth with water
   b. Gargle with mouthwash

4. Antihistamines are used to treat all of the following EXCEPT
   a. Rhinitis   c. Rash
   b. Conjunctivitis   d. Asthma

5. Side effects of first-generation antihistamines, e.g., Benadryl, can include all of the following EXCEPT
   a. Dizziness   c. Urinary frequency
   b. Mucus plugs   d. Sedation

CHAPTER REVIEW QUIZ

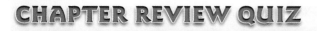

Match the medication in the first column with the condition in the second column that it is used to treat. Conditions may be used more than once.

Medication	**Condition**
1. _____ Allegra	**A.** Bronchospasm (anticholinergic)
2. _____ Habitrol	**B.** Chronic asthma
3. _____ Guaifenesin	**C.** Asthma (adrenergic)
4. _____ Xopenex	**D.** Asthma (prophylactic)
5. _____ Spiriva	**E.** Allergies
6. _____ Tessalon	**F.** Smoking cessation
7. _____ Cromolyn sodium	**G.** Bronchitis (unproductive cough)
8. _____ Accolate	
9. _____ Zyban	

Choose the correct answer.

10. All of the following are *possibilities* with inhalers EXCEPT:
    a. increased systemic effects   c. breath-actuated
    b. dry powder formulations   d. metered-dose

11. Adrenergic bronchodilators, for example Alupent, could cause all of the following side effects EXCEPT:
    a. Nervousness   c. Hypertension
    b. Hypoglycemia   d. Tachycardia

12. Anticholinergic bronchodilators, for example Atrovent, could cause all of the following side effects EXCEPT:
    a. Dried secretions   c. Bradycardia
    b. Confusion   d. Dizziness

13. Singulair is appropriate for all of the following EXCEPT:
    a. Asthma prophylaxis   c. Young children
    b. MDI inhalations   d. Chronic asthma

14. Patient education for inhaled corticosteroid treatment would include all of the following EXCEPT:
    a. Rinse equipment after   c. Expect dry mouth
    b. Use before a bronchodilator d. Rinse mouth after

15. The following statements are true about quaifenesin, found in many cough syrups, EXCEPT:
    a. Can cause runny nose   c. Increases secretions
    b. Helps expel sputum   d. Stops the cough

519 Respiratory System Drugs and Antihistamines

16. The following statements are true of Claritin, EXCEPT:
   a. For allergies
   b. Less sedation
   c. For rhinitis
   d. For asthma

17. Decongestants should only be used short term. Which of the following is NOT a decongestant?
   a. Diphenhydramine
   b. Afrin
   c. Neosynephrine
   d. Sudafed

18. Antitussives frequently contain controlled substances. Which one of the following medicines is available OTC?
   a. Hycodan
   b. Dextromethorphan
   c. Robitussin AC
   d. Organidin NR

19. Cough and cold medications containing antihistamines are only appropriate when the cause of the cough is
   a. Asthma
   b. Allergic rhinitis
   c. Emphysema
   d. Smoking

20. Nicorette would be an appropriate treatment for one with which condition?
   a. Arrhythmia
   b. Dentures
   c. Pregnancy
   d. COPD

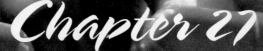

Chapter 21
Drugs and Older Adults

Key Terms

Absorption

Cumulative effects

Distribution

Excretion

Gray List drugs

Mental impairment

Motor impairment

Metabolism

Polypharmacy

Objectives

Upon completion of this chapter, the learner should be able to

1. Define the Key Terms

2. List at least 15 drugs that are inappropriate for older people

3. Describe four factors that may lead to cumulative effects in older adults

4. Name at least five categories of drugs that frequently cause adverse side effects in older adults

5. List at least 10 drugs that can cause mental problems in older adults

6. Describe the dangers and side effects associated with NSAID therapy

7. List side effects and cautions for gastrointestinal (GI) drugs

8. Explain patient education for nonsteroidal anti-inflammatory drugs (NSAIDs) and GI drugs

9. Describe patient education for all patients on long-term drug therapy

10. List the responsibilities of health care personnel in preventing complications of drug therapy

Today, people are living longer and are taking more medications. Consequently, there has also been an increase in serious complications resulting from adverse drug reactions. It has been estimated that more than 200,000 adults over the age of 60 are hospitalized yearly as the result of adverse drug effects. In 2000, it was estimated that medication-related problems caused 106,000 deaths annually.

Therefore, it is imperative that members of the health care community work together to reverse this dangerous trend.

The aging process is an individualized matter. Because of genetic or environmental factors or good health practices, for example, exercise, healthy diet, and mental stimulation, some older individuals may not feel or appear particularly different. However, we need to realize that there are gradual changes in body composition and organ function as we grow older. These changes can affect the reaction to drugs and make the individual more sensitive to a wide variety of medications.

A study by Harvard Medical School researchers looked at medicines prescribed for individuals over 65 years of age. The panel of experts in geriatrics and pharmacology found "a disturbingly high level of potentially inappropriate prescribing for older people. Over the course of one year, almost one quarter of older Americans were unnecessarily exposed to potentially hazardous prescribing."

CUMULATIVE EFFECTS OF DRUGS

Complex changes of aging involve both anatomic and physiological factors that affect how drugs are processed in the body (see Chapter 3). The four processes that drugs undergo in the body—that is, **absorption, distribution, metabolism** (biotransformation), and **excretion**—are all altered as the body ages. The end result of this slowed process can be a buildup of drugs in the system, leading to dangerous or toxic levels.

Cumulative effects of drugs in older adults can be due to:

Inadequate absorption—slowed GI motility or reduced fluid intake

Impaired distribution—circulatory dysfunction

Slower metabolism—hepatic dysfunction

Impaired excretion—renal dysfunction, constipation, or poor exchange of gases in the lungs

Absorption

As we age, several things happen to our GI tract. Not only does the gastric motility decrease, but the gastric pH also increases, causing a more alkaline environment, which affects the absorption process.

Antacids are used frequently by older persons. Calcium, magnesium, and aluminum form insoluble and nonabsorbable complexes that are passed out of the body in the feces. Some of the drugs that are affected by antacids are quinolone antibiotics, tetracycline, iron salts, ketoconazole, and isoniazid. Therefore, it is recommended that these, and other drugs as well, not be taken within two hours of taking antacids.

Decreased gastric motility, especially when taking anticholinergic drugs, for example, the tricyclic antidepressants or the antispasmodics, can cause adverse effects. Gastric slowing will lead to increased time for other drugs to be dissolved and absorbed.

Additionally, it has been determined that as many as 30% of adults over 50 have diminished gastric acid production. Many adults also take medication that reduces gastric acid, for example, Zantac or Prilosec. (See Chapter 16, Gastrointestinal Drugs.)

Distribution

Once drugs are absorbed and enter the circulation, many of them bind to proteins. Albumin is the principal protein used to bind drugs. As we age, the liver produces less albumin, especially in conditions such as malnutrition, cancer, diabetes, surgery, burns, and liver disease.

Phenytoin (Dilantin) is an example of a drug that responds quite noticeably to drops in plasma albumin levels. Older clients need to be monitored frequently with laboratory studies, especially with symptoms such as sleepiness, confusion, nystagmus, diplopia, and ataxia. Other drugs that are highly protein-bound include warfarin (Coumadin), aspirin, naproxen, tolbutamide (Orinase), and valproate (Depakene). When any of these drugs is used in the older person, the best advice is to start at the lowest effective dose and increase slowly to avoid adverse effects.

Because the older person has less body water, drugs that are water soluble may become concentrated and cause adverse reactions, with additive effects over time.

Metabolism

As we age, the mass of functional liver tissue and blood flow to the liver decreases. The ability of the liver to break down drugs declines, and drugs remain in the body longer. Repeated dosing can result in the accumulation of the drug and increase the risk for toxicity. Some drugs that can produce toxic effects when poorly metabolized are caffeine, diazepam, chlordiazepoxide, lidocaine, theophylline, meperidine, hydromorphone, warfarin, phenytoin, diphenhydramine (Benadryl), and propranolol.

Long-acting benzodiazepines have been implicated in falls and hip fractures. These drugs build up with repeated administration and cause *side effects,* such as daytime sedation, dizziness, lethargy, and ataxia. Therefore, it is safer to use *shorter-acting sedatives,* for example lorazepam (Ativan) in doses no higher than 3 mg, and hypnotics, such as zolpidem (Ambien).

Cimetidine (Tagamet) inhibits liver enzymes from breaking down the long-acting benzodiazepines and prolongs the drug's duration of action. It is therefore preferable to use antiulcer medications such as famotidine (Pepcid) or nizatidine (Axid), rather than Tagamet.

Excretion

In the older person, kidney size, blood flow, and glomerular filtration all decrease, resulting in a decline in creatinine clearance. Illnesses such as hypertension, heart failure, and diabetes add to the age-related loss and further reduce creatinine clearance. Consequently, drug by-products normally eliminated through the kidneys can accumulate, with toxic effects. *Nephrotoxic* drugs, such as the aminoglycosides, can prove particularly dangerous to older people with reduced renal function. Acute renal failure and irreversible damage to the eighth cranial nerve (auditory and vestibular branches) are possible.

Meperidine (Demerol) poses great risks to older adults with impaired renal function. Morphine is a safer choice.

Older persons are more likely to have *adverse drug reactions to anticholinergics.* (See Chapter 13.) The resulting *side effects* are blurred vision, confusion, disorientation, dry mouth, dry eyes, constipation, palpitations, worsening of glaucoma, and urinary retention. Men with prostate problems are at extreme risk for acute urinary retention.

Drugs that produce significant anticholinergic effects include:

- Antipsychotic agents, such as chlorpromazine (Thorazine), thioridazine (Mellaril), and perphenazine (Trilafon)

- Antidepressants, such as tricyclics, amitriptyline (Elavil), doxepin (Sinequan), and nortriptyline (Pamelor)

- Antiparkinson agents, such as benztropine (Cogentin) and trihexyphenidyl (Artane)

- Antispasmodics, such as dicyclomine (Bentyl) and hyoscyamine (Levsin)

- Antihistamines, such as diphenhydramine (Benadryl) and promethazine (Phenergan)

Because the increase in the amount of a drug circulating in the system is often gradual, the consequences of an "overdose" may not be recognized. Family, friends, and even patients themselves may conclude that their symptoms are just due to "aging."

Some medicines that are perfectly safe for a 30-year-old person may produce unexpected results in a person over age 50 or 60. An example is *digoxin (Lanoxin)*. An older person still on the same dose that was appropriate 10 or 20 years earlier may experience *side effects* such as loss of appetite, weakness, personality changes, nightmares, confusion, or even hallucinations. Older adults should receive no more than 0.125 mg per day of digoxin for an extended period of time unless an arrhythmia is being treated. In addition, digoxin can interact with many other drugs, sometimes slowing clearance of the drug from the system, which could result in cumulative effects, including possible dangerous arrhythmias.

POTENTIALLY INAPPROPRIATE MEDICATION USE IN OLDER ADULTS

A group of physicians led by Dr. Mark Beers conducted a national survey of geriatrics experts in 1997 to determine the most *inappropriate* drugs for ambulatory nursing home residents and adults 65 or older. The results of this survey came to be called *The Gray List* (**Gray List drugs**).

The Beers study was updated and revised by another panel of experts and the results were published in 2003 under the title, *Updating the Beers Criteria for Potentially Inappropriate Medication Use in Older Adults*. A summary of the results from both of these studies can be found in the following Table 27-1.

Table 27-1 Potentially Inappropriate Medications for Older Adults

Adults over 65 should avoid these drugs completely unless noted otherwise.

GENERIC NAME	TRADE NAME	COMMENTS
Sedative-Hypnotics		
long-acting benzodiazepines—Prolonged daytime effects: sedation, dizziness, ataxia		
chlordiazepoxide	Librium, Limbitrol, Librax	
diazepam	Valium	
flurazepam	Dalmane	
meprobamate	Miltown	
short-acting benzodiazepines—Avoid long-term use; can be habit forming.		
alprazolam	Xanax	No dose greater than 2 mg; do not exceed daily max
lorazepam	Ativan	No dose greater than 3 mg; do not exceed daily max
oxepam	Serax	No dose greater than 60 mg; do not exceed daily max
temazepam	Restoril	No dose greater than 15 mg; do not exceed daily max
triazolam	Halcion	No dose greater than 0.25 mg; do not exceed daily max
Antidepressants		
amitriptyline	Elavil	Anticholinergic effects
doxepin	Sinequan	Anticholinergic effects
fluoxetine	Prozac	Long half-life; potential for agitation
		Safer alternatives
Antipsychotics		
haloperidol	Haldol	Doses >3 mg/day should be avoided (patients with known psychotic disorders may receive higher doses)
thioridazine	Mellaril	Avoid doses >30 mg/day (unless known psychotic disorder)
Antihypertensives		
hydrochlorothiazide	Esidrix HydroDIURIL	Avoid >50 mg doses
methyldopa	Aldomet	
propranolol	Inderal	Other beta-blockers offer less CNS penetration
reserpine	Serpasil	
clonidine	Catapress	Potential for CNS adverse effects and orthostatic hypotension.
Antiarrhythmic		
disopyramide	Norpace	May induce heart failure in older adults Anticholinergic; better alternatives
NSAIDs		
indomethacin	Indocin	Other NSAIDs cause less CNS and GI toxic reactions than these drugs
ketorolac	Toradol	
phenylbutazone	Butazolidin	
Oral Hypoglycemics		
chlorpropamide	Diabinese	Causes SIADH*

Table 27-1 continued

Adults over 65 should avoid these drugs completely unless noted otherwise.

GENERIC NAME	TRADE NAME	COMMENTS
Analgesics		
meperidine	Demerol	May cause confusion
		Better alternative, for example, morphine
propoxyphene	Darvon	Adverse CNS effects potentiated in older adults
	Darvocet N	
pentazocine	Talwin	
Platelet Inhibitors		
dipyridamole	Persantine	Only avoid short-acting; ER acceptable
Histamine-2 Blockers		
cimetidine	Tagamet	Avoid doses >900 mg/day
		CNS effects
Anti-infective		
nitrofurantoin	Macrodantin	Potential for renal impairment
		Safer alternatives available
Antihistamines—*Nonanticholinergic* antihistamines are preferred for older adults (see Chapter 26 *Respiratory Drugs*)		
chlorpheniramine	Chlor-Trimeton	All of these drugs have anticholinergic effects; use
		short-term only for conditions other than allergies
diphenhydramine	Benadryl, Tylenol PM	
hydroxyzine	Vistaril, Atarax	
promethazine	Phenergan	
Decongestants		
oxymetazoline	Afrin, Dristan, others	Avoid daily use >2 wk
phenylephrine	Neo-Synephrine	Avoid daily use >2 wk
pseudoephedrine	Sudafed	Avoid daily use >2 wk
Iron	Ferrous sulfate	Avoid doses >325 mg/day
Antispasmodics—Avoid long-term use; potential for toxicity greater than potential benefit		
hyoscyamine	Cytospaz, Levsin, Levsinex	All of these have anticholinergic effects
belladonna alkaloids	Donnatal and others	
dicyclomine	Bentyl	
oxybutynin	Ditropan	Does not apply to Ditropan XL
tolterodine	Detrol	Does not apply to Detrol LA
Muscle Relaxants—All cause anticholinergic adverse side effects		
cyclobenzaprine	Flexeril	
orphenadrine	Norflex	
methocarbamol	Robaxin	
carisoprodol	Soma	
Antiemetics		
trimethobenzamide	Tigan	Can cause extrapyramidal effects

*SIADH, syndrome of inappropriate antidiuretic hormone secretion.

DRUGS THAT MAY CAUSE MENTAL IMPAIRMENT

Many medications can cause mental problems in older people. One government study found that more than 150,000 older adults had experienced *serious mental impairment either caused or worsened by drugs.* Many medications can have CNS *side effects,* such as anxiety, depression, confusion, disorientation, forgetfulness, hallucinations, nightmares, or impaired mental clarity, *especially in older adults.* Some drugs that can cause **mental impairment** in older adults include:

Aldomet	Mellaril
Artane	Pamelor
Benadryl	Phenergan
Bentyl	Prednisone
Cogentin	Pro-Banthine
Compazine	Quinidine
Corgard	Reglan
Dalmane	Sinemet
Desyrel	Sinequan
Dilantin	Tagamet
Ditropan	Tegretol
Donnatal	Tenormin
Elavil	Thorazine
Halcion	Timoptic
Haldol	Tofranil
Inderal	Xanax
Lopressor	

Other CNS drugs also impair mental function. This is a representative list of the most frequently used drugs. In addition, all antipsychotics can cause tardive dyskinesia and/or parkinsonism. Alcohol can also potentiate adverse effects of many drugs.

Many CNS drugs and antihypertensives can also cause dizziness or **motor impairment,** which increases the risk of falls. These drugs can also impair sexual functioning, reducing the quality of life for some older adults.

NONSTEROIDAL ANTI-INFLAMMATORY DRUGS

Many older people suffer from arthritis and take over-the-counter nonsteroidal anti-inflammatory drugs (NSAIDs), frequently without adequate supervision. Anyone taking NSAIDs should be cautioned about the real danger of serious complications. Every year there are over 70,000 hospitalizations and more than 7,000 deaths from drug-induced bleeding ulcers or perforations. Particularly in older adults, there may be no warning signs of pain and the first symptoms of trouble may be a "silent" bleed that could lead to fatal GI hemorrhage.

Side effects of NSAIDs and corticosteroids (e.g., prednisone) can include:

✳ Indigestion, heartburn, abdominal pain

　Nausea, vomiting, and anorexia

　Flatulence, diarrhea, or constipation

✳ Silent ulceration (no symptoms of GI problems)

Other possible side effects of NSAIDs (including aspirin):

✳ Prolonged bleeding time

　Liver toxicity and kidney dysfunction

　Bronchospasm (especially with asthma)

　Visual or hearing problems (e.g., tinnitus)

The newer NSAID, the COX-2 inhibitor Celebrex, has a lower risk of gastric problems, GI bleeding, or other bleeding problems than the other nonselective NSAIDs.

✳ However, studies have indicated *increased risk of cardiovascular problems* with the use of some COX-2 inhibitors. Vioxx and Bextra were taken off the market because of these risks. Therefore, caution should be exercised in the use of any drug in this category. Consultation with the physician should include consideration of whether the benefits outweigh the risks.

Misoprostol (Cytotec) is sometimes given for the prevention of NSAID-induced gastric ulcers, but may cause severe diarrhea.

Patient Education

Patients receiving NSAID therapy should be instructed regarding:

Administration with food

Not exceeding dosage prescribed by physician

Not taking aspirin, alcohol, or any other drugs at the same time because they may potentiate GI or bleeding problems

The possibility of "silent" bleeding

Reducing dosage of NSAIDs and substituting acetaminophen for pain, if possible, at least part of the time

Trying exercise and heat for pain control, as approved by physician

See Chapter 21 for a list of NSAIDs and interactions.

GI problems, for example indigestion, heartburn, and constipation, are frequent complaints of older adults. Consequently, a common practice is the taking of over-the-counter (OTC) remedies without adequate awareness of potential side effects or implications.

Patient Education

Patients receiving GI medicines should be instructed regarding:

Side effects of antacids, including constipation (with aluminum or calcium carbonate products), diarrhea (with magnesium antacids); acid rebound, belching, or flatulence (with calcium carbonate)

Avoiding prolonged use (no longer than two weeks) of OTC antacids without medical supervision because of the danger of masking symptoms of GI bleeding or GI malignancy

Avoiding taking antacids within two hours of any other drug because of numerous interactions (see Chapter 16)

Antiulcer drugs, for example Tagamet, can lead to mental confusion, especially in older adults.

Avoiding frequent use of strong cathartics, which can lead to laxative dependence and loss of normal bowel function. Instead, increase fluids and high-fiber diet and regular bowel habits. If laxatives are necessary, use bulk laxatives (e.g., psyllium) or stool softeners.

POLYPHARMACY

Individuals at any age, but especially older adults, may be the victims of **polypharmacy,** that is, excessive use of drugs or prescriptions or many drugs given at one time (see Figure 27-1). Polypharmacy increases the risk of dangerous interactions, with potentially serious adverse side ef-

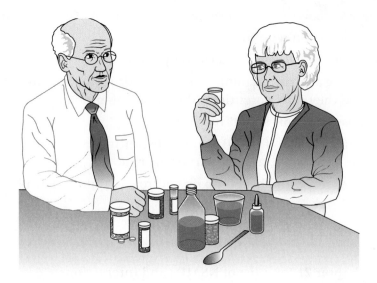

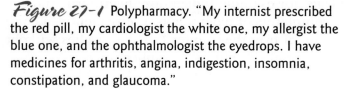

Figure 27-1 Polypharmacy. "My internist prescribed the red pill, my cardiologist the white one, my allergist the blue one, and the ophthalmologist the eyedrops. I have medicines for arthritis, angina, indigestion, insomnia, constipation, and glaucoma."

fects. Health care workers should take every opportunity to educate their patients regarding their medicines, the purpose for them, possible side effects, potential dangers, and interactions between medicines. Anyone receiving medicines should be monitored on an ongoing basis to determine continuing effectiveness and possible cumulative or adverse effects. Medicines should be reviewed regularly to determine feasibility of reducing dosage, possibly substituting a more effective or safer medicine, or discontinuing some of the medicines.

Patient Education

Older patients should be instructed regarding:

Making a list of *all* medicines (with dosage). Include pain medicine, eyedrops, OTC medicines, vitamins and herbal remedies, and topical medications. This list should be carried in wallet and/or be readily available at all times.

The purpose for their medicines, side effects, and interactions

Reporting side effects to physician immediately

The importance of seeing their physician on a regular basis, every six months to a year or more often, to reevaluate the need for and effectiveness of the drug

Not stopping the medicine or changing the dose without consulting the physician. Abrupt withdrawal can be dangerous with some medicines.

Asking the physician to prescribe a generic or less expensive alternative if the cost of the medicine is prohibitive. Sometimes social service departments can assist the patient in securing expensive medicines that are imperative to the patient's health.

If there is a problem with remembering to take medicines, ask the pharmacist to recommend a pillbox organizer.

All health care workers must be aware of their responsibilities in preventing complications of drug therapy in patients of any age, but especially the old and the very young, who are more vulnerable. The following guidelines should be helpful:

- Educate yourself, your patients, and their families regarding adverse side effects, cumulative effects, and interactions.
- With each newly prescribed drug, note diagnoses, allergies, and other medications.
- Monitor long-term drug use for effectiveness and physiological or mental changes. Do periodic laboratory tests as appropriate (e.g., digoxin levels).
- *Question* any inappropriate medicine or dosage. You have a moral, ethical, and legal responsibility to do what is best for the patient.
- Document all adverse side effects, calls to the physician, and action taken.

REFERENCES

Beers, M., M.D.; Fick, D., Ph.D., R.N.; Cooper, J., Ph.D., R.Ph.; Wade, W., Pharm.D., FASHP, FCCP; Waller, J., Ph.D.; Maclean, R., M.D. (2003). Updating the Beers Criteria for Potentially Inappropriate Medication Use in Older Adults. *Archives of Internal Medicine* [Dec. 8.]

Beers, Mark, M.D. (1997). Explicit criteria for determining potentially inappropriate medication use by the elderly. *Archives of Internal Medicine* [July 28].

Terrie, Yvette C., B.S.Pharm., R.Ph. (2004). Understanding and managing polypharmacy in the elderly. *Pharmacy Times* [Dec. 15].

Wick, J., R.Ph., M.B.A.; and Zanni, G. (2004). Geriatric pharmacology. *Pharmacy Times* [Nov. 15].

Wiseman, Rebecca, R.N., Ph.D. (2000). Polypharmacy in the elderly population. *Vital Signs* [Vol. X, No. 20, Oct. 24].

A. Case Study for Drugs and Older Adults

Harry Elder, a 75-year-old man, has a diagnosis of hypertension, angina, arteriosclerosis, GERD (gastroesophageal reflux disease), colitis, and BPH. He is receiving Lanoxin, Inderal, Xanax, Lopressor, Pepcid, and Halcion.

1. He is at risk for cumulative effects with his diagnoses and the following conditions EXCEPT
   a. Impaired excretion
   b. Hepatic dysfunction
   c. Circulatory dysfunction
   d. Increased GI motility

2. Side effects of Lanoxin can include the following EXCEPT
   a. Confusion
   b. Weakness
   c. Palpitations
   d. Anorexia

3. All of the drugs he is taking have the potential for causing mental impairment, depression, or confusion EXCEPT
   a. Inderal
   b. Xanax
   c. Lopressor
   d. Pepcid

4. All of the drugs he is taking have the potential for causing weakness or dizziness EXCEPT
   a. Lanoxin
   b. Halcion
   c. Pepcid
   d. Xanax

5. Serious interactions with toxicity are possible with his drugs and the following EXCEPT
   a. Antihistamines
   b. Antacids
   c. Alcohol
   d. Analgesics

B. Case Study for Drugs and Older Adults

Grace Grey, an 83-year-old resident of a nursing home, has a diagnosis of arthritis, diabetes, organic brain syndrome, and gastritis. Her medicines include prednisone, Naprosyn, Diabinese, Haldol, Tagamet, Ditropan, Metamucil, and Compazine PRN.

1. Side effects of corticosteriod and/or NSAIDs can include all of the following conditions EXCEPT
   a. GI distress
   b. Incontinence
   c. Bleeding
   d. Ulcers

2. Her medicines that could cause confusion include the following EXCEPT
   a. Diabinese
   b. Tagamet
   c. Ditropan
   d. Compazine

3. Haldol can cause all of the following EXCEPT
   a. Confusion
   b. Depression
   c. Weakness
   d. Diarrhea

4. Which oral antidiabetic agent is contraindicated for older adults?
   a. Micronase
   b. Tolinase
   c. Diabinese
   d. Glucotrol

5. Which is the only laxative that should be taken daily?
   a. Dulcolax
   b. Mineral oil
   c. Milk of Magnesia
   d. Metamucil

Note: A **Comprehensive Review Exam** for Part II can be found at the end of the text following the Summary.

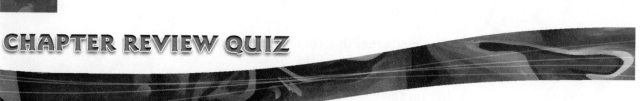

CHAPTER REVIEW QUIZ

Choose the correct answer.

1. Polypharmacy can result in the following EXCEPT:
   a. Better patient compliance
   b. More medication errors
   c. Overdose
   d. Dangerous interactions

2. Older adults should be instructed to do all of the following EXCEPT:
   a. Use pillbox organizer
   b. Stop medications abruptly
   c. List medicines
   d. Report problems

3. Older adults should be cautioned that adverse effects of NSAIDs are potentiated when taking with the following EXCEPT:
   a. Aspirin
   b. Alcohol
   c. Food
   d. Prednisone

4. Unless an arrhythmia is being treated, what is the maximum extended daily dose of digoxin for older adults?
   a. 0.25 mg
   b. 0.5 mg
   c. 0.125 mg
   d. 1.25 mg

5. Which problem of many nursing home residents is not potentiated by anticholinergic medications?
   a. Blurred vision
   b. Urinary frequency
   c. Constipation
   d. Confusion

6. Which one of these is an appropriate medication to treat arthritis pain for older adults?
   a. Indocin
   b. Toradol
   c. Acetaminophen
   d. Darvon

7. Which one of these is an appropriate medication to treat allergies in older adults?
   a. Benadryl
   b. Claritin
   c. Chlor-Trimeton
   d. Vistaril

8. Which one of these is an appropriate pain medication for older adults after surgery?
   a. Morphine
   b. Darvon
   c. Demerol
   d. Talwin

9. Which one of these anti-infectives should *not* be used to treat urinary infections in older adults?
   a. Macrodantin
   b. Keflex
   c. Trimpex
   d. Biaxin

10. Which one of these antihypertensives should *not* be used to treat older adults?
    a. Cozaar
    b. Calan
    c. Inderal
    d. Tenormin

11. Which of these cardiac drugs is *not* appropriate for older adults?
    a. Norpace
    b. Vasotec
    c. Procardia XL
    d. Apresoline

12. Which one of these is an appropriate antidepressant to treat older adults?
    a. Prozac
    b. Elavil
    c. Sinequan
    d. Wellbutrin

13. Which statement is *not* true of Tagamet?

    a. Prolongs drug effects   c. Speeds metabolism

    b. Inhibits liver enzymes   d. Possible CNS effects

14. Which statement is *not* true of short-acting sedatives, for example, Xanax?

    a. Can be habit forming   c. Dosage limited

    b. Short-term use only   d. Long half-life

15. Which statement is *not* true of antispasmodics, for example, Ditropan?

    a. Short-term use only   c. Potential toxicity

    b. Cholinergic effects   d. Long-acting preferable

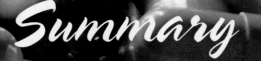

Summary

The health care worker has a great responsibility in the administration of medications and when advising others regarding drug therapy. As the older adult population increases and many more new drugs are developed and prescribed, more knowledge is required regarding cumulative effects and interactions. Moral, ethical, and legal issues of drug therapy are raised with increasing frequency. Therefore, it is imperative that the health care worker keep abreast of changes in drug therapy practices. Complete knowledge and good judgment are necessary for effective administration and adequate patient education.

The following guidelines should prove useful for safe drug therapy:

- Always research new drugs before administration to determine side effects, interactions, and cautions.

- Assess the patient before administration for allergies, general condition, and possible contraindications, and after administration for results and adverse effects.

- Question any inappropriate drugs, dosages, or possible interactions.

- Responsibilities of drug administration and medication errors are discussed further in Chapter 7.

- Reduce the risk of medication errors by checking the spelling of each medicine very carefully. Many drug names look and/or sound alike, but act differently. See appendix for *USP Quality Review* report, *Use Caution—Avoid Confusion,* which lists many similar drug names that have led to medication errors.

- Check the patient's diagnosis to be sure the medication is appropriate.

Comprehensive Review Exam for Part 1

1. Drug standards regulate all of the following factors in drug preparation EXCEPT
   a. Strength
   b. Purity
   c. Color
   d. Quality

2. All of the following facts are true of the Pure Food and Drug Act EXCEPT
   a. For consumer protection
   b. Listed approved drugs
   c. Set minimal standards
   d. Passed in 1776

3. The Food and Drug Administration regulates all of the following drug factors EXCEPT
   a. Prescription labeling
   b. Shape of tablet
   c. Effectiveness
   d. Safety

4. Which of the following drugs is *not* a controlled substance?
   a. Marijuana
   b. Valium
   c. Codeine
   d. Benadryl

5. Which statement is *not* true of controlled drugs?
   a. Listed by schedule
   b. Refilled PRN
   c. May cause dependence
   d. Sometimes illegal

6. Which is *not* a good source of drug information?
   a. PDR
   b. USP/DI
   c. Drug insert
   d. News magazine

7. Which statement is true of the generic name of a drug?
   a. Assigned by drug company
   b. Written in capital letters
   c. Common name
   d. Same as trade name

8. The term OTC refers to drugs:
   a. Often times controlled
   b. Requiring prescription
   c. For sale to anyone
   d. Officially certified

9. Which of the following conditions is *not* commonly listed as a *contraindication* for drug administration?
   a. Obesity
   b. Allergy
   c. Pregnancy
   d. Lactation

10. Before giving a new drug, you must know all of the following EXCEPT
    a. Interactions
    b. Contraindications
    c. Side effects
    d. Usual price

11. An antibiotic with *photosensitivity* listed as a side effect could cause
    a. Deafness
    b. Sunburn
    c. Blindness
    d. Kidney damage

12. Which is *not* a source of drugs?
    a. Minerals
    b. Gases
    c. Animals
    d. Laboratory

13. Which is *not* a process that drugs go through in the body?
    a. Tolerance
    b. Distribution
    c. Metabolism
    d. Excretion

14. Which of the following patient characteristics is *not* a factor affecting the processing of drugs in the body?
    a. Weight
    b. Age
    c. Mental state
    d. Skin color

15. Drug toxicity from cumulative effects may result from all of the following EXCEPT
    a. Low metabolism
    b. Poor circulation
    c. High blood pressure
    d. Kidney malfunction

16. Which term does *not* describe an adverse or unexpected result from a drug?
    a. Idiosyncrasy
    b. Anaphylaxis
    c. Placebo effect
    d. Teratogenic effect

17. Which route of administration is used most often?
    a. Topical
    b. Sublingual
    c. Injection
    d. Oral

18. Which is *not* a form of parenteral administration?
    a. Inhalation
    b. Rectal
    c. Dermal patch
    d. Injection

19. Which type of medication can be crushed and mixed with food to facilitate administration?
    a. Timed-release capsule
    b. Lozenge
    c. Scored tablet
    d. Enteric-coated tablet

20. Which is *not* a topical form of administration?
    a. Ointment
    b. Intradermal
    c. Eyedrops
    d. Vaginal cream

21. Which is the most rapid form of administration?
    a. PO
    b. IV
    c. IM
    d. subQ

22. Which is the least accurate system for measuring medication?
    a. Metric   c. Household
    b. Apothecary

23. Which is the most frequently used system for measuring medicine?
    a. Apothecary   c. Household
    b. Metric

24. Medication orders must contain all of the following EXCEPT
    a. Dosage   c. Medication name
    b. Route   d. Patient's address

25. The prescription blank for a controlled substance must contain all of the following EXCEPT
    a. Physician's DEA number   c. Frequency
    b. Name of drug company   d. Number of refills

26. Which type of equipment is least accurate in measuring medicine?
    a. Medicine cup   c. Teaspoon
    b. Minim glass   d. Syringe

27. Responsibilities of the health care worker include all of the following EXCEPT
    a. Patient education   c. Judgment
    b. Current information   d. Prescribing

28. Which is *not* appropriate action after administration of medication?
    a. Assessment   c. Evaluation
    b. Research concerning   d. Documentation
        meals

29. Which is the *least* helpful information in dispensing medication?
    a. Allergies   c. Health history
    b. Handicaps   d. Patient's occupation

30. If a medication error is made, all of the following actions are required EXCEPT
    a. Report to physician   c. Note on patient record
    b. File incident report   d. Apologize to patient

31. Before giving any medicine, it is essential to review the five Rights of Medication Administration, including all of the following EXCEPT
    a. Right amount   c. Right drug company
    b. Right drug   d. Right time schedule

32. Documentation of a controlled drug given PRN for pain requires all of the following EXCEPT
    a. Note on narcotic record   c. Note of effectiveness
    b. Note of trade name   d. Note on patient record

33. Which is *not* used for administration by the gastrointestinal route?
    a. Nasogastric tube   c. Rectal suppository
    b. Oral inhaler   d. Timed-release capsule

34. Which is *not* an advantage of the oral route over other routes?
    a. Speed   c. Economy
    b. Safety   d. Convenience

35. If a medication is ordered PO and the patient is NPO, which action is *most* appropriate?

a. Give medication by injection

b. Give medication rectally

c. Omit medication and note on chart

d. Consult the person in charge

36. Oral medications are usually best administered with which fluid?

a. Fruit juice

b. Milk

c. Water

d. Hot tea

37. When preparing cough syrup, which is the most appropriate action?

a. Shake the bottle

b. Dilute with liquid

c. Hold bottle label side down

d. Hold medicine cup at eye level

38. Which of the following is *not* required for administration of rectal suppository?

a. Lubricant

b. Privacy

c. Bed elevated

d. Disposable glove

39. Which parenteral route is *least* likely to be used for systemic effects?

a. Transdermal

b. Topical

c. Sublingual

d. Inhalation

40. Which route has the slowest action?

a. Transcutaneous

b. Inhalation

c. Sublingual

d. Injection

41. After instilling eyedrops, which is the most appropriate action?

a. Rub eyelid vigorously

b. Press inner canthus

c. Close eyelid quickly

d. Discard eyedropper

42. Which is *not* appropriate for intradermal injection?

a. Tuberculin syringe

b. 21-gauge, 1-inch needle

c. Wheal formation on skin

d. 0.1–0.2 ml solution

43. Which is *not* true of intramuscular injections?

a. Skin held taut

b. 1½-inch needle usual

c. 45-degree angle of needle

d. Can be Z-track

44. Which one of these intramuscular injection sites is used for infants?

a. Dorsogluteal

b. Ventrogluteal

c. Deltoid

d. Vastus lateralis

45. Before administering medication via NG tube, which step should be taken to verify placement?

a. Inject 10 ml water

b. Attach NG to suction

c. X-ray abdomen

d. Check pH of gastric juice

46. What is the first step to take if a two-year-old swallows several children's aspirin tablets?

a. Administer ipecac

b. Give activated charcoal

c. Call Poison Control

d. Give 8 oz of milk

47. If there is doubt about the type of poison, toxicology tests will be done on all of the following EXCEPT

a. Urine

b. Stool

c. Blood

d. Emesis

48. Which group is *least* at risk of accidental poisoning?

a. Infants

b. Older adults

c. Healthy adults

49. Patient education to prevent poisoning includes all of the following advice EXCEPT

    a. Label all medications and poisons

    b. Discard medications in toilet

    c. Always read medicine labels

    d. Keep medications at bedside

Calculate the correct dosage for administration in the following problems. Label your answers. Remember that syringes are not marked in fractions; therefore, when computing dosages for administration, you must convert all fractions to decimals and round off to one decimal place.

50. You are to give 7,500 units of heparin SubQ. The vial is labeled 10,000 units/ml. How many milliliters should you give?

51. You are to give 10 ml of Phenergan cough syrup with codeine. The bottle is labeled 10 mg of codeine in 5 ml of cough syrup. How much codeine would the patient receive in each prescribed dose?

52. The medicine bottle label states that the strength of each tablet in the bottle is 0.25 mg. The physician has ordered that the patient is to receive 0.5 mg. How many tablets should you give?

53. The physician has ordered 20 mg of meperidine to be given. On hand is medication containing 50 mg/ml. How many milliliters should you give?

54. To convert pounds to kilograms (kg), you would divide the number of pounds by what number?

Comprehensive Review Exam for Part 2

1. Deficiency of potassium may result in
   a. Diarrhea
   b. Petechiae
   c. Cardiac arrhythmias
   d. GI bleeding

2. Which would be *least* likely to require vitamin or mineral supplements?
   a. Executive secretary
   b. Nursing mother
   c. Adolescent
   d. Alcoholic

3. The following statements are true of vitamin C EXCEPT
   a. Destroyed by heat
   b. Unstable with antacids
   c. Found in citrus fruits
   d. Large supplements helpful

4. Which condition will slow absorption of topical medication?
   a. Heat
   b. Moisture
   c. Macerated skin
   d. Callused skin

5. The following statements are true of resistance to antibiotics EXCEPT
   a. Caused by too frequent use
   b. Caused by incomplete treatment
   c. Decreased with use of combination drugs
   d. Decreased with use of antacids concurrently

6. All of the following drugs are used in the initial treatment program for tuberculosis EXCEPT
   a. Isoniazid
   b. Rifampin
   c. Fluconazole
   d. Pyrazinamide

7. Unless ordered otherwise, antibiotics are best administered:
   a. With fruit juice
   b. With antacids
   c. 1 h ac
   d. ½ h pc

8. Allergic hypersensitivity can be manifested in all of the following ways EXCEPT
   a. Diarrhea
   b. Rash
   c. Hives
   d. Anaphylaxis

9. Which of the following would be most likely to develop a penicillin reaction?
   a. Premature infant
   b. Cancer patient
   c. Diabetic
   d. Allergic asthmatic

10. The following statements are true of atropine EXCEPT
    a. Used as a mydriatic
    b. Used as a cycloplegic
    c. Treatment for glaucoma
    d. Can cause blurred vision

11. The following statements are true of corticosteroid ophthalmic ointment EXCEPT
    a. Can delay healing
    b. Used short term
    c. Anti-inflammatory
    d. Used for infections

12. The following instructions are appropriate for those taking loop diuretics, for example, Lasix or Bumex, EXCEPT
    a. Avoid alcohol
    b. Report rash
    c. Take at bedtime
    d. Limit exposure to sun

13. The following side effects are possible with thiazide diuretics EXCEPT
    a. Hypokalemia
    b. Hypoglycemia
    c. Increased uric acid
    d. Muscle weakness

14. The thiazides are used to treat all of the following conditions EXCEPT
    a. Hypertension
    b. Congestive heart failure
    c. Gout
    d. Edema

15. Which term does *not* describe a purpose for antineoplastic drugs?
    a. Cytotoxic
    b. Analeptic
    c. Palliative
    d. Remission

16. Which is *not* a frequent side effect of antineoplastic drugs?
    a. Jaundice
    b. Diarrhea
    c. Ulcers of mucosa
    d. Nausea and vomiting

17. Which side effect is *not* associated with atropine?
    a. Diaphoresis
    b. Confusion
    c. Blurred vision
    d. Urinary retention

18. Which side effect is *not* associated with epinephrine?
    a. Palpitations
    b. Lethargy
    c. Tachycardia
    d. Tremor

19. Which is *not* an action of cholinergic drugs?
    a. Increased peristalsis
    b. Lowered intraocular pressure
    c. Reduced salivation
    d. Bladder contraction

20. Drugs that can cause mental impairment in older adults include all of the following EXCEPT
    a. Tagamet
    b. Naprosyn
    c. Benadryl
    d. Ditropan

Jim J. is admitted to the emergency room with a history of insecticide poisoning (cholinergic action). Questions 21 and 22 relate to Jim's situation:

21. Jim's symptoms might include all of the following EXCEPT
   a. Facial flushing   c. Diarrhea
   b. Diaphoresis   d. Nausea

22. His treatment would most likely include which drug?
   a. Prostigmin   c. Atropine
   b. Adrenalin   d. Isuprel

23. Which statement is *not* true of Lomotil?
   a. Slows peristalsis   c. Has drying effect
   b. Contains atropine   d. Used for food poisoning

24. Which laxative would be used for chronic constipation?
   a. Milk of Magnesia   c. Senokot
   b. Dulcolax   d. Metamucil

25. Which medication is *not* an antiemetic?
   a. Phenergan   c. Dramamine
   b. Imodium   d. Compazine

26. The most likely prescription for frequent gas pains is:
   a. Milk of Magnesia   c. Simethicone
   b. Colace   d. Metamucil

27. Which statement is *not* true of the nonsteroidal anti-inflammatory drugs?
   a. Alleviate pain of arthritis   c. Used long term sometimes
   b. Raise prostaglandin levels   d. Reduce joint swelling

28. Which drug is *not* a muscle relaxant?
   a. Robaxin   c. Naprosyn
   b. Valium   d. Flexeril

29. Which is *not* a likely side effect with opioid analgesics?
   a. Constipation   c. Urinary retention
   b. Tachycardia   d. Blurred vision

30. Which drug does *not* potentiate the CNS depression effect of analgesics and hypnotics?
   a. Alcohol   c. Corticosteroids
   b. Antihistamines   d. Muscle relaxants

31. Which is the most common side effect of prolonged use of haldoperidol (Haldol)?
   a. Hypertension   c. Diaphoresis
   b. Diarrhea   d. Parkinsonism

32. Which statement is *not* true of the tricyclic antidepressants?
   a. Rapidly effective   c. Tranquilizing effect
   b. Cause dry mouth   d. Anticholinergic action

33. Which statement is *not* true of the minor tranquilizers?
   a. For psychosomatic disorders   c. May cause photosensitivity
   b. Relieve nausea and vomiting   d. Useful long term

34. Adjuvant drugs that can enhance analgesic effect when combined with opioids include all of the following EXCEPT
   a. Neurontin   c. Tegretol
   b. Effexor   d. Tofranil

35. All of the following have GI bleeding as a possible side effect EXCEPT
   a. Ibuprofen   c. Prednisone
   b. Prilosec   d. Naprosyn

36. Which medication is used to treat febrile convulsions in children?
   a. Dilantin   c. Zarontin
   b. Depakote   d. Phenobarbital

37. Which is a purpose of the anticonvulsants?
   a. Reduce seizures   c. Cure epilepsy
   b. Sedate the patient   d. Treat parkinsonism

38. Which is *not* an antiparkinsonian drug?
   a. Cimetidine   c. Sinemet
   b. Cogentin   d. Symmetrel

39. Which condition is *not* treated with estrogen?
   a. Female hypogonadism   c. Threatened abortion
   b. Prostatic cancer   d. Atrophic vaginitis

40. Which condition is *not* treated with testosterone?
   a. Enuchoidism   d. Metastatic breast cancer
   b. Androgen deficiency   e. Prostate cancer
   c. Cryptorchidism

41. Which is *not* a possible side effect of corticosteroids?
   a. Delayed healing   c. Reduced resistance to infection
   b. Peptic ulcer formation   d. Hypoglycemia

42. Midazolam (Versed), a preoperative medication, can cause all of the following EXCEPT
   a. Slow respiration   c. Amnesia
   b. Tachycardia   d. Sedation

43. The following statements are true of isoproterenol (Isuprel) EXCEPT
   a. May cause hypoglycemia   c. May be given sublingually
   b. May cause palpitations   d. Used with inhaler

44. The following statements are true of codeine used as an antitussive EXCEPT
   a. May depress respirations   c. May be addictive
   b. Useful with COPD   d. Controlled substance

45. Which of the following respiratory drugs would not have tachycardia as a possible side effect?
   a. Alupent   c. Theophylline
   b. Atrovent   d. Singulair

46. Which is *not* a symptom of hypoglycemia?
   a. Tremor   d. Confusion
   b. Dry skin   e. Drowsiness
   c. Irritability

47. Which is *not* a symptom of hyperglycemia?
   a. Polyuria   d. Sweating
   b. Dehydration   e. Excessive thirst
   c. Lethargy

48. Which antihistamine is *least* likely to cause sedation?

    a. Benadryl   c. Chlor-Trimeton

    b. Phenergan   d. Claritin

49. All of the following might be a symptom of digitalis toxicity EXCEPT

    a. Cardiac arrhythmia   c. Urinary retention

    b. Blurred vision   d. GI disturbance

50. Which of the following antihypertensives is *least* likely to cause bradycardia?

    a. Procardia   c. Apresoline

    b. Inderal   d. Catapres

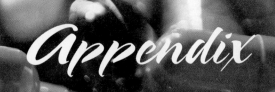

Appendix

A Publication of the USP Center for the Advancement of Patient Safety

APRIL 2004   No. 79

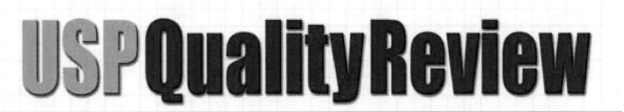

Use Caution—Avoid Confusion

This updated resource now includes reports submitted to both USP medication error reporting programs—MEDMARX℠ and the USP Medication Errors Reporting (MER) Program—from their inception through December 31, 2002. Similarity of drug names involves confusion between look-alike and/or sound-alike brand names, generic names, and brand to generic names. This confusion is compounded by illegible handwriting, lack of knowledge of drug names, newly available products, similar packaging or labeling, and incorrect selection of a similar name from a computerized product list.

Below is a list of similar drug names reported to MEDMARX and MER. It is important to remember that these names may not sound alike as you read them or look alike in print, but when handwritten or communicated verbally, these names have caused or could cause confusion. (**Brand names are *italicized*** and **new entries are highlighted in red.**)

Accolate	*Accupril*	*Acyclovir*	Famciclovir	*Altace*	*Accupril*
Accolate	*Accutane*	*Adalat CC*	*Aldomet*	*Altace* ..... *Amaryl* ... *Amerge*	
Accupril	*Aciphex*	*Adalat CC*	*Allegra*	*Altace*	*Artane*
Accupril	*Accolate*	*Adderall*	*Inderal*	*Altace*	*Norvasc*
Accupril	*Accutane*	Adenosine	Adenosine Phosphate	*Alupent*	*Atrovent*
Accupril	*Altace*	Adenosine Phosphate	Adenosine	Amantadine	Amiodarone
Accupril	*Aricept*	*Adipex-P*	*Aciphex*	Amantadine .. Ranitidine .. Rimantadine	
Accupril	*Monopril*	*Adriamycin*	*Aredia*	*Amaryl* .... *Altace* .... *Amerge*	
Accutane	*Accolate*	*Adriamycin*	*Idamycin*	*Amaryl*	*Avandia*
Accutane	*Accupril*	*Advair*	*Advicor*	*Amaryl*	*Reminyl*
Acebutolol	Albuterol	*Advicor*	*Advair*	*Amaryl*	*Symmetrel*
Acetaminophen and Codeine	Acetaminophen and Hydrocodone	*Aggrastat*	*Aggrenox*	*Ambien*	*Amen*
Acetaminophen and Codeine	Acetaminophen and Oxycodone	*Aggrastat*	*Argatroban*	*Ambien*	*Ativan*
		Aggrenox	*Aggrastat*	*Ambien*	*Coumadin*
Acetaminophen and Hydrocodone	Acetaminophen and Codeine	*Akarpine*	*Atropine*	*Amen*	*Ambien*
Acetaminophen and Oxycodone	Acetaminophen and Codeine	Albuterol	Acebutolol	*Amerge* .... *Altace* .... *Amaryl*	
		Aldara	*Alora*	*Amicar*	*Amikin*
Acetazolamide	Acetohexamide	Aldesleukin	Oprelvekin	Amikacin	Anakinra
Acetazolamide	Acetylcysteine	*Aldomet*	*Adalat CC*	*Amikin*	*Amicar*
Acetazolamide	Acyclovir	*Alkeran*	*Leukeran*	Amiloride	Amlodipine
Acetohexamide	Acetazolamide	*Allegra*	*Adalat CC*	Aminophylline	Amitriptyline
Acetylcysteine	Acetazolamide	*Allegra*	*Allegra-D*	Amiodarone	Trazodone
Aciphex	*Accupril*	*Allegra*	*Asacol*	Amiodarone	Amantadine
Aciphex	*Adipex-P*	*Allegra*	*Viagra*	Amiodarone	Amlodipine
Aciphex	*Aricept*	*Allegra-D*	*Allegra*	Amiodarone	Amrinone (Former nomenclature for Inamrinone)
Aciphex	*Vioxx*	*Allegra-D*	*Allerx-D*		
Activase	*Retavase*	*Allerx-D*	*Allegra-D*		
Actonel	*Actos*	Allopurinol	*Apresoline*	Amitriptyline	Aminophylline
Actos	*Actonel*	*Alora*	*Aldara*	Amitriptyline	Imipramine
Acular	Ocular Lubricants	Alprazolam	Clonazepam	Amitriptyline	Nortriptyline
Acyclovir	Acetazolamide	Alprazolam	Diazepam	Amlodipine	Amiloride
		Alprazolam	Lorazepam	Amlodipine	Amiodarone

USP   U.S. PHARMACOPEIA
The Standard of Quality℠

Amlodipine . . . . Felodipine
Amoxicillin . . . . *Amoxil*
Amoxicillin . . . . *Ampicillin*
Amoxicillin . . . . *Atarax*
Amoxicillin . . . . *Augmentin*
Amoxil . . . . Amoxicillin
Amphotericin B, ... Amphotericin B,
Lipid Complex   Liposomal
Amphotericin B, ... Amphotericin B,
Liposomal   Lipid Complex
Ampicillin . . . . Amoxicillin
Ampicillin . . . . *Augmentin*
Ampicillin . . . . Oxacillin
Amrinone . . . . Amiodarone
(Former nomenclature
for Inamrinone)
Anaflex . . . . *Zanaflex*
Anakinra . . . . Amikacin
Anaprox . . . . *Avapro*
Anaspaz . . . . *Antispas*
Anbesol . . . . *Anusol*
Ansaid . . . . *Asacol*
Antacid . . . . *Atacand*
Antispas . . . . *Anaspaz*
Anusol . . . . *Anbesol*
Anusol . . . . *Anusol-HC*
Anusol-HC . . . . *Anusol*
Anzemet . . . . *Aricept*
Apresoline . . . . Allopurinol
Apresoline . . . . *Priscoline*
Aredia . . . . *Adriamycin*
Argatroban . . . . *Aggrastat*
Argatroban . . . . *Orgaran*
Aricept . . . . *Accupril*
Aricept . . . . *Aciphex*
Aricept . . . . *Anzemet*
Artane . . . . *Altace*
Asacol . . . . *Allegra*
Asacol . . . . *Ansaid*
Asacol . . . . *Os-Cal*
Asparaginase . . . . Pegaspargase
Atacand . . . . Antacid
Atacand . . . . *Avandia*
Atarax . . . . Amoxicillin
Atarax . . . . *Ativan*
Atenolol . . . . Metoprolol
Atgam . . . . *Ratgam*
                  (Synonym for
                  Thymoglobulin)
Ativan . . . . *Ambien*
Ativan . . . . *Atarax*
Atorvastatin . . . . Pravastatin
Atropine . . . . *Akarpine*
Atrovent . . . . *Alupent*
Atrovent . . . . *Azmacort*
Atrovent . . . . *Flovent*
Atrovent . . . . *Natru-Vent*
Atrovent . . . . *Serevent*
Attenuvax . . . . *Meruvax*

Augmentin . . . . Amoxicillin
Augmentin . . . . Ampicillin
Avandia . . . . *Amaryl*
Avandia . . . . *Atacand*
Avandia . . . . *Avelox*
Avandia . . . . *Coumadin*
Avandia . . . . *Prandin*
Avapro . . . . *Anaprox*
Avapro . . . . *Avelox*
Avelox . . . . *Avandia*
Avelox . . . . *Avapro*
Avelox . . . . *Cerebyx*
Avinza . . . . *Invanz*
Avonex . . . . *Lovenox*
Azithromycin . . . . Erythromycin
Azithromycin . . . . Vancomycin
Azithromycin . . . . Aztreonam
Azmacort . . . . *Atrovent*
Azmacort . . . . *Nasacort*
Aztreonam . . . . Azithromycin
Bactrim . . . . *Biaxin*
Bactrim DS . . . . *Bancap HC*
Bancap HC . . . . *Bactrim DS*
Baycol . . . . *Bellergal*
Beclovent . . . . *Beconase*
Beconase . . . . *Beclovent*
Beconase . . . . *Beconase AQ*
Beconase AQ . . . . *Beconase*
Bellergal . . . . *Baycol*
Benadryl . . . . Benazepril
Benadryl . . . . *Bentyl*
Benadryl . . . . *Benylin*
Benazepril . . . . *Benadryl*
Benazepril . . . . Benzonatate
Benazepril . . . . Donepezil
Benazepril . . . . Lisinopril
Bentyl . . . . *Benadryl*
Bentyl . . . . *Bumex*
Bentyl . . . . *Proventil*
Benzonatate . . . . Benazepril
Benzonatate . . . . Benztropine
Benztropine . . . . Benzonatate
Bepridil . . . . *Prepidil*
Betagan . . . . *Betoptic*
Betapace . . . . *Betapace AF*
Betapace AF . . . . *Betapace*
Betoptic . . . . *Betagan*
Betoptic . . . . *Betoptic S*
Betoptic S . . . . *Betoptic*
Biaxin . . . . *Bactrim*
Bisacodyl . . . . Bisoprolol
Bisacodyl . . . . *Visicol*
Bisoprolol . . . . Bisacodyl
Bisoprolol . . . . Fosinopril
Boost bar . . . . *Buspar*
Brevibloc . . . . *Brevital*

Brevital . . . . *Brevibloc*
Bumex . . . . *Bentyl*
Bumex . . . . *Buprenex*
Bumex . . . . *Nimbex*
Bumex . . . . *Permax*
Bupivacaine . . . . Ropivacaine
Buprenex . . . . *Bumex*
Bupropion . . . . Buspirone
Buspar . . . . *Boost bar*
Buspirone . . . . Bupropion
Butalbital, ... Butalbital,
Acetaminophen,   Aspirin, and
and Caffeine   Caffeine
Butalbital, ... Butalbital,
Aspirin, and   Acetaminophen,
Caffeine   and Caffeine
Cafergot . . . . *Carafate*
Calan . . . . *Calan SR*
Calan . . . . *Colace*
Calan SR . . . . *Calan*
Calan SR . . . . *Cardizem CD*
Calan SR . . . . *Cardizem SR*
Calciferol . . . . Calcitriol
Calcitriol . . . . Calciferol
Calcium Acetate . . . . . . Calcium Carbonate
Calcium Carbonate . . . Calcium Acetate
Calcium Carbonate . . . Calcium Gluconate
Calcium Chloride . . . . . Calcium Gluconate
Calcium Gluconate . . . . Calcium Carbonate
Calcium Gluconate . . . Calcium Chloride
Capoten . . . . *Catapres*
Captopril . . . . Carvedilol
Carafate . . . . *Cafergot*
Carbatrol . . . . *Carbrital*
(Carbamezapine   (Pentobarbitone
in U.S.)   Sodium in Australia)
Carbidopa . . . . Levodopa and
                  Carbidopa
Carboplatin . . . . Cisplatin
Carbrital . . . . *Carbatrol*
(Pentobarbitone   (Carbamezapine
Sodium in Australia)   in U.S.)
Cardene . . . . *Cardizem*
Cardene . . . . *Cardura*
Cardene . . . . Codeine
Cardene SR . . . . *Cardizem SR*
Cardiem . . . . *Cardizem*
Cardizem . . . . *Cardene*
Cardizem . . . . *Cardiem*
Cardizem . . . . *Cardizem SR*
Cardizem . . . . Clonidine
Cardizem CD . . . . *Calan SR*
Cardizem CD . . . . *Cardizem SR*
Cardizem SR . . . . *Calan SR*
Cardizem SR . . . . *Cardene SR*
Cardizem SR . . . . *Cardizem*
Cardizem SR . . . . *Cardizem CD*
Cardura . . . . *Cardene*
Cardura . . . . *Cordarone*
Cardura . . . . *Coumadin*

Issued 4/04

USP Quality Review

April 2004

Cardura . . . . K-Dur	Cefpodoxime . . . . Cefixime	Chlorpromazine . . . . . . Thioridazine
Cardura . . . . Ridaura	Cefprozil . . . . Cefazolin	Chlorpropamide . . . . Chlorpromazine
Carteolol . . . . Carvedilol	Cefprozil . . . . Cefuroxime	Chlorthalidone . . . . Chlorpromazine
Cartia . . . . Cartia XT	Ceftazidime . . . . Cefazolin	Cipro . . . . Ceftin
(Aspirin in (Diltiazem in U.S.)	Ceftazidime . . . . Cefotaxime	Ciprofloxacin . . . . Cephalexin
New Zealand)	Ceftazidime . . . . Cefotetan	Ciprofloxacin . . . . Levofloxacin
Cartia XT . . . . Diltia XT	Ceftazidime . . . . Ceftizoxime	Ciprofloxacin . . . . Ofloxacin
Cartia XT . . . . Procardia XL	Ceftazidime . . . . Ceftriaxone	Cisplatin . . . . Carboplatin
Cartia XT . . . . Cartia	Ceftazidime . . . . Cefuroxime	Citracal . . . . Citrucel
(Diltiazem in U.S.) (Aspirin in	Ceftin . . . . Cefotan	Citrucel . . . . Hydrocil
New Zealand)	Ceftin . . . . Cefzil	Citrucel . . . . Citracal
Carvedilol . . . . Captopril	Ceftin . . . . Cipro	Claforan . . . . Cefotan
Carvedilol . . . . Carteolol	Ceftin . . . . Rocephin	Claritin . . . . Claritin-D
Cataflam . . . . Catapres	Ceftizoxime . . . . Cefazolin	Claritin-D . . . . Claritin
Catapres . . . . Capoten	Ceftizoxime . . . . Cefotaxime	Clinoril . . . . Clozaril
Catapres . . . . Cataflam	Ceftizoxime . . . . Cefotetan	Clinoril . . . . Oruvail
Ceclor . . . . Ceclor CD	Ceftizoxime . . . . Ceftazidime	Clomiphene . . . . Clomipramine
Ceclor CD . . . . Ceclor	Ceftizoxime . . . . Cefuroxime	Clomipramine . . . . Clomiphene
Cefaclor . . . . Cephalexin	Ceftriaxone . . . . Cefazolin	Clomipramine . . . . Desipramine
Cefazolin . . . . Cefepime	Ceftriaxone . . . . Cefotaxime	Clonapam . . . . Corlopam
Cefazolin . . . . Cefotaxime	Ceftriaxone . . . . Cefotetan	(Clonazepam (Fenoldopam
Cefazolin . . . . Cefotetan	Ceftriaxone . . . . Cefoxitin	in Canada) in U.S.)
Cefazolin . . . . Cefoxitin	Ceftriaxone . . . . Ceftazidime	Clonazepam . . . . Alprazolam
Cefazolin . . . . Cefprozil	Ceftriaxone . . . . Cefuroxime	Clonazepam . .Clonidine . . Klonopin
Cefazolin . . . . Ceftazidime	Ceftriaxone . . . . Cefotan	Clonazepam . . . . Clorazepate
Cefazolin . . . . Ceftizoxime	Cefuroxime . . . . Cefazolin	Clonazepam . . . . Diazepam
Cefazolin . . . . Ceftriaxone	Cefuroxime . . . . Cefotaxime	Clonazepam . . . . Lorazepam
Cefazolin . . . . Cefuroxime	Cefuroxime . . . . Cefprozil	Clonidine . . . . Colchicine
Cefazolin . . . . Cephalexin	Cefuroxime . . . . Ceftazidime	Clonidine . . . . Cardizem
Cefepime . . . . Cefazolin	Cefuroxime . . . . Ceftizoxime	Clonidine . . Klonopin . . Clonazepam
Cefepime . . . . Cefotetan	Cefuroxime . . . . Ceftriaxone	Clorazepate . . . . Clonazepam
Cefepime . . . . Cefotan	Cefuroxime . . . . Cephalexin	Clozaril . . . . Clinoril
Cefixime . . . . Cefpodoxime	Cefuroxime . . . . Deferoxamine	Clozaril . . . . Colazal
Cefobid . . . . Celecoxib	Cefuroxime . . . . Cefoxitin	Codeine . . . . Cardene
Cefobid . . . . Levbid	Cefzil . . . . Cefol	Codeine . . . . Iodine
Cefol . . . . Cefzil	Cefzil . . . . Ceftin	Codeine . . . . Lodine
Cefotan . . . . Ceftin	Cefzil . . . . Kefzol	Codiclear DH . . . . Codimal DH
Cefotan . . . . Claforan	Celebrex . . . Celexa . . . Cerebyx	Codimal DH . . . . Codiclear DH
Cefotan . . . . Cefepime	Celebrex . . . Celexa . . . Cerebra	Cognex . . . . Corgard
Cefotan . . . . Ceftriaxone	Celecoxib . . . . Cefobid	Colace . . . . Calan
Cefotaxime . . . . Cefazolin	Celexa . . . . Zyprexa	Colace . . . . Peri-Colace
Cefotaxime . . . . Cefotetan	Celexa . . . . . Celebrex . . Cerebra	Colace . . . . Colace
Cefotaxime . . . . Cefoxitin	Celexa . . . . . Cerebyx . . Celebrex	(Docusate Sodium) (Glycerin
Cefotaxime . . . . Ceftazidime	Cephalexin . . . . Cefaclor	suppository)
Cefotaxime . . . . Ceftizoxime	Cephalexin . . . . Cefazolin	Colace . . . . Colace
Cefotaxime . . . . Ceftriaxone	Cephalexin . . . . Cefuroxime	(Glycerin suppository) (Docusate Sodium)
Cefotaxime . . . . Cefuroxime	Cephalexin . . . . Ciprofloxacin	Colazal . . . . Clozaril
Cefotetan . . . . Cefazolin	Cerebra . . . . Celebrex . . Celexa	Colchicine . . . . Clonidine
Cefotetan . . . . Cefepime	Cerebyx . . . . Avelox	Combivir . . . . Epivir
Cefotetan . . . . Cefotaxime	Cerebyx . . . . Celebrex . . Celexa	Cordarone . . . . Cardura
Cefotetan . . . . Cefoxitin	Cetirizine . . . . Cyclobenzaprine	Cordarone . . . . Coumadin
Cefotetan . . . . Ceftazidime	Chlordiazepoxide . . . . . Chlorpromazine	Corgard . . . . Cognex
Cefotetan . . . . Ceftizoxime	Chlorhexidine . . . . Chlorpromazine	Corgard . . . . Cozaar
Cefotetan . . . . Ceftriaxone	Chlorpromazine . . . . Chlordiazepoxide	Corlopam . . . . Clonapam
Cefoxitin . . . . Cefazolin	Chlorpromazine . . . . . . Chlorhexidine	(Fenoldopam (Clonazepam in
Cefoxitin . . . . Cefotaxime	Chlorpromazine . . . . . . Chlorpropamide	in U.S.) Canada)
Cefoxitin . . . . Cefotetan	Chlorpromazine . . . . . . Chlorthalidone	Cortane . . . . Cortane-B
Cefoxitin . . . . Ceftriaxone	Chlorpromazine . . . . Prochlorperazine	Cortane-B . . . . Cortane
Cefoxitin . . . . Cefuroxime		Cortef . . . . Lortab
		Cortisone . . . . Hydrocortisone

Issued 4/04

Cortisporin (Ophthalmic)	Cortisporin (Otic)
Cortisporin (Otic)	Cortisporin (Ophthalmic)
Cosopt	Trusopt
Coumadin	Avandia
Coumadin	Cardura
Coumadin	Cordarone
Coumadin	Ambien
Covera	Provera
Cozaar	Corgard
Cozaar	Hyzaar
Cozaar	Zocor
Cyclobenzaprine	Cetirizine
Cyclobenzaprine	Cyproheptadine
Cyclophosphamide	Cyclosporine
Cycloserine	Cyclosporine
Cyclosporine	Cyclophosphamide
Cyclosporine	Cycloserine
Cyproheptadine	Cyclobenzaprine
Cytarabine .. Cytosar	Cytoxan
CytoGam	Gamimune N
Cytosar	Cytovene
Cytosar ... Cytoxan	Cytarabine
Cytosar-U	Neosar
Cytotec	Cytoxan
Cytovene	Cytosar
Cytoxan ... Cytosar	Cytarabine
Cytoxan	Cytotec
Danazol	Dantrium
Danocrine	Dantrium
Dantrium	Danazol
Dantrium	Danocrine
Darvocet	Percocet
Darvocet-N	Darvon
Darvocet-N	Darvon-N
Darvon	Darvocet-N
Darvon	Diovan
Darvon-N	Darvocet-N
Datril	Detrol
Daunorubicin	Doxorubicin
Deferoxamine	Cefuroxime
Demadex	Demerol
Demeclocycline	Dicyclomine
Demerol	Demadex
Demerol	Desyrel
Demerol	Dilaudid
Denavir	Indinavir
Depakene	Depakote
Depakote	Depakene
Depakote	Senokot
Depakote (Delayed Release)	Depakote ER (Extended Release)
Depakote ER (Extended Release)	Depakote (Delayed Release)
Depo-Estradiol	Depo-Testadiol
Depo-Medrol	Depo-Provera
Depo-Provera	Depo-Medrol
Depo-Testadiol	Depo-Estradiol

Deseril (Methysergide Maleate in Australia)	Desyrel (Trazodone in U.S.)
Desferal	DexFerrum
Desipramine	Imipramine
Desipramine	Clomipramine
Desipramine	Nortriptyline
Desyrel	Demerol
Desyrel (Trazodone in U.S.)	Deseril (Methysergide Maleate in Australia)
Detrol	Datril
Detrol	Dextrostat
DexFerrum	Desferal
Dextroamphetamine	Dextroamphetamine and Amphetamine
Dextroamphetamine and Amphetamine	Dextroamphetamine
Dextrostat	Detrol
DiaBeta	Zebeta
Diamox	Dobutrex
Diastix	Keto-Diastix
Diatex (Diazepam in Mexico)	Diatx (Multivitamin in U.S.)
Diatx (Multivitamin in U.S.)	Diatex (Diazepam in Mexico)
Diazepam	Alprazolam
Diazepam	Clonazepam
Diazepam	Ditropan
Diazepam	Ditropan XL
Diazepam	Lorazepam
Diazepam	Midazolam
Dicloxacillin	Doxycycline
Dicyclomine	Demeclocycline
Dicyclomine	Diphenhydramine
Dicyclomine	Doxycycline
Diflucan	Dilantin
Diflucan	Diprivan
Digoxin	Doxepin
Dilantin	Diflucan
Dilaudid	Demerol
Diltia XT	Cartia XT
Dimetapp	Donnatal
Diovan	Darvon
Diovan	Zyban
Diphenhydramine	Dicyclomine
Diphenhydramine	Dipyridamole
Diphtheria and Tetanus Toxoid	Tetanus Toxoid
Diprivan	Diflucan
Diprivan	Ditropan
Dipyridamole	Diphenhydramine
Ditropan	Diazepam
Ditropan	Diprivan
Ditropan XL	Diazepam
Dobutamine	Dopamine
Dobutrex	Diamox
Dobutrex	Dopamine
Docetaxel	Paclitaxel

Docusate Calcium	Docusate Sodium
Docusate Sodium	Docusate Calcium
Dolobid	Slo-bid
Donepezil	Benazepril
Donepezil	Doxazosin
Donnatal	Dimetapp
Donnatal	Donnatal Extentabs
Donnatal Extentabs	Donnatal
Dopamine	Dobutrex
Dopamine	Dobutamine
Doxazosin	Terazosin
Doxazosin	Donepezil
Doxepin	Digoxin
Doxepin	Doxycycline
Doxorubicin	Daunorubicin
Doxorubicin	Doxorubicin Liposomal
Doxorubicin	Idarubicin
Doxorubicin Liposomal	Doxorubicin
Doxycycline	Dicloxacillin
Doxycycline	Dicyclomine
Doxycycline	Doxepin
Duratuss	Duratuss-G
Duratuss-G	Duratuss
Dynabac	DynaCirc
Dynacin	DynaCirc
DynaCirc	Dynabac
DynaCirc	Dynacin
Edecrin	Eulexin
Efavirenz	Nelfinavir
Effexor	Effexor XR
Effexor XR	Effexor
Efudex	Eurax
Elavil	Enbrel
Elavil	Oruvail
Elavil	Plavix
Eldepryl	Enalapril
Eldopaque Forte	Eldoquin Forte
Eldoquin Forte	Eldopaque Forte
Elidel	Eligard
Eligard	Elidel
Elmiron	Imuran
Enalapril	Eldepryl
Enalapril	Lisinopril
Enbrel	Elavil
Enoxacin	Enoxaparin
Enoxaparin	Enoxacin
Entex LA	Eulexin
Entuss	Entuss-D
Entuss-D	Entuss
Ephedrine	Epinephrine
Epinephrine	Ephedrine
Epinephrine	Neo-Synephrine
Epinephrine	Norepinephrine
Epivir	Combivir
Epogen	Neupogen
Equagesic	EquiGesic
EquiGesic	Equagesic

Issued 4/04

USP Quality Review   **April 2004**

Erex	Urex
Erythrocin	Ethmozine
Erythromycin	Azithromycin
Eskalith	Estratest
Esmolol	Osmitrol
Esomeprazole	Omeprazole
Estrace	Evista
Estraderm	Testoderm
Estradiol	Ethinyl Estradiol
Estradiol	Risperdal
Estramustine	Exemestane
Estratab	Estratest
Estratest	Eskalith
Estratest	Estratab
Estratest	Estratest HS
Estratest HS	Estratest
Ethinyl Estradiol	Estradiol
Ethinyl Estradiol . . . . . . and Levonorgestrel	Ethinyl Estradiol and Norgestrel
Ethinyl Estradiol . . . . . . and Norgestrel	Ethinyl Estradiol and Levonorgestrel
Ethmozine	Erythrocin
Etidronate	Etomidate
Etomidate	Etidronate
Eulexin	Edecrin
Eulexin	Entex LA
Eurax	Efudex
Evista	Estrace
Evista	E-Vista (Monograph in Nursing Drug References)
E-Vista . . . . (Monograph in Nursing Drug References)	Evista
Exemestane	Estramustine
Famciclovir	Acyclovir
Famotidine	Fluoxetine
Famotidine	Furosemide
Felodipine	Amlodipine
Felodipine	Nifedipine
Felodipine	Ranitidine
Fentanyl Citrate	Sufentanil Citrate
Fer-In-Sol	Poly-Vi-Sol
Fioricet	Fiorinal
Fioricet	Florinef
Fiorinal	Fioricet
Fleet Enema	Fleet Phospho-Soda
Fleet Phospho-Soda . .	Fleet Enema
Flomax	Flonase
Flomax	Flovent
Flomax	Fosamax
Flomax	Volmax
Flonase	Flomax
Flonase	Flovent
Florinef	Fioricet
Florinef	Fluoride
Flovent	Atrovent
Flovent	Flomax

Flovent	Flonase
Flucytosine	Fluorouracil
Fludara	FUDR
Fludarabine	Flumadine
Flumadine	Fludarabine
Fluocinolone	Fluocinonide
Fluocinonide	Fluocinolone
Fluocinonide	Fluorouracil
Fluoride	Florinef
Fluorouracil	Flucytosine
Fluorouracil	Fluocinonide
Fluoxetine	Fluphenazine
Fluoxetine	Fluvoxamine
Fluoxetine	Famotidine
Fluoxetine	Fluvastatin
Fluoxetine	Furosemide
Fluoxetine	Paroxetine
Fluphenazine	Fluoxetine
Fluphenazine	Perphenazine
Fluphenazine	Trifluoperazine
Flurazepam	Temazepam
Fluvastatin	Fluoxetine
Fluvoxamine	Fluoxetine
FML Forte	FML S.O.P.
FML S.O.P.	FML Forte
Folic Acid	Folinic Acid
Folinic Acid	Folic Acid
Foltex PFS	FOLTX
FOLTX	Foltex PFS
Foradil	Toradol
Fortovase	Invirase
Fosamax	Flomax
Fosinopril	Bisoprolol
Fosinopril	Furosemide
Fosinopril	Lisinopril
Fosinopril	Minoxidil
Fosphenytoin	Phenytoin
FUDR	Fludara
Furosemide	Famotidine
Furosemide	Fluoxetine
Furosemide	Fosinopril
Furosemide	Torsemide
Gamimune N	CytoGam
Gemzar	Zinecard
Gengraf	Prograf
Gentamicin	Tobramycin
Gentamicin	Vancomycin
Glipizide	Glyburide
Glucophage	Glucophage XR
Glucophage	Glucotrol
Glucophage	Glutofac
Glucophage . . Glucophage XR . . Glucotrol
Glucophage XR	Glucotrol XL
Glucophage XR	Glucophage
Glucophage XR . . . Glucotrol . . . Glucophage
Glucotrol . . Glucophage . . Glucophage XR
Glucotrol	Glucophage
Glucotrol	Glucotrol XL

Glucotrol	Glyburide
Glucotrol XL	Glucophage XR
Glucotrol XL	Glucotrol
Glutofac	Glucophage
Glyburide	Glipizide
Glyburide	Glucotrol
Glycerin	Nitroglycerin
Granulex	Regranex
Guaifenesin	Guanfacine
Guanfacine	Guaifenesin
Halcion	Haldol
Haldol	Halcion
Haldol	Haldol Decanoate
Haldol	Inderal
Haldol	Stadol
Haldol Decanoate	Haldol
Haloperidol	Halotestin
Halotestin	Haloperidol
Hemoccult	Seracult
Heparin	Levaquin
Heparin	Hespan
Herceptin	Perceptin
Hespan	Heparin
Humalog	Humalog Mix
Humalog Mix	Humalog
Humalog, Insulin Human	Humulin, Insulin Human
Humulin 70/30	Humulin N
Humulin 70/30	Humulin R
Humulin L	Humulin N
Humulin L . . . . (Lente)	Humulin U (Ultralente)
Humulin N	Humulin 70/30
Humulin N	Humulin R
Humulin N	Humulin U
Humulin N	Novolin N
Humulin N	Humulin L
Humulin R	Humulin 70/30
Humulin R	Humulin N
Humulin R	Humulin U
Humulin R	Novolin R
Humulin U	Humulin N
Humulin U	Humulin R
Humulin U . . . . (Ultralente)	Humulin L (Lente)
Humulin, Insulin Human	Humalog, Insulin Human
Hydralazine	Hydrochlorothiazide
Hydralazine	Hydrocortisone
Hydralazine	Hydroxyzine
Hydrochlorothiazide . .	Hydralazine
Hydrochlorothiazide . .	Hydroxychloroquine
Hydrocil	Citrucel
Hydrocodone	Hydrocortisone
Hydrocodone and Acetaminophen	Oxycodone and Acetaminophen
Hydrocodone and Acetaminophen	Hydromorphone
Hydrocortisone	Cortisone

Issued 4/04

USP Quality Review

Hydrocortisone	Hydralazine
Hydrocortisone	Hydrocodone
Hydromorphone	Hydrocodone and Acetaminophen
Hydromorphone	Morphine
Hydroxychloroquine	Hydrochlorothiazide
Hydroxyurea	Hydroxyzine
Hydroxyzine	Hydralazine
Hydroxyzine	Hydroxyurea
Hypergel	MPM GelPad Hydrogel Saturated Dressing
Hyzaar	Cozaar
Idamycin	Adriamycin
Idarubicin	Doxorubicin
IMDUR	Imuran
IMDUR	Inderal LA
IMDUR	K-Dur
Imipenem	Meropenem
Imipenem	Omnipen
Imipramine	Amitriptyline
Imipramine	Desipramine
Imodium	Indocin
Imovax	Imovax I.D.
Imovax I.D.	Imovax
Imuran	Elmiron
Imuran	IMDUR
Imuran	Tenormin
Inapsine	Lanoxin
Inderal	Adderall
Inderal	Haldol
Inderal	Isordil
Inderal	Toradol
Inderal LA	IMDUR
Indinavir	Denavir
Indocin	Imodium
Infliximab	Rituximab
Insulin	Integrilin
Insulin Human	Lispro, Insulin Human
Insulin Human	Isophane, Insulin Human
Integrilin	Insulin
Invanz	Avinza
Invirase	Fortovase
Iodine	Codeine
Iodine	Lodine
Ismo	Isordil
Isophane, Insulin Human	Insulin Human
Isopto Carpine	Propine
Isordil	Inderal
Isordil	Ismo
Isosorbide Dinitrate	Isosorbide Mononitrate
Isosorbide Mononitrate	Isosorbide Dinitrate
Kaletra	Keppra
Kaopectate	Kayexalate
Kayexalate	Kaopectate

Kayexalate	Potassium Acetate
K-Dur	Cardura
K-Dur	IMDUR
K-Dur	K-Lor
Keflex	Kefzol
Keflex	Norflex
Kefurox	Kefzol
Kefzol	Cefzil
Kefzol	Keflex
Kefzol	Kefurox
Kenalog	Ketalar
Keppra	Kaletra
Ketalar	Kenalog
Keto-Diastix	Diastix
Ketorolac	Ketotifen
Ketotifen	Ketorolac
Klonopin . . Clonidine . .	Clonazepam
K-Lor	K-Dur
K-Lor	K-Lyte
K-Lyte	K-Lor
K-Lyte	K-Lyte Cl
K-Lyte Cl	K-Lyte
Kogenate	Kogenate-2
Kogenate-2	Kogenate
K-Phos Neutral	Neutra-Phos-K
Labetolol	Lamictal
Lacrilube	Surgilube
Lamicel	Lamisil
Lamictal	Labetolol
Lamictal	Lamisil
Lamictal	Lomotil
Lamictal	Ludiomil
Lamisil	Lamicel
Lamisil	Lamictal
Lamisil	Lomotil
Lamivudine	Lamotrigine
Lamivudine	Zidovudine
Lamotrigine	Lamivudine
Lanoxin	Levothyroxine
Lanoxin	Inapsine
Lanoxin . . . . Lasix	Lomotil
Lanoxin	Levoxyl
Lanoxin	Levsin
Lanoxin	Lonox
Lanoxin	Lovenox
Lanoxin	Xanax
Lantus, Insulin	Lente, Insulin Human
Lasix . . . . . Lomotil	Lanoxin
Lasix	Luvox
L-Dopa . . . . Levodopa . . .	Methyldopa
Lente, Insulin Human	Lispro, Insulin Human
Lente, Insulin Human	Lantus, Insulin Human
Leucovorin . . Leukine . .	Leukeran
Leucovorin	Levothyroxine
Leukeran	Alkeran
Leukeran . . Leucovorin . .	Leukine

Leukine . . . Leukeran . .	Leucovorin
Levaquin	Heparin
Levaquin	Lovenox
Levaquin	Tequin
Levbid	Cefobid
Levbid	Lithobid
Levbid	Lopid
Levbid	Lorabid
Levlen	Tri-Levlen
Levobunolol	Levocabastine
Levocabastine	Levobunolol
Levocarnitine	Levofloxacin
Levodopa . . L-Dopa . . .	Methyldopa
Levodopa and . . . . Carbidopa	Carbidopa
Levofloxacin	Ciprofloxacin
Levofloxacin	Levocarnitine
Levothyroxine	Lanoxin
Levothyroxine	Leucovorin
Levothyroxine	Liothyronine
Levoxyl	Lanoxin
Levoxyl	Luvox
Levsin	Lanoxin
Lexapro	Loxapine
Librax	Librium
Librium	Librax
Lioresal	Lotensin
Liothyronine	Levothyroxine
Lipitor	Zocor
Lisinopril	Benazepril
Lisinopril	Enalapril
Lisinopril	Fosinopril
Lisinopril	Quinapril
Lisinopril	Risperdal
Lispro, Insulin Human	Insulin Human
Lispro, Insulin Human	Lente, Insulin Human
Lithobid	Levbid
Lithobid	Lithostat
Lithostat	Lithobid
Lodine	Codeine
Lodine	Iodine
Lomotil	Lamictal
Lomotil	Lamisil
Lomotil . . . Lanoxin . . .	Lasix
Loniten	Lotensin
Lonox	Lanoxin
Loperamide	Lorazepam
Lopid	Levbid
Lopid . . . . . Lorabid . . .	Slo-bid
Lorabid	Levbid
Lorabid	Lortab
Lorabid . . . . Slo-bid . . .	Lopid
Loratadine	Losartan
Lorazepam	Alprazolam
Lorazepam	Clonazepam
Lorazepam	Diazepam
Lorazepam	Loperamide

Issued 4/04

Lorazepam	Midazolam	Methadone	Meperidine	Molindone	Midodrine
Lorazepam	Temazepam	Methadone	Methylphenidate	Monoket	Monopril
Lorcet	Lortab	Methazolamide	Methimazole	Monopril	Accupril
Lortab	Cortef	Methazolamide	Metronidazole	Monopril	Minoxidil
Lortab	Lorabid	Methimazole	Methazolamide	Monopril	Monoket
Lortab	Lorcet	Methohexital	Methotrexate	Morphine	Hydromorphone
Lortab	Luride	Methotrexate	Methohexital	Morphine	Meperidine
Losartan	Loratadine	Methotrexate	Metolazone	Moxapen (Amoxacillin Trihydrate in Thailand)	Maxipime (Cefepime Hydrochloride in U.S.)
Losartan	Valsartan	Methyldopa . . L-Dopa . . Levodopa			
Lotensin	Lioresal	Methylphenidate	Methadone		
Lotensin	Loniten	Methylprednisolone	Medroxyprogesterone	MPM GelPad Hydrogel Saturated Dressing	Hypergel
Lotensin	Lovastatin	Methylprednisolone	Prednisone		
Lotrimin	Lotrisone	Metoclopramide	Metolazone	MS Contin	OxyContin
Lotrisone	Lotrimin	Metoclopramide	Metoprolol	Murocel	Murocoll-2
Lotronex	Lovenox	Metoclopramide	Metronidazole	Murocoll-2	Murocel
Lotronex	Protonix	Metolazone	Medroxyprogesterone	Mycelex	Mycolog
Lovastatin	Lotensin	Metolazone	Metaxalone	Mycolog	Mycelex
Lovenox	Avonex	Metolazone	Methotrexate	Mycophenolate	Meclofenamate
Lovenox	Lanoxin	Metolazone	Metoclopramide	Mylanta	Mylicon
Lovenox	Levaquin	Metolazone	Metoprolol	Myleran	Melphalan
Lovenox	Lotronex	Metoprolol	Atenolol	Mylicon	Mylanta
Lovenox	Luvox	Metoprolol	Metoclopramide	Naprelan	Naprosyn
Loxapine	Lexapro	Metoprolol	Metolazone	Naprosyn	Naprelan
Loxitane	Soriatane	Metoprolol	Metronidazole	Naprosyn	Niaspan
Ludiomil	Lamictal	Metoprolol	Misoprostol	Narcan	Norcuron
Luride	Lortab	Metoprolol Succinate	Metoprolol Tartrate	Narcan	Nubain
Luvox	Lasix			Nasacort	Azmacort
Luvox	Levoxyl	Metoprolol Tartrate	Metoprolol Succinate	Nasalcrom	Nasalide
Luvox	Lovenox			Nasalide	Nasalcrom
Magnesium Citrate	Magnesium Sulfate	MetroGel	MetroGel-Vaginal	Nasarel	Nizoral
		MetroGel-Vaginal	MetroGel	Natru-Vent	Atrovent
Magnesium Sulfate	Magnesium Citrate	Metronidazole	Metformin	Navane	Norvasc
		Metronidazole	Methazolamide	Nebcin	Nubain
Maxipime (Cefepime Hydrochloride in U.S.)	Moxapen (Amoxacillin Trihydrate in Thailand)	Metronidazole	Metoclopramide	Nefazodone	Nelfinavir
		Metronidazole	Metoprolol	Nelfinavir	Efavirenz
		Metronidazole	Miconazole	Nelfinavir	Nefazodone
Meclofenamate	Mycophenolate	Miacalcin	Micatin	Nelfinavir	Nevirapine
Medigesic	Medi-Gesic	Micatin	Miacalcin	Neoral	Neurontin
Medi-Gesic	Medigesic	Miconazole	Metronidazole	Neoral	Nizoral
Medroxyprogesterone	Methylprednisolone	Micro-K	Micronase	Neosar	Cytosar-U
Medroxyprogesterone	Metolazone	Micronase	Micro-K	Neo-Synephrine	Epinephrine
Mefloquine	Meloxicam	Micronase	Microzide	Neo-Synephrine	Neo-Synephrine 12-Hour
Megace	Reglan	Microzide	Micronase		
Mellaril	Melphalan	Midazolam	Diazepam	Neo-Synephrine	Norepinephrine
Meloxicam	Mefloquine	Midazolam	Lorazepam	Neo-Synephrine 12-Hour	Neo-Synephrine
Melphalan	Mellaril	Midodrin	Midrin		
Melphalan	Myleran	Midodrine	Molindone	Nephrox	Niferex
Meperidine	Methadone	Midrin	Midodrin	Neumega	Neupogen
Meperidine	Morphine	Mifepristone	Misoprostol	Neupogen	Epogen
Mepron (Atovaquone in U.S.)	Mepron (Meprobamate in Australia)	Minoxidil	Fosinopril	Neupogen	Neumega
		Minoxidil	Monopril	Neurontin	Neoral
Meropenem	Imipenem	MiraLax	Mirapex	Neurontin	Noroxin
Meruvax	Attenuvax	Mirapex	MiraLax	Neutra-Phos	Neutra-Phos-K
Mesalamine	Sulfasalazine	Misoprostol	Metoprolol	Neutra-Phos-K	K-Phos Neutral
Metadate CD	Metadate ER	Misoprostol	Mifepristone	Neutra-Phos-K	Neutra-Phos
Metadate ER	Metadate CD	Mitomycin	Mitoxantrone	Nevirapine	Nelfinavir
Metaxalone	Metolazone	Mitoxantrone	Mitomycin	Niacin	Niaspan
Metformin	Metronidazole	Moban	Mobic	Niaspan	Naprosyn
		Mobic	Moban		

Issued 4/04

Niaspan	Niacin
Nicardipine .. Nifedipine .. Nimodipine	
Nicoderm	Nitroderm
NicoDerm CQ	Nitro-Dur
Nifedipine	Felodipine
Nifedipine .. Nicardipine .. Nimodipine	
Niferex	Nephrox
Nimbex	Bumex
Nimbex	Revex
Nimodipine .. Nicardipine .. Nifedipine	
Nitro-Bid	Nitro-Dur
Nitroderm	Nicoderm
Nitro-Dur	NicoDerm CQ
Nitro-Dur	Nitro-Bid
Nitro-Dur	NitroQuick
Nitroglycerin	Glycerin
NitroQuick	Nitro-Dur
Nizatidine	Tizanidine
Nizoral	Nasarel
Nizoral	Neoral
Nolvadex	Norvasc
Norcuron	Narcan
Norepinephrine	Epinephrine
Norepinephrine	Neo-Synephrine
Norepinephrine	Phenylephrine
Norflex	Keflex
Norflex ... Noroxin ... Norfloxacin	
Norflex	Norvasc
Norfloxacin .. Norflex ... Noroxin	
Noroxin	Neurontin
Noroxin .... Norflex ... Norfloxacin	
Norpramin	Nortriptyline
Nortriptyline	Amitriptyline
Nortriptyline	Desipramine
Nortriptyline	Norpramin
Norvasc	Altace
Norvasc	Navane
Norvasc	Nolvadex
Norvasc	Norflex
Norvasc	Vasotec
Norvir	Retrovir
Novolin 70/30	Novolin N
Novolin L	Novolin N
Novolin N	Humulin N
Novolin N	Novolin 70/30
Novolin N	Novolin L
Novolin N	Novolin R
Novolin R	Humulin R
Novolin R	Novolin N
Nubain	Narcan
Nubain	Nebcin
Nutropin	Nutropin AQ
Nutropin AQ	Nutropin
Ocufen	Ocuflox
Ocufen	Ocupress
Ocuflox	Ocufen
Ocular Lubricants	Acular
Ocumycin	Ocu-Mycin

Ocu-Mycin	Ocumycin
Ocupress	Ocufen
Ofloxacin	Ciprofloxacin
Olanzapine	Oxcarbazepine
Omeprazole	Esomeprazole
Omnipen	Imipenem
Opium Tincture, Deodorized	Opium, Camphorated
Opium, Camphorated	Opium Tincture, Deodorized
Oprelvekin	Aldesleukin
Organan	Argatroban
Ortho Tri-Cyclen	Ortho-Cyclen
Ortho Tri-Cyclen	Tri-Levlen
Ortho-Cept	Ortho-Cyclen
Ortho-Cept	Ortho-Est
Ortho-Cyclen	Ortho-Cept
Ortho-Cyclen	Ortho Tri-Cyclen
Ortho-Est	Ortho-Cept
Oruvail	Clinoril
Oruvail	Elavil
Os-Cal	Asacol
Osmitrol	Esmolol
Oxacillin	Ampicillin
Oxazepam	Oxycodone
Oxazepam	Temazepam
Oxcarbazepine	Olanzapine
Oxybutynin	OxyContin
Oxycodone	Oxazepam
Oxycodone	OxyContin
Oxycodone and Acetaminophen	Hydrocodone and Acetaminophen
Oxycodone and Acetaminophen	Oxycodone and Aspirin
Oxycodone and Aspirin	Oxycodone and Acetaminophen
OxyContin	MS Contin
OxyContin	Oxybutynin
OxyContin	Oxycodone
Paclitaxel	Docetaxel
Paclitaxel	Paroxetine
Paclitaxel	Paxil
Pamelor	Panlor SS
Panlor SS	Pamelor
Papaverine	Propafenone
Parafon Forte DSC	Profen Forte
Paraplatin	Platinol
Parlodel	Pindolol
Parlodel	Provera
Paroxetine	Fluoxetine
Paroxetine	Paclitaxel
Paroxetine	Pyridoxine
Paxil	Paclitaxel
Paxil	Plavix
Paxil	Taxol
Pediapred	Pediazole
Pediapred	Risperdal
Pediazole	Pediapred
Pegaspargase	Asparaginase

Penicillamine	Penicillin
Penicillin	Penicillamine
Penicillin G Potassium	Penicillin G Procaine
Penicillin G Procaine	Penicillin G Potassium
Pentobarbital	Phenobarbital
Pepcid	Prevacid
Perative	Periactin
Perceptin	Herceptin
Percocet	Darvocet
Percocet	Percodan
Percocet	Procet
Percodan	Percocet
Percodan	Peri-Colace
Percodan	Vicodin
Periactin	Perative
Peri-Colace	Colace
Peri-Colace	Percodan
Peri-Colace	Procardia
Permax	Bumex
Permethrin	Pyrethrins, Piperonyl Butoxide
Perphenazine	Fluphenazine
Phenazopyridine	Promethazine
Phenobarbital	Pentobarbital
Phenylephrine	Norepinephrine
Phenylephrine	Phenytoin
Phenytoin	Fosphenytoin
Phenytoin	Phenylephrine
Physostigmine	Pyridostigmine
Pilocar	Polocaine
Pilocarpine	Proparacaine
Pindolol	Parlodel
Pindolol	Plendil
Pioglitazone	Rosiglitazone
Pitocin	Pitressin
Pitressin	Pitocin
Platinol	Paraplatin
Plavix	Elavil
Plavix	Paxil
Plendil	Pindolol
Plendil	Pletal
Plendil	Prilosec
Plendil	Prinivil
Pletal	Plendil
Pneumococcal Vaccine, 23-Valent (Polyvalent)	Pneumococcal Vaccine, 7-Valent
Pneumococcal Vaccine, 7-Valent	Pneumococcal Vaccine, 23-Valent (Polyvalent)
Polocaine	Pilocar
Poly-Vi-Sol	Fer-In-Sol
Potassium	Prednisone
Potassium Acetate	Kayexalate
Potassium Acetate	Potassium Chloride
Potassium Bicarbonate and Potassium Chloride	Potassium Bicarbonate and Potassium Citrate

Issued 4/04

USP Quality Review

Potassium Bicarbonate and Potassium Citrate ... Potassium Bicarbonate and Potassium Chloride

Potassium Chloride ... Potassium Acetate

Potassium Chloride ... Potassium Citrate

Potassium Chloride ... Sodium Chloride

Potassium Citrate ..... Potassium Chloride

Potassium Phosphates ... Sodium Phosphates

Prandin .... Avandia

Pravachol .... Prevacid

Pravachol .... Prinivil

Pravachol .... Propranolol

Pravastatin .... Atorvastatin

Prazosin .... Terazosin

Precare .... Precose

Precose .... Precare

Prednisolone .... Prednisone

Prednisone .... Methylprednisolone

Prednisone .... Potassium

Prednisone .... Prednisolone

Prednisone .... Prilosec

Prednisone .... Primidone

Prednisone .... Pseudoephedrine

Premarin .... Prempro

Premarin .... Prevacid

Premarin .... Primaxin

Premarin .... Provera

Premphase .... Prempro

Premphase .... Vancenase

Prempro .... Premarin

Prempro .... Premphase

Prepidil .... Bepridil

Prevacid .... Prinivil

Prevacid .... Pepcid

Prevacid .... Pravachol

Prevacid .... Premarin

Prevacid .... Prilosec

Preven .... Preveon

Preveon .... Preven

Prilosec .... Plendil

Prilosec .... Prednisone

Prilosec .... Prevacid

Prilosec .... Prinivil

Prilosec .... Prozac

Primacor .... Primaxin

Primatene .... ProAmantine

Primaxin .... Premarin

Primaxin .... Primacor

Primidone .... Prednisone

Prinivil .... Plendil

Prinivil .... Pravachol

Prinivil .... Prevacid

Prinivil .... Prilosec

Prinivil .... Prinzide

Prinivil .... Proventil

Prinzide .... Prinivil

Priscoline .... Apresoline

ProAmantine .... Primatene

Probenecid .... Procanbid

Procainamide .... Prochlorperazine

Procan SR .... Proscar

Procanbid .... Probenecid

Procardia .... Peri-Colace

Procardia .... Provera

Procardia XL .... Cartia XT

Procet .... Percocet

Prochlorperazine ...... Chlorpromazine

Prochlorperazine ..... Procainamide

Prochlorperazine ..... Promethazine

Proctocort .... Proctocream HC

Proctocream HC ...... Proctocort

Profen .... Profen II ... Profen LA

Profen Forte .... Parafon Forte DSC

Profen II ... Profen ... Profen LA

Profen LA .. Profen ... Profen II

Prograf .... Gengraf

Promethazine .... Phenazopyridine

Promethazine .... Prochlorperazine

Promethazine VC ..... Promethazine w/ Codeine

Promethazine VC ..... Promethazine w/ Codeine w/ Codeine

Promethazine .... Promethazine VC w/ Codeine w/ Codeine

Promethazine .... Promethazine VC w/ Codeine

Propafenone .... Papaverine

Proparacaine .... Pilocarpine

Propine .... Isopto Carpine

Propranolol .... Pravachol

Propranolol .... Propulsid

Propulsid .... Propranolol

Propylthiouracil ...... Purinethol

Proscar .... Procan SR

Proscar .... ProSom

Proscar ... ProSom ... Prozac

Proscar .... Provera

ProSom .... Proscar

ProSom ... Prozac .... Proscar

Protonix .... Lotronex

Proventil .... Bentyl

Proventil .... Prinivil

Provera .... Covera

Provera .... Parlodel

Provera .... Premarin

Provera .... Procardia

Provera .... Proscar

Prozac .... Prilosec

Prozac ..... Proscar ... ProSom

Pseudoephedrine ..... Prednisone

Pulmicort .... Pulmozyme

Pulmozyme .... Pulmicort

Purinethol .... Propylthiouracil

Pyrazinamide .... Pyridostigmine

Pyrethrins, ... Permethrin Piperonyl Butoxide

Pyridium .... Pyridoxine

Pyridostigmine .... Physostigmine

Pyridostigmine .... Pyrazinamide

Pyridostigmine .... Pyridoxine

Pyridoxine .... Paroxetine

Pyridoxine .... Pyridium

Pyridoxine .... Pyridostigmine

Pyridoxine .... Pyrimethamine

Pyrimethamine .... Pyridoxine

Quibron ... Quibron-T ... Quibron-T/SR

Quibron-T ... Quibron ... Quibron-T/SR

Quibron-T/SR ... Quibron ... Quibron-T

Quinacrine .... Quinidine

Quinapril .... Lisinopril

Quinidine .... Quinacrine

Quinidine .... Quinine

Quinine .... Quinidine

Raloxifene .... Ropinirole

Ramipril .... Rifampin

Ranitidine .. Amantadine .. Rimantadine

Ranitidine .... Felodipine

Ratgam .... Atgam (Synonym for Thymoglobulin)

ReFresh .... Refresh (breath drops) (lubricant eye drops)

Refresh .... ReFresh (lubricant eye drops) (breath drops)

Reglan .... Megace

Reglan .... Renagel

Reglan .... Robitussin

Reglan .... Zofran

Regranex .... Granulex

Relafen .... Rezulin

Remegel .... Renagel

Remeron .... Restoril

Remeron .... Zemuron

Reminyl .... Amaryl

Reminyl .... Robinul

Renagel .... Reglan

Renagel .... Remegel

Reno-60 .... Renografin-60

Renografin-60 .... Reno-60

Reopro .... Rheomacrodex

Repaglinide .... Rosiglitazone

Requip .... Risperdal

Reserpine .. Risperdal .. Risperidone

Restoril .... Remeron

Restoril .... Risperdal

Restoril .... Vistaril

Retavase .... Activase

Retrovir .... Norvir

Retrovir .... Ritonavir

Revex .... Nimbex

Revex .... ReVia

ReVia .... Revex

Rezulin .... Relafen

Rheomacrodex .... Reopro

Ridaura .... Cardura

Rifabutin .... Rifampin

Rifadin .... Rifater

Issued 4/04

Rifampin . . . . Ramipril
Rifampin . . . . Rifabutin
Rifater . . . . Rifadin
Rimantadine . . Amantadine . . Ranitidine
Risedronate . . . . Risperidone
Risperdal . . . . Estradiol
Risperdal . . . . Lisinopril
Risperdal . . . . Pediapred
Risperdal . . . . Requip
Risperdal . . . Reserpine . . . Risperidone
Risperdal . . . . Restoril
Risperidone . . . Reserpine . . . Risperdal
Risperidone . . . . Risedronate
Risperidone . . . . Ropinirole
Ritalin . . . . Ritalin SR
Ritalin SR . . . . Ritalin
Ritonavir . . . . Retrovir
Rituximab . . . . Infliximab
Robinul . . . . Reminyl
Robitussin . . . . Reglan
Robitussin . . . . Robitussin DM
Robitussin AC . . . . Robitussin DAC
Robitussin AC . . . . Robitussin DM
Robitussin DAC . . . . . . Robitussin AC
Robitussin DM . . . . Robitussin
Robitussin DM . . . . Robitussin AC
Robitussin DM . . . . Rondec DM
Rocephin . . . . Ceftin
Rondec DM . . . . Robitussin DM
Ropinirole . . . . Raloxifene
Ropinirole . . . . Risperidone
Ropivacaine . . . . Bupivacaine
Rosiglitazone . . . . Pioglitazone
Rosiglitazone . . . . Repaglinide
Roxanol . . . . Roxicet
Roxanol . . . . Roxicodone
Roxanol . . . . Roxicodone
Intensol
Roxicet . . . . Roxanol
Roxicet . . . . Roxicodone
Roxicodone . . . . Roxanol
Roxicodone . . . . Roxicet
Roxicodone . . . . Roxicodone
Intensol
Roxicodone Intensol . . Roxanol
Roxicodone Intensol . . Roxicodone
Rynatan . . . . Rynatuss
Rynatuss . . . . Rynatan
Salagen . . . . Selegiline
Salbutamol . . . . Salmeterol
(Albuterol in
other countries)
Salmeterol . . . . Salbutamol
(Albuterol in other
countries)
Salsalate . . . . Sulfasalazine
Sarafem . . . . Serophene
Selegiline . . . . Salagen
Selegiline . . Serentil . . Sertraline . . Serzone
Selegiline . . . . Sertraline

Senna . . . . Soma
Senokot . . . . Depakote
Senokot . . . . Sinemet
Seracult . . . . Hemoccult
Serentil . . Selegiline . . Sertraline . . Serzone
Serentil . . . . Seroquel
Serentil . . . . Serzone
Serentil . . . . Sinequan
Serevent . . . . Atrovent
Serevent . . . . Serevent Diskus
Serevent Diskus . . . . . Serevent
Serophene . . . . Sarafem
Seroquel . . . . Serentil
Seroquel . . Serzone . . Sinequan
Seroquel . . . . Symmetrel
Seroquel . . . . Sertraline
Sertraline . . Selegiline . . Serentil . . Serzone
Sertraline . . . . Seroquel
Serzone . . Seroquel . . Sinequan
Serzone . . Sertraline . . Selegiline . . Serentil
Sinemet . . . . Senokot
Sinemet . . . . Sinemet CR
Sinemet CR . . . . Sinemet
Sinequan . . . . Serentil
Sinequan . . . Seroquel . . . Serzone
Sinequan . . . . Singulair
Singulair . . . . Sinequan
Slo-bid . . . . Dolobid
Slo-bid . . . . Lopid . . . Lorabid
Slow Fe . . . . Slow-K
Slow-K . . . . Slow Fe
Sodium . . . . Sodium Chloride
Bicarbonate
Sodium Chloride . . . . . Potassium
Chloride
Sodium Chloride . . . . . Sodium
Bicarbonate
Sodium Phosphates . . . Potassium
Phosphates
Solu-Cortef . . . . Solu-Medrol
Solu-Medrol . . . . Depo-Medrol
Solu-Medrol . . . . Solu-Cortef
Soma . . . . Senna
Soma . . . . Soma Compound
Soma Compound . . . . . Soma
Soriatane . . . . Loxitane
Sotalol . . . . Subdue
Stadol . . . . Haldol
Stadol . . . . Toradol
Subdue . . . . Sotalol
Sufentanil Citrate . . . . . Fentanyl Citrate
Sulfadiazine . . . . Sulfasalazine
Sulfasalazine . . . . Mesalamine
Sulfasalazine . . . . Salsalate
Sulfasalazine . . . . Sulfadiazine
Sulfasalazine . . . . Sulfisoxazole
Sulfisoxazole . . . . Sulfasalazine
Sumatriptan . . . . Zolmitriptan
Suprax . . . . Surfak

Surfak . . . . Suprax
Surgilube . . . . Lacrilube
Symmetrel . . . . Amaryl
Symmetrel . . . . Seroquel
Symmetrel . . . . Synthroid
Synagis . . . . Synvisc
Synthroid . . . . Symmetrel
Synvisc . . . . Synagis
Tambocor . . . . Temodar
Tamiflu . . . . Tamoxifen
Tamiflu . . . . Theraflu
Tamoxifen . . . . Tamiflu
Tamoxifen . . . . Tamsulosin
Tamsulosin . . . . Tamoxifen
Taxol . . . . Paxil
Taxol . . . . Taxotere
Taxotere . . . . Taxol
Tegretol . . . . Toradol
Tegretol . . . . Trental
Tegretol . . . . Trileptal
Tegretol-XR . . . . Toprol-XL
Temazepam . . . . Flurazepam
Temazepam . . . . Lorazepam
Temazepam . . . . Oxazepam
Temodar . . . . Tambocor
Tenormin . . . . Imuran
Tenormin . . . . Thiamine
Tenormin . . . . Trovan
Tequin . . . . Levaquin
Tequin . . . . Ticlid
Terazosin . . . . Prazosin
Terazosin . . . . Doxazosin
Testoderm . . . . Estraderm
Tetanus Toxoid . . . . . . Diphtheria and
Tetanus Toxoid
Tetracycline . . . . Tetradecyl Sulfate
Tetradecyl Sulfate . . . . Tetracycline
Thalitone . . . . Thalomid
Thalomid . . . . Thalitone
Theraflu . . . . Tamiflu
Thiamine . . . . Tenormin
Thioridazine . . . . Chlorpromazine
Thorazine . . . . Thioridazine
Thioridazine . . . . Thorazine
Tiagabine . . . . Tizanidine
Tiazac . . . . Tigan
Tiazac . . . . Ziac
Ticlid . . . . Tequin
Tigan . . . . Tiazac
Timoptic . . . . Timoptic-XE
Timoptic-XE . . . . Timoptic
Tizanidine . . . . Nizatidine
Tizanidine . . . . Tiagabine
TNKase . . . . t-PA
(Synonym for
Alteplase,
recombinant)
Tobradex . . . . Tobrex
Tobramycin . . . . Gentamicin

Issued 4/04

Tobrex	Tobradex	
Tolazamide	Tolbutamide	
Tolbutamide	Tolazamide	
Tolcapone	Tolterodine	
Tolterodine	Tolcapone	
Topamax	Toprol-XL	
Topiramate	Torsemide	
Toprol-XL	Tegretol-XR	
Toprol-XL	Topamax	
Toradol	Foradil	
Toradol	Inderal	
Toradol	Stadol	
Toradol	Tegretol	
Toradol	Torecan	
Toradol	Tramadol	
Torecan	Toradol	
Torsemide	Furosemide	
Torsemide	Topiramate	
t-PA	TNKase	
(Synonym for		
Alteplase, recombinant)		
Tramadol	Toradol	
Tramadol	Trandolapril	
Tramadol	Trazodone	
Tramadol	Voltaren	
Trandate	Trental	
Trandate	Tridrate	
Trandolapril	Tramadol	
Trazodone	Amiodarone	
Trazodone	Tramadol	
Trental	Tegretol	
Trental	Trandate	
Triad	Triad	
(Butalbital/	(topical)	
Acetaminophen/		
Caffeine)		
Triad	Triad	
(topical)	(Butalbital/	
	Acetaminophen/	
	Caffeine)	
Triamterene	Trimethoprim	
Tridrate	Trandate	
Trifluoperazine	Fluphenazine	
Trifluoperazine	Trihexyphenidyl	
Trihexyphenidyl	Trifluoperazine	
Trileptal	Tegretol	
Tri-Levlen	Levlen	
Tri-Levlen	Ortho Tri-Cyclen	
Trimethoprim	Triamterene	
Tri-Nasal	Triphasil	
Tri-Norinyl	Triphasil	
Triphasil	Tri-Nasal	
Triphasil	Tri-Norinyl	
Trovan	Tenormin	
Trusopt	Cosopt	
Tylenol	Tylenol w/ Codeine	
Tylenol Children's	Tylenol w/ Codeine	
Tylenol w/ Codeine ...	Tylenol	
Tylenol w/ Codeine ...	Tylenol Children's	
Ultane	Ultram	

Ultracef	Ultracet
(Cefadroxil in	(Acetaminophen/
other countries)	Tramadol
	Hydrochloride
	in U.S.)
Ultracet	Ultracef
(Acetaminophen/	(Cefadroxil in
Tramadol	other countries)
Hydrochloride in U.S.)	
Ultram	Ultane
Ultram	Voltaren
Unasyn	Zosyn
Uniretic	Univasc
Univasc	Uniretic
Univasc	Urispas
Urex	Erex
Uridon	Vicodin
Urised	Urocit-K
Urispas	Univasc
Urispas	Uro-Mag
Urocit-K	Urised
Uro-Mag	Urispas
Valacyclovir	Valgancyclovir
Valcyte	Valtrex
Valgancyclovir	Valacyclovir
Valium	Versed
Valium	Vicodin
Valsartan	Losartan
Valtrex	Valcyte
Vancenase	Premphase
Vancenase	Vanceril
Vancenase AQ	Vanceril DS
Vanceril	Vancenase
Vanceril DS	Vancenase AQ
Vancomycin	Azithromycin
Vancomycin	Gentamicin
Vancomycin	Vecuronium
Vancomycin	Vibramycin
Vantin	Ventolin
Vasocon	Vasocon A
Vasocon A	Vasocon
Vasotec	Norvasc
Vecuronium	Vancomycin
Ventolin	Benylin
Ventolin	Vantin
Vepesid	Versed
Verapamil	Verelan
Verelan	Verapamil
Verelan	Virilon
Versed	Valium
Versed	Vepesid
Versed	Vistaril
Vexol	VoSol
Viagra	Allegra
Vibramycin	Vancomycin
Vicodin	Percodan
Vicodin	Uridon
Vicodin	Valium
Vicodin	Vicodin ES
Vicodin	Vioxx

Vicodin ES	Vicodin
Vinblastine	Vincristine
Vincristine	Vinblastine
Vioxx	Aciphex
Vioxx	Vicodin
Vioxx	Zyvox
Viracept	Viramune
Viramune	Viracept
Virilon	Verelan
Visicol	Bisacodyl
Vistaril	Restoril
Vistaril	Versed
Vistaril	Zestril
Vitamin C	Vitamin E
Vitamin D	Vitamin E
Vitamin E	Vitamin C
Vitamin E	Vitamin D
Volmax	Flomax
Voltaren	Tramadol
Voltaren	Ultram
VoSol	Vexol
Wellbutrin	Wellbutrin SR
Wellbutrin SR	Wellbutrin
Xalatan	Xalcom
	(Latanoprost/
	Timolol in other
	countries)
Xalcom	Xalatan
(Latanoprost/	
Timolol in other	
countries)	
Xanax	Lanoxin
Xanax	Zanaflex
Xanax	Zantac
Xanax .... Zantac	Zyrtec
Xigris	Zydis
	(Dosage Form
	Trademark)
Yocon	Zocor
Zagam	Zyban
Zaleplon	Zolpidem
Zanaflex	Anaflex
Zanaflex	Xanax
Zantac	Xanax
Zantac .... Xanax	Zyrtec
Zantac	Zofran
Zaroxolyn	Zyprexa
Zebeta	DiaBeta
Zemuron............	Remeron
Zerit	Zestril
Zestril	Vistaril
Zestril	Zerit
Zestril	Zocor
Zestril	Zyrtec
Ziac	Tiazac
Ziac	Zocor
Zidovudine	Lamivudine
Zidovudine	Zidovudine and
	Lamivudine
Zidovudine	Ziprasidone

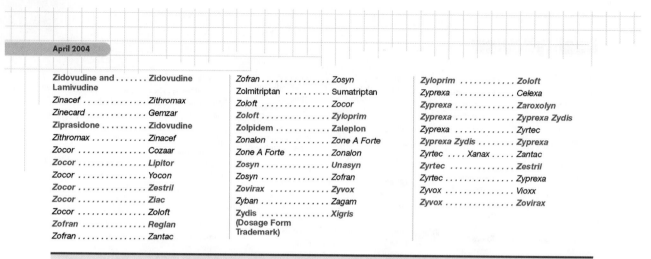

April 2004

Zidovudine and . . . . Zidovudine Lamivudine	Zofran . . . . Zosyn	Zyloprim . . . . Zoloft
Zinacef . . . . Zithromax	Zolmitriptan . . . . Sumatriptan	Zyprexa . . . . Celexa
Zinecard . . . . Gemzar	Zoloft . . . . Zocor	Zyprexa . . . . Zaroxolyn
Ziprasidone . . . . Zidovudine	Zoloft . . . . Zyloprim	Zyprexa . . . . Zyprexa Zydis
Zithromax . . . . Zinacef	Zolpidem . . . . Zaleplon	Zyprexa . . . . Zyrtec
Zocor . . . . Cozaar	Zonalon . . . . Zone A Forte	Zyprexa Zydis . . . . Zyprexa
Zocor . . . . Lipitor	Zone A Forte . . . . Zonalon	Zyrtec . . . . Xanax . . . . . Zantac
Zocor . . . . Yocon	Zosyn . . . . Unasyn	Zyrtec . . . . Zestril
Zocor . . . . Zestril	Zosyn . . . . Zofran	Zyrtec . . . . Zyprexa
Zocor . . . . Ziac	Zovirax . . . . Zyvox	Zyvox . . . . Vioxx
Zocor . . . . Zoloft	Zyban . . . . Zagam	Zyvox . . . . Zovirax
Zofran . . . . Reglan	Zydis . . . . Xigris	
Zofran . . . . Zantac	(Dosage Form Trademark)	

**Wall posters and pocket references of this resource will be available
in June 2004 for purchase at http://store.usp.org.**

Online reporting to the USP Medication Errors Reporting (MER) Program is available through the Internet at
www.usp.org/patientSafety/reporting/mer.html. Report forms may also be requested by phone at 1-800-23-ERROR
(1-800-233-7767). The MER Program is presented in cooperation with the Institute for Safe Medication Practices.

USP CENTER FOR THE ADVANCEMENT OF PATIENT SAFETY
12601 TWINBROOK PARKWAY, ROCKVILLE, MD 20852 • 800-23-ERROR • http://www.usp.org/patientSafety • uspcaps@usp.org

PSF032G

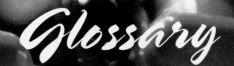

Glossary

Abbreviations. Symbols used for medication orders.

Absence epilepsy. Absence of convulsions characterized by a sudden 10–30 second loss of consciousness with no falling; formerly called petit mal.

Absorption. Passage of a substance through a body surface into body fluids or tissues.

Acetylcholine. Mediator of nerve impulses in the parasympathetic system.

Action. A description of the cellular changes that occur as a result of a drug.

Addiction. Physical and/or psychological dependence on a substance, especially alcohol or drugs, with use of increasing amounts (tolerance) and withdrawal reactions.

Adjunct. Addition to the course of treatment to increase the efficacy.

Adjuvant. A drug added to a prescription to hasten or enhance the action of a principal ingredient.

Adrenal. Glands located adjacent to the kidneys that secrete hormones called corticosteroids.

Adrenergic. Sympathomimetic drug that mimics the action of the sympathetic nervous system.

Adsorbent. Substance that leads readily to absorption.

Adverse effects. Harmful unintended reactions to a drug.

Adverse reaction. A list of possible unpleasant or dangerous secondary effects, other than the desired effect.

Allergic reaction. Response of the body resulting from hypersensitivity to a substance (e.g., rash, hives, and anaphylaxis).

Alopecia. Loss or absence of hair.

Apha-blockers. Drugs that block the alpha-1 receptors found in smooth muscle in the bladder neck and prostate, causing them to relax.

Alzheimer's disease. Dementia characterized by a devastating, progressive decline in cognitive function, followed by increasingly severe impairment in social and occupational functioning.

Aminoglycosides. Drugs used in combination with other antibiotics that treat many infections caused by gram-negative and gram-positive bacteria.

Amnesia. Loss of memory.

Ampule. Glass container with drug for injection, must be broken at the neck to withdraw drug in solution.

Analeptic. A drug used to stimulate the central nervous system, especially with poisoning by CNS depressants.

Analgesic. Medication that alleviates pain.

Anaphylaxis. Allergic hypersensitivity reaction of the body to a foreign substance or drug. Mild symptoms include rash, itching, and hives. Severe symptoms include dyspnea, chest constriction, cardiopulmonary collapse, and death.

Androgens. Male hormones that stimulate the development of male characteristics.

Angina pectoris. Severe chest pain resulting from decreased blood supply to the heart muscle.

Angiogenesis. Development of new blood vessels.

Anorexia. Loss of appetite.

Antacid. Agent that neutralizes gastric hydrochloric acid.

Antagonism. Opposing action of two drugs in which one decreases or cancels out the effect of the other.

Antiandrogen. A gonadotropin-releasing hormone analog that is used to treat prostate cancer.

Antiarrhythmic. Drug that controls or prevents cardiac irregularities.

Anticholinergic. Drug that blocks the action of the parasympathetic nervous system.

Anticoagulants. Medications used to prevent formation of clots or decrease the extension of existing clots in such conditions as venous thrombosis, pulmonary embolism, and coronary occlusion.

Anticonvulsants. Medication used to reduce the number and/or severity of seizures in patients with epilepsy.

Antidepressant. Medication used to treat patients with various types of depression; sometimes called mood elevators.

Antidiabetic. Medication to lower blood glucose levels in those with impaired metabolism of carbohydrates, fats, and proteins.

Antidiarrhea. Medication that reduces the number of loose stools.

Antidote. Substance that neutralizes poisons or toxic substances.

Antiemetic. Drug that prevents or treats nausea, vomiting, or motion sickness.

Antiflatulent. Symptomatic treatment of gastric bloating or GI gas pain.

Antifungal. Medication used in the treatment of candidial and other specific susceptible fungi.

Antiglaucoma drugs. Medications used to lower intraocular pressure.

Antihistamines. Medications that provide symptomatic relief of allergic symptoms caused by histamine release.

Antihypertensives. Medications used in the treatment and management of all degrees of hypertension.

Anti-infective. Medication used in the treatment of infections; includes antibiotics, antifungals, and antivirals.

Anti-inflammatory. Medication used to relieve inflammation.

Antilipemic. Drug that lowers the serum cholesterol and low-density lipoproteins (LDLs) and increases the high-density lipoproteins (HDLs).

Antimuscarinics. Drugs that block cholinergic stimuli at muscarinic receptors. A type of anticholinergic. Also called parasympatholytics.

Antineoplastic. Agent that prevents the development, growth, or spreading of malignant cells.

Antioxidant. Agent that prevents or inhibits oxidation or cell destruction in damaged or aging tissues. A compound that fights against the destructive effects of free radical formation.

Antiparkinsonian drugs. Medications used in the treatment of Parkinson's disease to relieve symptoms and maintain mobility, but do not cure the disease.

Antipruritic. Products applied topically to alleviate itching.

Antipsychotic. Major tranquilizers used to relieve symptoms of psychoses or severe neuroses; sometimes called neuroleptics.

Antipyretic. Medication to reduce fever.

Antiseptic. Substances that inhibit the growth of bacteria.

Antispasmodics. Medications used to reduce the strength and frequency of contractions of the urinary bladder and to decrease gastrointestinal motility.

Antithyroid. Medication used to relieve the symptoms of hyperthyroidism in preparation for surgical or radioactive iodine therapy.

Antituberculosis agents. Medications used to treat asymptomatic infection, and to treat active clinical tuberculosis and prevent relapse.

Antitussive. Medication that suppresses coughing.

Antiulcer. Drug that reduces gastric acid secretion, or that acts to prevent or treat gastric or duodenal ulcers.

Antiviral. Medications used to treat viruses, for example, HIV and herpes.

Anxiolytics. Antianxiety medications (tranquilizers) used for the short-term treatment of anxiety disorders, neurosis, some psychosomatic disorders, and insomnia.

Appropriate. Reasonable under the circumstances for a specific patient.

Arteriosclerosis. A common arterial disorder characterized by thickening and loss of elasticity of the arterial walls, resulting in a decreased blood supply, especially to the cerebrum and lower extremities.

Asthma treatment. Medications used for prophylaxis and treatment of chronic asthma. Bronchodilators are used for acute asthmatic attacks.

Asymptomatic. No evidence of clinical disease.

Ataxia. Defective muscular coordination, especially with voluntary muscular movements (e.g., walking).

Atherosclerosis. A type of arteriosclerosis characterized by yellowish plaques of cholesterol, lipids, and cellular debris in the walls of large and medium-sized arteries, resulting in reduced circulation, the major cause of coronary heart disease, such as angina pectoris or myocardial infarction.

Atypical antipsychotics. A newer class of antipsychotics with less potential for adverse effects, such as extrapyramidal symptoms and tardive dyskinesia.

Autonomic. Automatic, self-governing, or involuntary nervous system.

Bactericidal. Destroying bacteria.

Bacteriostatic. Inhibiting or retarding bacterial growth.

Beta-blocker. Drug that blocks the action of the sympathetic nervous system.

565

Biotransformation. Chemical changes that a substance undergoes in the body.

Bipolar disorder. Manic-depressive mental disorder in which the mood fluctuates from mania to depression.

Blood dyscrasia. A condition in which any of the blood constituents are abnormal or are present in abnormal quantity.

BPH. Benign prostatic hypertrophy.

BPH therapy. Drug used to reduce prostate size and associated urinary obstruction and manifestations in patients with benign prostatic hypertrophy (BPH).

Bradycardia. Abnormally slow heartbeat.

Bradykinesia. Abnormally slow movement.

Broad spectrum. Antibiotic effective against a large variety of organisms.

Bronchodilators. Medications that relax the smooth muscles of the bronchial tree, thereby relieving bronchospasm and increasing the vital capacity of the lungs.

Buccal. In the cheek pouch.

C & S. Culture and sensitivity test to identify a causative infectious organism and the specific medicine to which it is sensitive.

Calculus. Stone.

Carbonic anhydrase inhibitors. Drugs that reduce the hydrogen and bicarbonate ions and have a diuretic effect (increasing the excretion of fluids from the body through the urine).

Cardiac glycosides. Medication used primarily in the treatment of congestive heart failure.

Cardiotonic. Increasing the force and efficiency of contractions of the heart muscle.

Cardioversion. Correcting an irregular heartbeat (arrhythmia). Usually accomplished by electrical shock (e.g., defibrillation).

Catecholamines. Mediators released at the sympathetic nerve endings (e.g., epinephrine and norepinephrine).

Cautions. Precautions; steps to take to prevent errors.

Cephalosporins. Semisynthetic antibiotic derivatives produced by a fungus.

Chemical dependency. Condition in which alcohol or drugs have taken control of an individual's life and affect normal functioning.

Chemotherapy. Chemicals (drugs) with specific and toxic effects upon disease-producing organisms.

Cholelithiasis. The presence of gallstones in the gallbladder.

Cholinergic. Parasympathomimetic drug that mimics the action of the parasympathetic nervous system.

Classification. Broad subcategory for drugs that affect the body in similar ways.

Clone. A copy.

Clonic. Spasm marked by alternate contraction (rigidity) and relaxation of muscles.

Coanalgesic. Nonopioid analgesic drugs that are combined with opioids for more effective analgesic action in relief of acute or chronic pain (e.g., NSAID or acetaminophen).

Coenzyme. Enzyme activator.

Comorbidities. Other serious conditions existing concurrently with the one under discussion.

Concomitant. Taking place at the same time.

Concurrent. Existing at the same time.

Contraceptives. Medications used for birth control.

Contraindication. Condition or circumstance that indicates that a drug should not be given.

Controlled substance. Drug controlled by prescription requirement because of the danger of addiction or abuse.

Conversion. Changing from one system of measurement to another.

COPD. Chronic obstructive pulmonary disease.

Coronary vasodilators. Medications used in the treatment of angina. See **Vasodilator.**

Corticosteroids. Hormones secreted by the adrenal glands that act on the immune system to suppress the body's response to infection or trauma; medications given for their anti-inflammatory and immunosuppressant properties.

COX-2 inhibitors. Anti-inflammatory drugs that do not inhibit clotting and cause fewer gastric problems and less GI bleeding than other NSAIDs.

Cryptorchidism. Undescended testicles.

Cumulative effect. Increased effect of a drug that accumulates in the body.

Cushing's syndrome. Excessive production or administration of adrenal cortical hormones, resulting in edema, puffy face, fatigue, weakness, and osteoporosis.

Cycloplegic. Drug that paralyzes the muscles of accommodation for eye examinations.

Cytotoxic. Destroys cells.

Decongestants. Drugs that constrict blood vessels in the respiratory tract, resulting in shrinkage of swollen mucous membranes and opened nasal airway passages.

Deficiency. Lacking adequate amount.

Demulcent. Medication used topically to protect or soothe minor dermatological conditions such as diaper rash, abrasions, and minor burns.

Dependence. Acquired need for a drug after repeated use; may be psychological with craving and emotional changes or physical with body changes and withdrawal symptoms.

Digitalization. The process of establishing the correct therapeutic dose of digitalis for maintaining optimal functioning of the heart without toxic effects.

Diplopia. Double vision.

Direct toxicity. Drug that results in tissue damage; may or may not be permanent.

Distribution. Circulation of drugs, after absorption, to the organs of the body.

Diuretic. Medication that increases urine excretion.

Documentation. Recording medication given to a patient on the patient's medical record, including the dose, time, route, and location of injections.

Dosage. Amount of drug given for a particular therapeutic or desired effect.

Dosage calculation. Using mathematical computation to determine the correct dosage to administer when a dosage ordered differs from the dose on hand.

Drug. Chemical substance taken into the body that affects body function.

Drug abuse. The use of a drug for other than therapeutic purposes.

Drug Enforcement Administration (DEA). A bureau of the Department of Justice that enforces the Controlled Substances Act.

Drug form. The type of preparation in which a drug is supplied.

Drug interactions. Response that may occur when more than one drug is taken. The combination may alter the expected response of each individual drug.

Drug processes. Four biological changes that drugs undergo within the body.

Drug standards. Federally approved requirements for the specified strength, quality, and purity of drugs.

Dyskinesia. An impairment of the ability to execute voluntary movements, frequently an adverse effect of prolonged use of some medications, for example, phenothiazines.

Dyslipidemia. Abnormal levels of various blood lipid fractions.

Dysphagia. Difficulty in swallowing.

Dystonic reaction. Spasm and contortion, especially of the head, neck, and tongue, as an adverse effect of antipsychotic medication.

Effects of drugs. Physiological changes that occur in response to drugs.

Emetic. Agent that induces vomiting.

Emollient. Medication used topically to protect or soothe minor dermatological conditions, such as diaper rash, abrasions, and minor burns.

Endocrine. Internal secretion (hormone) produced by a ductless gland that secretes directly into the bloodstream.

Endogenous. Produced or originating within a cell or organism.

Endorphin. Endogenous analgesics produced within the body.

Enteric coated. Tablet with a special coating that resists disintegration by the gastric juices and dissolves in the intestines.

Enuresis. Urinary incontinence; bed-wetting.

Epidural anesthesia. Local anesthetic solution injected into the epidural space just outside the spinal cord.

Epilepsy. A recurrent paroxysmal disorder of brain function characterized by sudden attacks of altered consciousness, motor activity, or sensory impairment.

Epistaxis. Nosebleed.

Estrogens. Female sex hormones responsible for the development of female secondary sexual characteristics; medications used for many conditions.

Eunuchism. Lack of male hormone, resulting in high-pitched voice and absence of beard and body hair.

Euphoria. Exaggerated feeling of well-being and elation.

Euthyroid. Normal thyroid function.

Excretion. Elimination of by-products of drug metabolism from the body, essentially through the kidneys, some from the intestines and lungs.

Exogenous. Originating outside the body or an organ or produced from external causes.

Expectorants. Drugs that increase secretions, reduce viscosity, and help to expel sputum.

Extrapyramidal. Disorder of the brain characterized by tremors, parkinsonlike symptoms, dystonic twisting of body parts, or tardive dyskinesia, sometimes associated with prolonged use of antipsychotic drugs and some other CNS drugs.

Fat-soluble. Vitamins A, D, E, and K.

Flatulence. Excessive gas in the digestive tract.

Follicle-stimulating hormone (FSH). Hormone that stimulates development of ovarian follicles in the female and sperm production in the testes of the male.

Food and Drug Administration (FDA). A department of Health and Welfare that enforces the provisions of the Federal

Food, Drug, and Cosmetic Act and amendments of 1951 and 1965.

Free radicals. Unbound compounds that attack and damage the cells or initiate growth of abnormal cells, resulting in conditions such as cancer or atherosclerosis.

Gastric tube administration. Medication administered through a tube in the abdomen to the stomach.

Gastroesophageal reflux disease (GERD). A backward flow of gastric secretions into the esophagus causing inflammation and discomfort. GERD is treated with drugs to accelerate gastric emptying.

Gastroparesis. Partial paralysis of the stomach.

Generic name. General, common, or nonproprietary name of a drug.

GERD. Gastroesophageal reflux disease.

Gingivitis. Inflammation of the gums characterized by redness, swelling, and tendency to bleed.

Glaucoma. Abnormal condition of the eye with increased intraocular pressure (IOP) due to obstruction of the outflow of aqueous humor.

Glossitis. Inflammation of the tongue.

Glycosuria. Sugar in the urine.

Goiter. Enlargement of the thyroid gland.

Gout. Form of arthritis in which uric acid crystals are deposited in and around joints.

Grand mal seizures. A form of epilepsy characterized by loss of consciousness, falling, and generalized tonic, followed by clonic contractions of the muscles.

Gray List. List of inappropriate drugs for nursing home residents based on a national survey of geriatric experts.

HAART. Highly active antiretroviral therapy for HIV infections.

Hematological. Concerned with the blood and its components.

Hematuria. Blood in the urine.

Hepatotoxicity. Damage to the liver as an adverse reaction to certain drugs.

Herbs. Any product intended for ingestion as a supplement to the diet.

Heterocyclics. Second-generation cyclic antidepressants with very different adverse effect profiles.

Homeostasis. Body balance, state of internal equilibrium.

Hormone replacement therapy (HRT). Estrogen with or without progestin used for osteoporosis prevention and treatment.

Hyperalimentation. The intravenous infusion of a hypertonic solution containing all of the necessary elements to sustain life. Usually infused through a subclavian catheter into the superior vena cava.

Hypercalcemia. Abnormally high blood calcium.

Hyperglycemia. Abnormally high blood glucose.

Hyperkalemia. Abnormally high potassium in the blood can lead to cardiac arrhythmias.

Hyperlipidemia. High lipid levels in the blood.

Hyperosmotic. Laxative to draw water from the tissues and stimulate evacuation.

Hyperpyrexia. Extreme elevation of body temperature.

Hypersensitivity. Allergic or excessive response of the immune system to a drug or chemical.

Hypertriglyceridemia. High triglyceride level in the blood.

Hyperuricemia. Abnormal amount of uric acid in the blood.

Hypnotic. Drug that promotes sleep.

Hypoglycemia. Abnormally low blood glucose.

Hypokalemia. Abnormally low blood potassium can lead to cardiac arrhythmias.

Hypotensive. Antihypertensive; medication used in the treatment of hypertension.

Hypothyroidism. Diminished or absent thyroid function.

Hypoxia. Deficiency of oxygen.

Idiopathic. Condition without a known cause.

Idiosyncracy. Unusual reaction to a drug, other than expected.

Immunosuppressive. Decreasing the production of antibodies and phagocytes and depressing the inflammatory reaction.

Indications. List of conditions for which a drug is meant to be used.

Infiltration anesthesia. Local anesthetic solution injected into the skin, subcutaneous tissue, or mucous membranes of the area to be anesthetized.

Ingestion. To take into the body by mouth through swallowing.

Inhalation therapy. Medications administered through a metered dose inhaler, small-volume nebulizer, or intermittent positive pressure breathing apparatus.

Interactions. Actions that occur when two or more drugs are combined, or when drugs are combined with certain foods. See **Drug interactions**.

Intra-articular (intracapsular). Injected into the joint.

Intradermal (ID). Injected into the layers of the skin.

Intramuscular (IM). Injected into the muscle.

Intravenous (IV). Injected into the vein.

Ischemia. Holding back of the blood; local deficiency of blood supply due to obstruction of circulation to a part (e.g., heart or extremities).

Keratolytic. An agent that promotes loosening or scaling of the outer layer of the skin.

Korsakoff's psychosis. Disorder characterized by polyneuritis, disorientation, mental deterioration, and ataxia with painful foot drop, usually associated with chronic alcoholism.

Lability. State of being unstable or changeable.

Laxatives. Drugs that promote evacuation of the intestine.

Legend drug. Available only by prescription.

Leukopenia. Abnormal decrease in white blood cells, usually below 5,000.

Local. Affecting one specific area or part.

Local anesthetic. Medication administered to produce temporary loss of sensation or feeling in a specific area.

Lozenge (troche). Tablet that dissolves slowly in the mouth for local effect.

Luteinizing hormone (LH). Hormone that works in conjunction with FSH to induce secretion of estrogen, ovulation, and development of corpus luteum.

Luteotropic hormone (LTH). Hormone that stimulates the secretion of progesterone by the corpus luteum and secretion of milk by the mammary gland.

Macrolides. Drugs used in many infections of the respiratory tract, for skin conditions such as acne, or for some sexually transmitted infections when the patient is allergic to penicillin.

Medication orders. The physician's prescription for administration of a drug; contains six parts.

Megadose. Abnormally large dose.

Melena. Blood in the stool.

Mental impairment. Decreased mental function in older adults frequently caused or worsened by drugs.

Metabolism. Physical and chemical alterations that a substance undergoes in the body.

Metric system. International standard for weights and measures.

Minerals. Chemical elements occurring in nature and in body fluids.

Miotic. Drugs that cause the pupil to contract.

Mixed seizure. Having more than one type of seizure.

Monoclonal antibodies. Chemotherapy designed to target only cancer cells, thereby sparing normal tissues.

Mortar and pestle. Glass cup with glass rod used to crush tablets.

Mucolytic. Medication that liquefies pulmonary secretions.

Myalgia. Tenderness or pain in the muscles.

Mydriatic. Drug that dilates the pupil.

Myelosuppression. Inhibiting bone marrow function.

Myopathy. Abnormal condition of skeletal muscle.

Nasogastric tube administration. Medication administered through a tube inserted through the nose and extending into the stomach.

Nebulizer (vaporizer). Apparatus for producing a fine spray or mist for inhalation.

Nephropathy. Disease of the kidneys.

Nephrotoxicity. Damage to the kidneys as an adverse reaction to certain drugs.

Neuropathy. Any disease of the nerves.

Neurotoxicity. Having the capability of harming nerve tissue.

Neurotransmitters. Substances that travel across the synapse to transmit messages between nerve cells.

Neutropenia. Abnormally small number of neutrophil leukocytes in the blood.

Nosocomial. Hospital-acquired infection.

NSAID. Nonsteroidal anti-inflammatory drug.

Nystagmus. Involuntary rhythmic movements of the eyeball.

Objective. Referring to symptoms observed or perceived by others.

Oligospermia. Deficient sperm production.

Onychomycosis. Toenail fungus.

Opioids. Analgesics, controlled substances, whose action is similar to opium in altering the perception of pain; can be natural or synthetic.

Opportunistic infections. Infections that occur because the immune system is compromised.

Oral medications. Medication administered by mouth.

Orphan drug. A drug or biological product for the diagnosis, treatment, or prevention of a rare disease or condition, that is, one affecting less than 200,000 persons in the United States, or greater than 200,000 persons where the cost of developing the drug is probably not recoverable in the United States.

Osmotic agents. Medications used to reduce intracranial or intraocular pressure.

Osteomalacia. Softening of the bones due to inadequate calcium and/or vitamin D.

Osteoporosis. Softening of the bone seen most often in older adults, especially postmenopausal women.

Osteoporosis therapy. Medications used to prevent or treat osteoporosis by increasing bone mineral density.

Ototoxicity. Damage to the eighth cranial nerve resulting in impaired hearing or ringing in the ears (tinnitus); adverse reaction to certain drugs.

Overdose. A higher than normal amount sufficient to cause toxicity.

Over-the-counter drug (OTC). Medication available without a prescription.

Oxytocin. Hormone that stimulates the uterus to contract, thus inducing childbirth.

Palliative. Referring to alleviation of symptoms, but not producing a cure.

Paradoxical. Opposite effect from that expected.

Paraphilia. A psychosexual disorder in which unusual or bizarre imagery or acts are necessary for realization of sexual excitement.

Parasympatholytics. Anticholinergics; medications that decrease the chemical that promotes bronchospasm.

Parenteral. Any route of administration not involving the gastrointestinal tract (e.g., injection, topical, and inhalation).

Paresthesia. Numbness, tingling, or a "pins and needles" feeling, especially in extremities.

Parkinson's disease. A chronic neurological disorder characterized by fine, slowly spreading muscle tremors, rigidity and weakness of muscles, and shuffling gait.

Pedophilia. Sexual attraction to children.

Pellagra. A disease caused by deficiency of niacin (nicotinic acid), characterized by skin, gastrointestinal, mucosal, neurological, and mental symptoms.

Penicillins. Antibiotics produced from certain species of a fungus.

Peripheral. Away from the center. Usually refers to the extremities.

Peripheral nerve block. Local anesthetic solution injected into or around nerves or ganglia supplying the area to be anesthetized.

Pharmacology. The study of drugs and their origin, nature, properties, and effects on living organisms.

Photosensitivity. Increased reaction to sunlight with danger of sunburn; adverse reaction to certain drugs.

Physiological dependence. Physical adaptation of the body to a drug and withdrawal symptoms after abrupt drug discontinuation.

Phytoestrogen. A plant substance with estrogen-like properties.

Placebo. Inactive substance given to simulate the effect of another drug; physical or emotional changes that occur reflect the expectations of the patient.

Placebo effect. Relief from pain as the result of suggestion without active medication.

Platelet inhibitor. A drug that inhibits platelet aggregation (clumping) to prevent clots.

Poison. Substance that is taken into the body by ingestion, inhalation, injection, or absorption that is toxic and can cause illness, injury, or death.

Polypharmacy. Excessive use of drugs or prescription of many drugs given at one time.

Postherpetic neuralgia. Nerve pain following an episode of shingles.

Potentiation. Increased effect; action of two drugs given simultaneously is greater than the effect of the drugs given separately.

Precautions. List of conditions or types of patients that warrant closer observation for specific side effects when given a drug.

Prevention of medication errors. Rules to follow to avoid making mistakes.

Priapism. Prolonged penile erection.

Prodrug. A newly developed group of chemicals that exhibit their pharmacological activity after biotransformation.

Progesterone. Hormone responsible for changes in uterine endometrium in the second half of the menstrual cycle in preparation for implantation of the fertilized ovum, development of maternal placenta after implantation, and development of mammary glands; medication with several uses.

Progestins. Synthetic drugs that exert progesterone-like activity.

Proliferation. Rapid reproduction.

Proportion. Two ratios that are equal.

Prototype. Model or type from which subsequent types arise (e.g., an example of a drug that typifies the characteristics of that classification).

Psychomotor epilepsy. Also known as temporal lobe epilepsy because of the area in the brain that is involved; characterized by temporary impairment of consciousness, confusion, loss of judgment, and abnormal acts, even crimes and hallucinations, but no convulsions.

Psychotropic. Any substance that acts on the mind.

Quinolones. Drugs used in adults for the treatment of some infections of the urinary tract, lower respiratory tract, gastrointestinal tract, skin, bones, and joints.

Ratio. A relationship between two numbers.

Rectal medications. Medication in suppository or liquid form administered as a retention enema.

Refractory. A disorder resistant to treatment.

REM. Rapid eye movement, or dream phase of sleep.

Reporting. Notifying the FDA of serious adverse events or product quality problems associated with medications (MEDWATCH).

Resistance. An organism's lack of response to antibiotics when they are used too often or treatment is incomplete.

Responsibility. Duty to administer drugs safely and accurately.

Rhabdomyolysis. An acute, sometimes fatal disease characterized by destruction of muscle leading to renal failure.

"Rights" of medication administration. Guidelines for giving medication that include the right medication, right amount, right time, right route, right patient, and right documentation.

Route of delivery. The way that drugs are taken into the body.

Scurvy. A vitamin C deficiency disease usually resulting from lack of fresh fruits and vegetables in diet. Symptoms include ulcerated gums and mouth, loose teeth, muscle cramps and weakness, poor healing, and bruising.

Sedatives. Controlled substances used to promote sedation in smaller doses and to promote sleep in larger doses.

Selective distribution. Affinity or attraction of a drug to a specific organ or cells.

Selective Serotonin Reuptake Inhibitors (SSRI). Antidepressants that block the reabsorption of the neurotransmitter serotonin, thus helping to restore the brain's chemical balance.

Skeletal muscle relaxants. Medication used to treat some musculoskeletal disorders associated with pain, spasm, abnormal contraction, or impaired mobility.

Smoking cessation aids. Medications used to slowly lower the level of nicotine while the patient participates in a behavior modification program for smoking cessation.

Somogyi effect. Hyperglycemic rebound, usually a result of frequent overdoses of insulin, which causes an accelerated release of glucagon.

Sources of drugs. Four ways that the drugs are obtained.

Spinal anesthesia. Local anesthetic solutions injected intrathecally (into the subarachnoid space of the spinal canal) either in the lumbar region or lower (saddle block), depending on the area to be anesthetized.

STD. Sexually transmitted diseases.

Status epilepticus. Continual attacks of convulsive seizures without intervals of consciousness.

Stomatitis. Inflammation of the mucous membranes of the mouth.

Subcutaneous (SubQ). Beneath the skin.

Subjective. Perceived by the individual, not observable by others.

Sublingual (SL). Under the tongue.

Sulfonamides. Anti-infectives used in combinations with other drugs to slow the development of resistance; used in treatment of urinary tract infections, enteritis, and opportunistic infections of AIDS.

Sulfonylurea. Oral antidiabetic drug for treatment of type II diabetes.

Superinfection. A new infection with different resistant bacteria or fungi. Usually associated with certain types of antibiotic therapy.

Supplement. Any product intended for ingestion as an addition to the diet.

Sympathomimetic. Adrenergic drug that mimics the action of the sympathetic nervous system.

Synergism. Action of two drugs working together for increased effect.

Synthetic. Prepared in the laboratory by artificial means.

Systemic. Affecting the whole body or system.

Tachycardia. Abnormally fast heartbeat.

Tachypnea. Abnormal rapidity of respiration.

Tardive dyskinesia (TD). Slow, rhythmical, stereotyped, involuntary movements such as tics.

Temporal lobe epilepsy. See **Psychomotor epilepsy.**

Teratogenic effect. Effect of a drug administered to the mother that results in abnormalities in the fetus.

Testosterone. Male hormone; medication used for replacement therapy and other uses.

Tetracyclines. Broad-spectrum antibiotics used in the treatment of infections caused by rickettsia, chlamydia, or some uncommon bacteria.

Thrombocytopenia. Abnormal decrease in number of blood platelets.

Thrombolytic agents. Medications used to dissolve clots after they have formed.

Timed-release capsules (sustained-release or extended-release). Capsules containing many small pellets that are dissolved over a prolonged period of time.

Tinnitus. Ringing in the ears.

Tolerance. Decreased response to a drug after repeated dosage; greater amounts of the drug are required for the same effect.

Tonic. A persistent, involuntary muscular contraction.

Topical. Applied to a specific area for a local effect to that area only (e.g., applied to skin or mucous membranes).

Topical anesthesia. Application of a local anesthetic directly to the surface of the area to be anesthetized.

Toxicity. Condition resulting from exposure to a poison or a dangerous amount of a drug.

Toxicology. Study and detection of toxic substances, establishing treatment and methods of prevention of poisoning.

Trade name. Name by which a pharmaceutical company identifies its product; brand name.

Transcutaneous. Transdermal. Medication is delivered to the body slowly by absorption through the skin.

Transdermal (transcutaneous) delivery system. Patch containing the medicine is applied to the skin; the drug is absorbed through the skin over a prolonged period of time.

Tricyclics. Antidepressants that elevate the mood, have a mild sedative effect, and increase appetite.

Unilateral seizures. Affect only one side of the body.

Uricosuric. Promoting urinary excretion of uric acid.

Urinary analgesic. Medication used to relieve burning, pain, and discomfort in the urinary tract mucosa.

Urinary anti-infectives. Drugs used for initial or recurrent urinary tract infections caused by susceptible organisms, usually bacteriostatic instead of bactericidal.

Urticaria. Hives.

Variables. Factors that affect the speed and efficiency of drugs processed by the body.

Vasconstrictor. Drug that narrows blood vessels resulting in increased blood pressure; used in the treatment of shock.

Vasodilator. A drug that expands the walls of the blood vessels, improving blood flow and resulting in a lowering of blood pressure.

Verify. Confirm the result of calculations with another professional, such as an instructor.

Vial. Glass container with rubber stopper that must be punctured with a needle to withdraw a drug solution or to reconstitute a drug in powdered form.

Water-soluble. B-complex vitamins and vitamin C.

Wernicke's syndrome. Mental disorder characterized by loss of memory, disorientation, and confusion, usually associated with old age or chronic alcoholism.

Withdrawal. Cessation of administration of a drug, especially a narcotic or alcohol, to which a person has become physiologically and/or psychologically addicted; withdrawal symptoms vary with the chemical used.

Xanthines. Medications that indirectly increase the chemical that causes bronchodilation; used particularly for treatment of acute asthmatic attacks.

Xerophthalmia. Dryness of the eyes.

Xerostomia. Dryness of the mouth.

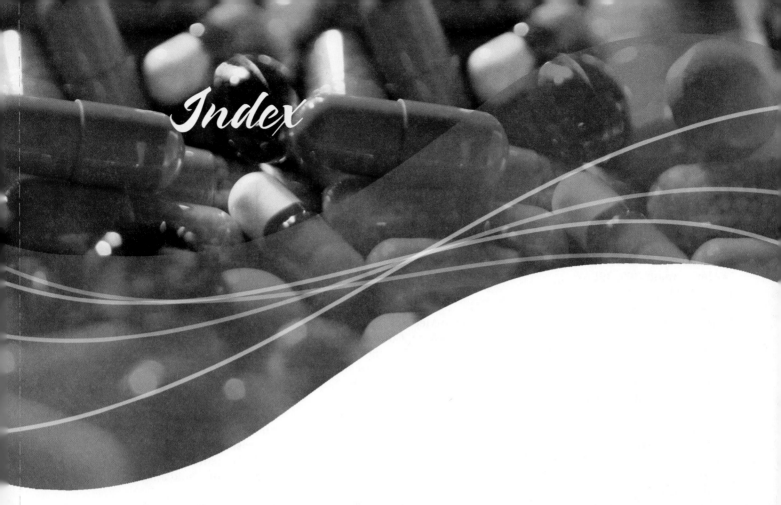

Index

Note: Italicized page numbers indicate illustrations.

577

588